T0146100

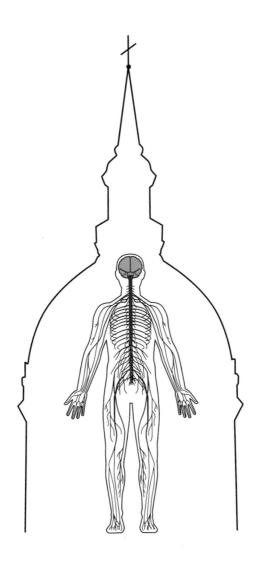

JOHNS HOPKINS
NEUROLOGY
—— HALF A CENTURY OF INNOVATION ——

Daniel B. Drachman, M.D., *Editor-in-Chief*

R. John Leigh, M.D., *Associate Editor*

Guy M. McKhann, M.D., *Founding Chair, Department of Neurology*

Justin C. McArthur, M.B.,B.S., M.P.H., *Chair, Department of Neurology*

Janet Farrar Worthington, *Writer/Editor*

Laura Hatcher, *Designer*

2019

© 2019 Johns Hopkins Department of Neurology

The Johns Hopkins University and The Johns Hopkins Health System Corporation,
All rights reserved.

www.hopkinsmedicine.org

Printed in the United States on acid-free paper by
Mount Royal Printing & Communications

Distributed by the Johns Hopkins University Press
2715 North Charles Street
Baltimore, Maryland 21218-4363

www.press.jhu.edu

Cataloging-in-Publication Data is available from the Library of Congress
Library of Congress Control Number 2019022740
A catalog record for this book is available from the British Library.

ISBN 978-1-4214-3675-3

Composed in Mercury serif typeface family designed by Jonathan Hoefler and Tobias Frere-Jones and the sans serif typeface Franklin Gothic developed by the type foundry American Type Founders (ATF) and credited to its head designer Morris Fuller Benton.

Editors: Daniel B. Drachman, M.D., R. John Leigh, M.D., Janet Farrar Worthington

Book Design: Laura LeBrun Hatcher

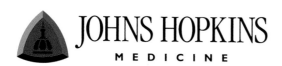

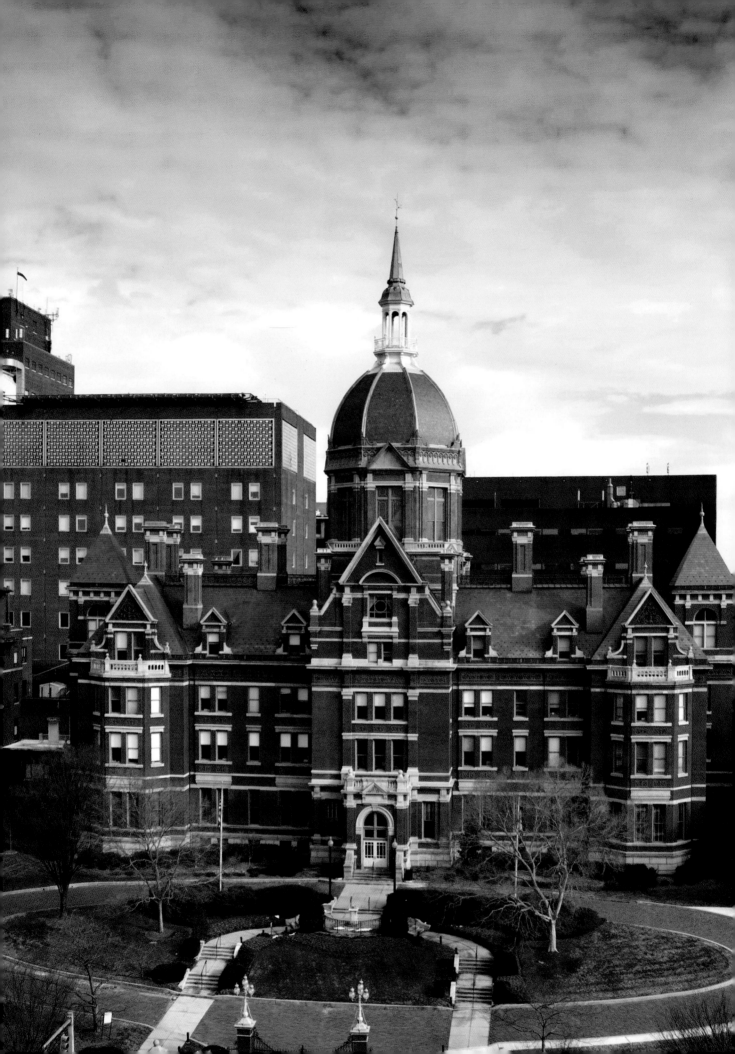

ACKNOWLEDGMENTS

We are grateful to the following individuals, who have contributed to the writing of chapters that are indicated by number in the parentheses following their names: Marilyn Albert (16), Jee Bang (7), Gregory Bergey (15), Jaishri Blakeley (8), Ari Blitz (12), David Clark (1), Tom Crawford (10), Daniel Drachman (3), Eric Drachman (cover concept), Peter Calabresi (6), Ted Dawson (7), Mahlon DeLong (7), John Freeman (1,14), Barry Gordon (16), Diane Griffin (5), Rebecca Gottesman (11), Daniel Hanley (17), Tony Ho (4), Ahmet Höke (4), John Krakauer (11), Eric Kossoff (15), John Laterra (8), John Leigh (9, 20), Richard Leigh (12), Mike Levy (6), Rafael Llinas (19), Ski Lower (17), Justin McArthur (5), Guy McKhann (2, 12, 14), Howard Moses (1,2), Ellen Mowry (6), Alexander Pantelyat (7), Donald Price (18), Daniel Reich (12), Jeff Rothstein (13), Nicoline Schiess (5), Harvey Singer (14) Charlotte Sumner (10), Klaus Toyka (3), Patti Vining (14), David Zee (9), and the Alumni of Johns Hopkins Neurology (21).

We are also grateful to Laura Hatcher for her inspired design of the book, to Timothy Wisniewski for archival assistance, and to Cecilia Young, Victoria Maranto, Sandy Vieyra, and Geordan Burton for administrative support.

We acknowledge the very generous philanthropic support of many individuals and families over the past 50 years. Their vision has helped create a platform for discovery and neurological care.

Daniel B. Drachman, M.D.

R. John Leigh, M.D.

Guy M. McKhann, M.D.

Justin C. McArthur, M.B., B.S., M.P.H

Janet Farrar Worthington

TABLE OF CONTENTS

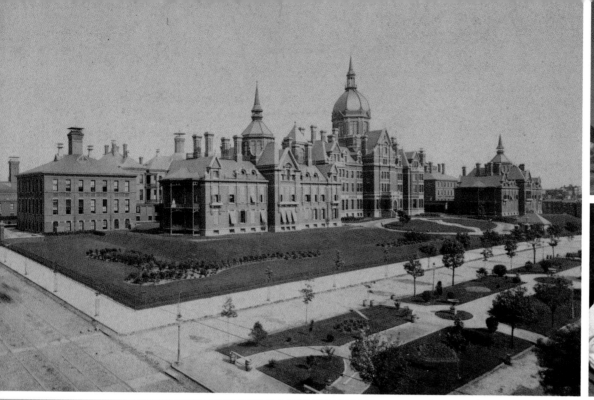
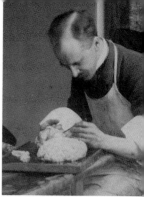
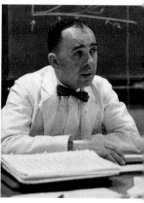
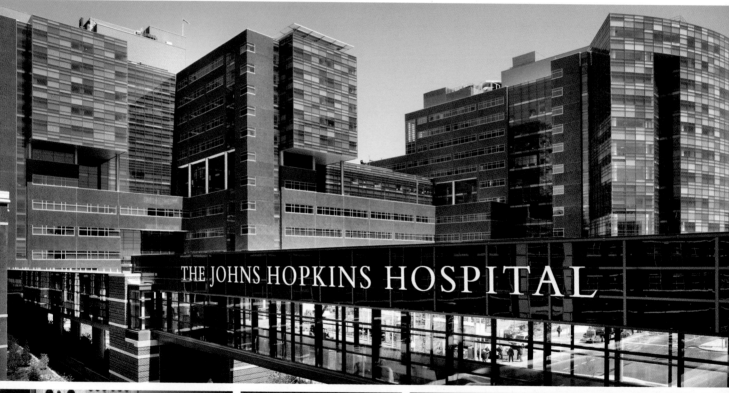

THE JOHNS HOPKINS HOSPITAL

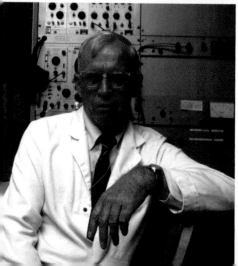
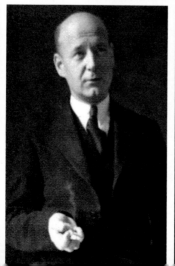
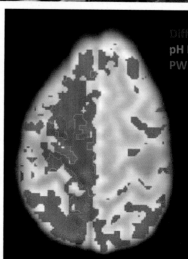
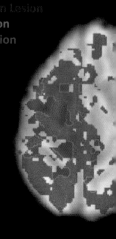

Diffusion Lesion
pH Lesion
PWI Lesion

IN JUST 50 YEARS...

The field of Neurology has changed so profoundly during the last 50 years – the blink of an eye in the perspective of time – that it is daunting even to attempt to describe the differences. Back in 1969, Neurology was a more or less leisurely descriptive specialty. Now it has become a dynamic, therapeutically oriented field, driven by technological advances and new concepts in multiple areas that were inconceivable in the early days. At Hopkins, we have been privileged to have participated in both the discovery of some of these advances, and in the application of many changes that now define this exciting specialty.

Imaging: Fifty years ago, it was virtually impossible to *see* what the nervous system of a live human looked like without opening the skull or spine. Imaging then consisted of skull X-rays, enhanced sometimes by the painful introduction of air into the ventricles, or by injection of dye into the blood vessels. Imaging has progressed through CT scans, MRIs and visualization of the brain, spinal cord, peripheral nerves, blood vessels and muscles. Perhaps imaging has been the most profound change in the practice of Neurology.

Immunology: The relationship between the immune system and the nervous system has played a remarkable role in our understanding and treatment of many diseases of the nervous system. Myasthenia gravis, multiple sclerosis, myositis, Guillain-Barré Syndrome and related neuropathies, neuromyelitis optica, autoimmune encephalitis, are a few of the examples of formerly deadly neurological diseases that now are often treatable by immunological strategies. Neuroimmunology is one of the triumphs of neurological progress.

Stroke: There have been remarkable changes in the treatment of strokes during this era. Dissolution of clots by tPA, endovascular removal of occlusions, and the use of stents to restore blood flow to the brain, provided that they are applied in time, have dramatically changed the prognosis of strokes.

Molecular Biology and Genetics: Genetic studies have revealed the underlying abnormalities and provided diagnostic criteria for many neurologic disorders, including muscular dystrophies, peripheral neuropathies, "neurodegenerative diseases" such as Huntington's, spinocerebellar degenerations, neurofibromatosis, some forms of ALS, and many others. As yet, few of the genetic abnormalities of these diseases have been correctable. However, we have seen remarkable results in treating spinal muscular atrophy by antisense oligonucleotides, and this bodes well for the future. The pathogenic effects of excessive numbers of nucleotide repeats in many of the genetic neurologic diseases is another important clue that may lead to novel treatments.

Neurology has always been part of medical care at Johns Hopkins, but it took many years and many attempts to establish an independent department.

Clockwise, from top left:

Johns Hopkins Hospital in 1889.

Sir William Osler, considered "by himself and others as a neurologist for adults and children."

David Bodian, whose research led to development of the polio vaccine.

The Hospital today.

MRI images of a right hemisphere stroke, comparing the extent of cell death (Diffusion Lesion), impaired vascular perfusion (PWI Lesion), and lactic acidosis in the penumbra (pH Lesion). Courtesy of Peter van Zijl, Jinyuan Zhou, Hye-Young Heo, Alan Huang, and Richard Leigh.

Frank Ford, outstanding neurological diagnostician and author of the 1937 landmark book: *Diseases of the Nervous System in Infancy, Childhood and Adolescence.*

Vernon Mountcastle, distinguished neurophysiologist and winner of the Lasker Award for his discovery of the columnar organization of the cerebral cortex. He also played a critical role in helping Neurology break away from the Department of Medicine.

Epilepsy: Seizure disorders are far more treatable now than they were 50 years ago, as a result of new anti-epileptic agents, the use of ketogenic diets, and surgical treatment of epilepsy.

Neurodegenerative Diseases: Some of the most devastating neurodegenerative diseases such as Parkinson's and Alzheimer's are under investigation at Hopkins and elsewhere, and this research is yielding exciting results.

Neurovirology: Neurovirology has undergone important progress, with remarkable therapeutic results in HIV encephalitis, understanding of the autoimmune nature of post-measles encephalopathies, and basic understanding of prion diseases.

Information Technology: Information technology has been keeping pace with the rapid growth of Neuroscience. The internet has made it enormously easier to access information about any clinical or research area. The practice of Neurology has been altered remarkably by the introduction of electronic methods of record-keeping. The ready availability of electronic records – instead of the frequently missing paper notes of 50 years ago – has changed Neurology, as well. While our current electronic version, Epic, may not be a pleasure to use, the electronic records are clearly better than paper. In addition, Neuroscience has contributed to computational techniques and artificial intelligence – both of which undoubtedly will play critical roles in the future.

Who are our Residents? Another striking difference has been the gender change in Neurology. Fifty years ago, Neurology was a virtually exclusive male specialty. Happily, that is no longer the case: there are now a great many women in Neurology. During the first five years of this department, all 30 residents were men; now (and for the last five years), two-thirds of our 66 residents are women.

For those of us who have watched and participated in the dramatic evolution of Neurology over the past half-century, these years have been filled with excitement and satisfaction. Neurology is poised for further extraordinary developments, especially in the fields of genetics, systems neuroscience, the discovery and therapy of neurodegenerative diseases, and the prediction and prevention of these manifest disorders.

Daniel B. Drachman, M.D.

W.W. Smith Charitable Trust Professor of Neuroimmunology
Professor of Neurology and Neuroscience

CHAPTER ONE

THE LONG ROAD TO INDEPENDENCE

1889-1969

Neurology has been strong at Johns Hopkins since its very beginning in 1889. In fact, so intrinsically a part of the Department of Medicine was neurology – its roots so deeply entwined with the work of Hopkins' first Professor of Medicine, William Osler, the faculty he hired and the gifted clinicians who succeeded them – that it was eighty years before Hopkins finally created a separate Department of Neurology.

Why couldn't Medicine let Neurology go? For many reasons, some philosophical and some not so lofty. In his book, *Looking Back: A Career in Child Neurology*, John Freeman, M.D., longtime Hopkins pediatric neurologist, noted that Osler "had trained with Gowers in England and other outstanding neurologists of the time and was considered, both by himself and others, as a neurologist for both adults and children. He wrote about cases of neurologic importance within both medicine and pediatrics, and there never seemed to be a need for a separate neurology department."

The interests of other departments spilled over into neurology, as well: Harvey Cushing, one of William Halsted's earliest surgical residents, created the field of neurosurgery and developed procedures to treat neurological conditions for which there previously had been little help. One of Cushing's most gifted residents, in turn, was Walter Dandy, who contributed greatly to the field of neurosurgery and also made breakthroughs in neuroimaging, with his development of ventriculography and pneumoencephalography – which made it possible to see brain tumors. Frank Walsh was a pioneer in neuro-ophthalmology, and neurovirologist and anatomist David Bodian performed critical research on the polio virus that led to development of the Salk and Sabin polio vaccines. Adolf Meyer, chief of psychiatry and a pioneer in the field, believed neurology and psychology were linked and envisioned combining them into one institute.

Well into the 1960s, the belief persisted that at Hopkins, neurology didn't need to be its own entity. And yet, Freeman wrote, "There was, according to Professor of Physiology Vernon Mountcastle, increasing agitation to have a Department of Neurology. Mountcastle, a neurophysiologist, realized the future for the neurosciences depended on a separate department." Backing up Mountcastle were Bodian and A. Earl Walker, professor of neurosurgery (not yet its own department, either). But A. McGehee "Mac" Harvey, chairman of Medicine, "remained vehemently opposed, claiming that since neuromuscular disease, his particular field of expertise, and brain infections were all part of internal medicine, there was no need for a neurology department."

He would soon change his mind. But why was the decision so long in coming? In fact, the idea of a separate Department of Neurology at Hopkins had been percolating since the 1920s. After World War I, when Osler had left Baltimore for England, the Hospital trustees began searching for a prestigious neurologist to lead a proposed Institute of Neurology. Somehow, the institute never happened. Over the years, subsequent committees were appointed to start a new search; great flurries of activity followed, with interviews and visits full of mutual enthusiasm that either petered out or ended more abruptly (see side stories). No director came, and neurology remained a division of internal medicine.

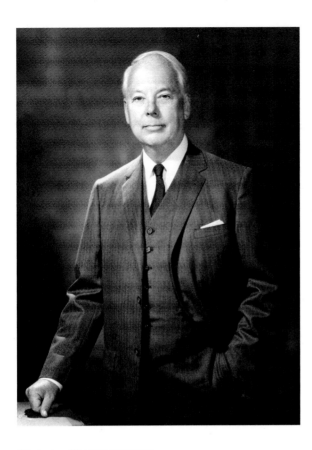

THOMAS B. TURNER
Turner, former Dean of the School of Medicine, noted that like many institutions, Hopkins had greater goals than it had depth of pockets to pay for them. Neurology was one of several proposed academic departments that "foundered on inability to attract able directors, probably mainly because of inadequate financing."

Vision Unfulfilled

In his Hopkins history, *Heritage of Excellence*, Thomas B. Turner, M.D., former Dean of the School of Medicine, pointed out that neurology was not alone in the category of "visions unfulfilled" at Hopkins, an institute that – like many others at the time – had greater goals than it had depth of pockets to pay for them. From the 1920s on, after remarkable expansion in other areas, "at least four new academic departments were projected... All these efforts ... foundered on inability to attract able directors, probably mainly because of inadequate financing."

In Osler's time, in addition to Osler himself, there was Henry Thomas (see side story), Osler's chief of Neurology and clinical professor of diseases of the nervous system from 1896 until his death in 1925. "Thomas had always been on the part-time staff," Turner wrote, with "his maximum salary from the Medical School never exceeding $1,000 annually." Frank R. Ford, a brilliant diagnostician who had trained under Thomas, stepped up to lead neurology after Thomas died. In 1932, Ford was officially made the head of the division. Ford was "undoubtedly the foremost clinical neurologist of the period in Baltimore," a pioneer in pediatric neurology and the author of the respected textbook, *Diseases of the Nervous System in Infancy, Childhood and Adolescence*. But he, too, was "never on more than a part-time status," added Turner.

But the lack of momentum was more complicated than just chronic lack of funding. Hopkins had been blessed with excellent part-time faculty who provided outstanding neurological care and hardly cost the institution anything. In this sense, the Department of Medicine was spoiled.

In 1921, one attempt to hire a neuropathologist failed, Turner said, "because of the low salary offered." In 1925, another committee was appointed to make recommendations concerning neurology. The committee concluded: "It is essential to select, as soon as possible, the future head of the Neurological Department,

Early Stars in Neurology at Hopkins

Before there was a Department of Neurology, there was excellent neurology at Hopkins – groundbreaking work done in multiple areas of the field. The early history of Johns Hopkins has been written about, very well, by A. McGehee Harvey, Thomas Turner, Alan Mason Chesney, and others, and is not the subject of this book. But briefly, here are three early bright stars in the Hopkins neurological firmament:

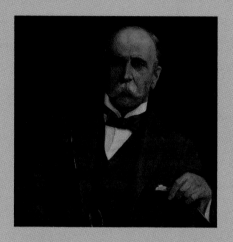

SIR WILLIAM OSLER

Books have been written about William Osler, the first Professor of Medicine at Johns Hopkins, so if you want to know more about him, there's plenty of good reading available. But many believe that Osler was actually Hopkins' first Professor of Neurology, as well. His interest in "the nervous diseases" spanned adult and pediatric neurology, and he wrote nearly 200 scientific papers on neurological subjects, including stroke, muscular dystrophy, cerebral palsy, and spinal cord disorders. His landmark textbook, *The Principles and Practice of Medicine*, included more than 16,000 neurological cases seen at Hopkins Hospital, and another work, *A System of Medicine*, written with Thomas McCrae, devoted an entire volume to diseases of the nervous system.

Left: Sir William Osler. Oil painting by Harry Herman Salomon.

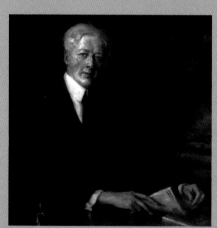

LEWELLYS BARKER

Barker, one of Osler's earliest residents, succeeded Osler as Professor of Medicine in 1905. He shared Osler's interest in neurology and wrote a groundbreaking work, *The Nervous System and Its Constituent Neurons* – the first major American textbook on neuroanatomy.

Left: Portrait of Lewellys Franklin Barker from MedChi archives.

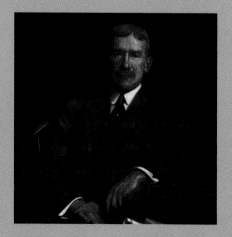

HENRY M. THOMAS, SR.

Thomas, a graduate of the University of Maryland School of Medicine, did further training in Europe and returned to Baltimore to study with Hopkins pathologist William Welch. Osler named him chief of his new division of clinical neurology in 1889, and Thomas contributed to the section on neurological diseases in Osler's *Principles and Practice of Medicine*. One of Thomas's first students was budding surgeon Harvey Cushing, who had a deep interest in neurology and would soon head the brand-new Division of Neurosurgery at Hopkins.

Left: Portraid of Henry M. Thomas Jr., M.D.

and having made this selection, to solicit funds for the proper development of this department." As Turner sadly noted: "Again we see confusion over what should come first."

Then, "while these plans were in the process of miscarrying," as Turner put it, another report was issued. This one, developed for the Johns Hopkins Half-Century Committee, proposed a University clinic and Institute of Neurology and included cost estimates for building and equipping the clinical facilities, and for funding faculty and research that totaled $2.75 million. "There can be little doubt," Turner said, "that this document reflected the opinion of the leaders of Hopkins of that day." In other words, they realized that Johns Hopkins needed to take its place among other world-class institutions in the field of neurology, and they really wanted this to happen. "The report also pointed out that Europe was in the lead in this field, with especially strong clinics and institutes in England and France. It is not altogether clear just what went wrong at Hopkins to frustrate these plans," Turner continued. "In retrospect, one may challenge the validity of a plan to attract an outstanding individual before adequate funds were in hand." Although the Rockefeller Foundation had expressed interest, "no promises had been made." Negotiations with other possible funding sources failed, and then the Great Depression "finally submerged the plans ... beneath a sea of hopelessness and eventual indifference."

Before this sinking, "while there was still hope," several top neurologists from around the world had considered taking the job. Among them was Professor Gordon Holmes, of London, "one of the most eminent neurologists in England and senior consultant at the National Hospital for Nervous Diseases in London, better known as Queen Square Hospital." Even as the Advisory Board voted to offer Holmes the job, "two qualifying notations were made in the minutes of the meeting: first, it was clear that although funds were in the offing, financing was not assured; and second, the question of the relationship of Neuro-Surgery to Neurology was one which need not be settled at the present time." Holmes said no. "He was at the height of his career in England, secure in his practice and enormously influential in neurological circles," Turner wrote. "Moreover, the largest full-time professional salary which Hopkins could offer was far below his current income."

Surely an important factor for Holmes, and anyone else who considered this position, was that there were no dedicated patient beds for neurological patients in the Hospital; there never had been any. In 1942, School of Medicine Dean Alan Mason Chesney wrote to Hospital President Isaiah Bowman that Neurology "is a sub-department of Medicine and a step-child" which, "lacking beds of its own, must rely for its clinical material upon the dispensary and the wards of the Baltimore City Hospitals."

In 1942, School of Medicine Dean Alan Mason Chesney wrote to Hospital President Isaiah Bowman that Neurology "is a sub-department of Medicine and a step-child" which, "lacking beds of its own, must rely for its clinical material upon the dispensary and the wards of the Baltimore City Hospitals."

FIEFDOMS: PEDIATRICS VS. MEDICINE

David B. Clark, a neurologist who left Hopkins in 1965 to become the founding chairman of Neurology at the University of Kentucky, offered a personal perspective on the critical time between World War II and the mid-1960s in his 1989 keynote speech at the celebration of the Hopkins Department of Neurology's 20th anniversary.

"This period was dominated by the personalities of two men, and the positions of two departments," Clark said. The men were Frank Ford and John Magladery. The Departments were Medicine and Pediatrics, neither of which "had yet accepted the premise of an independent Neurology. Neither saw the need for medical specialization based rather on physiological systems than on chronology. Neither, therefore, was able to see the need for a Department of Neurology which cared for the child and the adult. And neither was, in the fifties, willing to sacrifice its sovereignty of the neurological problems of its age group."

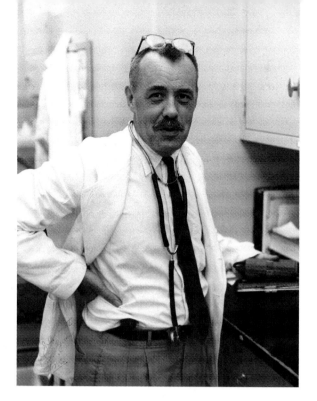

DAVID B. CLARK described neurology at Hopkins between World War II and the mid-1960s as being dominated by the personalities of two men, Frank Ford and John Magladery, and by the positions of Medicine and Pediatrics, "neither of which had yet accepted the premise of an independent Neurology," and neither "willing to sacrifice its sovereignty."

Ford and Magladery were vastly different in just about every way, Clark noted: Both were "intelligent, estimable men, kindly and concerned for patients, Hospital, and colleagues, good friends and sturdy enemies." But "beyond an interest in the nervous system, they had really nothing in common."

This was unfortunate, because the field of neurology was changing – and change was being led from without, rather than within, Hopkins. It was, Clark said, the time of the great expansion of Neurology, financed largely by the National Institute of Neurological Disease and Stroke (NINDS; see Chapter 2). "Independence, and control of bed services by developing programs in Neurology were very nearly obligatory if one expected NIH support. Neurology found itself in a genuine dilemma between funding source on the one hand, and established clinical empires on the other. It was into this (battlefield) that we were injected. And it was against this backdrop that the two strong personalities and two powerful departments met and clashed."

Ford was, as Clark described, one of the more outstanding members of a hospital staff well known for characters. After graduating from the Johns Hopkins School of Medicine just after World War I, Ford had designed his own neurology training program that was at least forty years before its time. This included a year of psychiatry with Adolf Meyer, a year of laboratory virology, a year of neurophysiology "in which, interestingly, he sought for evidence for circulating neurotoxins in the plasma of myasthenics, and finally a residency in neurology at Bellevue with Foster Kennedy. He returned to Hopkins as a resident Neurologist, just as the (fruitless) Institute search was beginning."

Clark points out that Ford's approach – just like that of Osler – was clinical, and "not of the laboratory. He told me once that when, after his years of waiting in the wings whilst foreign dignitaries visited, he was finally made Chief of Neurology, he considered his situation carefully. He decided he was neither a scientist nor a great leader. He could not give The Hopkins great neurology, but he could give it a great

An Unsuccessful Interview

In the 1920s, the Board of Trustees and the Medical Board decided that Hopkins should create an Institute of Neurosciences. "And there," recalled neurologist David Clark, "lay the seeds of battle." Clark, who arrived at Hopkins in 1947, heard many stories from colleagues who had been at Hopkins in earlier days. One of them was Sir Francis Walshe of Queen Square Hospital in London, who also shared with Clark some of his correspondence relating to his consideration for the post of director of this projected Institute.

The interviews were complicated by institutional politics, Clark said. "Neurosurgery, headed at that time by Walter Dandy and protected by Dean Lewis as a part of his surgical empire, found no enthusiasm for joining an endeavor which it would not control."

THERE HAD BEEN SO MANY INTERVIEWS. WOULD WALSHE BE THE ONE WHO WOULD FINALLY GET THE JOB?

"Throughout the twenties and into the early thirties this Institute scheme was the Neurological leit-motif of the Hospital," noted Clark. "It took form as a sort of neuro-recruiting quartan ague" (a recurring fever in malaria), "marked by recurrent periods of active recruitment." To Clark, it had assumed almost the nature of a ritual. "Every time another candidate ... would visit the Hospital – usually, in that distant quieter time, for a few weeks or a month, give lectures, be wined and dined, perhaps leave a paper in the Bulletin, and depart, presumably courteously to refuse appointment if proffered."

Into that environment came Walshe, who must have known something of what he was getting into; he had spent a year at Hopkins as a fellow in Medicine with William Sydney Thayer. The faculty did its best to smooth the way, Clark explained, but some alarm bells were ringing. "It was recognized that his visit could easily be complicated by brushes with Dr. Dandy. Walshe was a Londoner of Londoners. Dandy ... was an Anglophobe of malignant proportion. Further, he was then riding the crest of his discovery of ventriculography (one of two procedures Dandy invented using air, injected into the brain, to provide a contrast that helped brain tumors show up on x-rays), which in a sense was the MRI of its day. Young Dr. (Frank) Ford, who used to tell this tale with relish, was given the task of assuring Dr. Dandy's good behavior. He was able to extract a grudging promise of courtesy, then waited with some apprehension for the first encounter."

It went better than anyone had expected, until the very end. "Dandy asked, 'Now, Dr. Walshe, is there anything you would like me to show you while you're here?'" Walshe airily replied, "Oh, no, I think not. Oh, yes there is! I'd like to see you do that air squirt of yours sometime!" Ford told Clark that he was able to separate the two men, but just barely.

Later that day, Ford encountered Dandy, "who said grimly, 'You know, Ford, I knew I wasn't going to like that man.'"

The position of Director of the planned Institute remained unfilled.

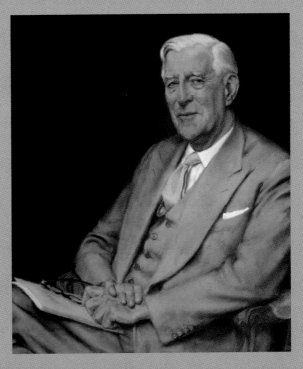

SIR FRANCES WALSHE sailed through his interview at Hopkins, until he said the wrong thing to Walter Dandy – unfortunately referring to his ventriculography as "that air squirt of yours." Seen here in a 1963 portrait that hangs in the National Hospital for Neurology and Neurosurgery, Queen Square, London.

Reproduced with permission from University College London Hospital (UCLH) Arts and Heritage, UCLH NHS Foundation Trust.

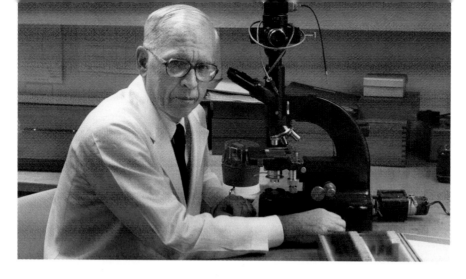

VERNON MOUNTCASTLE long an advocate for a separate neurology department at Hopkins, finally made Mac Harvey see the light.

neurologist. He set out to do exactly that, and his career is outstanding evidence of his success. He was, I think, one of the three or four finest neurological diagnosticians I have ever seen.

"With this enormous ability, he combined little or no desire to develop Neurology and made few demands on the Hospital. He was exactly what was wanted after the decade of search for an Institute director. He filled the role to perfection. It was his tragedy that the needs of The Hopkins grew beyond what he alone could provide."

In 1946, Mac Harvey, new in his role as Department of Medicine chairman, brought in Magladery to help develop the Division of Neurology. From a standpoint of sheer personality compatibility, it was an ill-fated move: Magladery and Ford clashed repeatedly. Clark, an eyewitness to many of these battles, viewed both sides with compassion: Magladery came after serving in the British Army, "and a more complete antithesis to Ford and the Neurology he represented could not be imagined. Irish by extraction, Canadian by birth and education, he had studied pathology with Aschoff, and neurophysiology, especially muscle and spinal reflex physiology, at Oxford before doing a registrarship at Queen Square, where he found his role model, Dr. Arnold Carmichael."

"Like Ford, an incredibly kindly man, and like Ford, an incredibly stubborn one, Magladery had his own tragedy, that being a total lack of humor. I do not believe he ever encountered a situation which he found genuinely funny. As a clinician he shared a trait of Arnold Carmichael's: he took a superb history, did a meticulous examination – he examined patients beautifully – then added up his findings to (an initial) diagnosis that was almost always wrong. Where Ford would ask two questions and elicit one reflex to come up with the right answer, Magladery would labor for hours, to end up as often as not in error."

Although both men made a sincere effort to work together, Clark continued, "an administrative failure (on Harvey's part) to clarify responsibility, plus their own personal incompatibilities, was simply too much. At a time when developing Neurology needed all its strength and cohesiveness for the evolving struggle for its Departmental identity, there was always a strong element of divisiveness. Old and dear friends, especially Frank Walsh, did their best, but the differences ran too deep."

Somehow, though, neurology at Hopkins kept going, providing excellent care, and training future neurologists, despite the drama. In fact, said Clark, "the residency program was a genuine jewel, and Magladery's abilities as a recruiter of young people became more and more visible. *This is not the record of a failing program. Nor were we lacking in other achievements.* Grant support for the time was good. Publications, by number and journal, were more than adequate." But Hopkins could not take neurology to the next level. "We lacked the base – the beds, the service structure, the identity – to attempt any of the larger programs readily available in those times. We remained a consultative service, with all this implies, and always with the feeling of a second-class citizenship. Recruitment went well, and by the late fifties we numbered six on the faculty, four in adult and two in child Neurology."

So things were good and yet not so good; trouble was brewing.

Ford retired in 1958, and Hopkins neurology reached its crisis point in the mid-1960s. Even describing the situation more than 20 years after the fact, Clark still felt the misery of it. "One cannot live in an atmosphere of that sort of emotional stress indefinitely," he said. "One by one, we began to realize that, whatever the right or the wrong of it, wherever justice or injustice lay, the reality was that with the dramatis personae of Neurology, Medicine, and Pediatrics, independent status for Neurology was an impossibility." The faculty began to dwindle. "Luttrell left first, I followed, then John Menkes. The blow to Magladery was tremendous. He felt, I think, betrayed and deserted, and we were none of us ever really able to change that, nor really to convince either Ford or Magladery what they had meant to us. Those were painful days."

It was Mountcastle who finally made Harvey see the light. John Freeman told the story well: "Finally, after one committee meeting chaired by Mountcastle, he and Harvey walked out together. Mountcastle said in his laconic fashion, 'You know, Mac, this isn't about brain infections or about neuromuscular disease; it isn't even about clinical neurology. It's about the science of the brain and about the science of behavior.'"

Harvey said, "Oh!" followed by: "Then neurology needs to be a department."

And boom, the walls of opposition fell down. With Harvey on board, the trustees soon voted to create a department – also motivated by the knowledge that Hopkins-trained neurology residents weren't joining other academic departments, and weren't making their own mark in research or the training of new neurologists. This was a sensitive point, noted Freeman: "Hopkins prided itself on creating future leaders of departments at other schools." A third cause of this sea change was serendipity: Dean Turner had just secured two new professorships for the School, one named for John F. Kennedy, the other for Dwight D. Eisenhower, sponsored by the Joseph P. Kennedy Foundation and the Cerebral Palsy Foundation.

"Finally," Harvey wrote in his Hopkins history, *A Model of Its Kind,* "space could be had in the planned Traylor Building for research, and beds were available in the hospital for the care of patients with neurological disorders."

No one was happier than those who had loved Hopkins neurology and mourned its time of turmoil. "The French tell us parting is to die a little," wrote Clark. "I would put it to you, parting from The Hopkins is to die more than just a little. Personally, I did not begin to recover until the spring of 1967, when Vernon Mountcastle wired me – down in the wilds of Kentucky – that the trustees had authorized the Department, that the endowed professorships, to be held by Dr. (Guy) McKhann and Dr. (Richard) Johnson, were authorized, and that Neurology at The Hopkins was again under way – that the winter of our discontent was gone."

"Finally, after one committee meeting chaired by Mountcastle, he and Harvey walked out together. Mountcastle said, 'You know, Mac, this isn't about brain infections or about neuro-muscular disease; it isn't even about clinical neurology. It's about the science of the brain and about the science of behavior.'" Harvey said, "Oh! Then neurology needs to be a department." And boom, the walls of opposition fell down.

The Days of Ford and Magladery

Frank Ford and John Magladery: two good men, fine neurologists and, from all accounts, two very different personalities. Former Hopkins neurologist David Clark described them as polar opposites – oil and water – and even compared the Hopkins neurology environment from the mid-1940s to mid-1960s as being like that of Bosworth Field, the last major battleground of the War of the Roses, England's civil war.

Civil war, really? Undoubtedly, there was tension, and in such an environment, it is difficult not to choose a side; it is also stressful to walk on eggshells. Clark tried hard to see both sides, and so did Howard Moses, who was on the faculty in the Division of Neurology, and who left Hopkins to become founding chief of neurology at Greater Baltimore Medical Center in 1965. In 2000, Moses wrote an account of neurology during those days; he also wrote an obituary for Magladery, who died in 1977.

Frank Rodolph Ford started his private practice of neurology in 1927 at the Medical Arts Building, said Moses. He happened to know the specific year because he bought Ford's furniture after he died in 1969 and "found the original engraving plate announcing the opening of his practice."

FORD SHARED OFFICES WITH INTERNIST JOSIAH MOORE, WHO ONCE TREATED THE NOTORIOUS GANGSTER, AL CAPONE, FOR SYPHILIS.

Ford was known at Hopkins as "The Judge," Moses wrote, "an eccentric person who patronized the arts," whose wife was an artist, and who did not drive. Ford, with neurosurgeon Walter Dandy and neuro-ophthalmologist Frank Walsh, "formed a strong triumvirate in the 1940s covering Johns Hopkins and Baltimore City Hospitals." Quiet and shy, Ford smoked cigars in the clinic where he sometimes taught; over the course of Frank Walsh's two-hour neuro-ophthalmology rounds, he would smoke two Optimo Admirals. "During World War II, he commuted to Johns Hopkins Hospital on a horse-drawn milk truck."

Despite his idiosyncrasies, Ford was an astute clinician and everyone who watched him examine a patient and come to a diagnosis learned from him – but "if he had a fellow or any teaching program, it did not amount to very much," noted Moses.

When Department of Medicine chair A. McGehee (Mac) Harvey decided to strengthen neurology academically, it was a time when several internists "were doing some neurology," as well, said Moses, and the lines for who did what were not very clear. In fact, Harvey himself studied myotonia and kept a herd of Barbary goats on the roof of the School of Hygiene. To head the brand-new Division, Harvey hired Magladery, a Rhodes Scholar who had trained at the University of Western Ontario and served in the African campaign under Montgomery in World War II.

MAGLADERY "OFTEN SPOKE OF HIS (WARTIME) GENERAL MEDICAL DISPENSARY WORK. HIS FAMILIAR GREETINGS TO HIS COLLEAGUES, 'HEIGH HO,' AND 'BUNGO HO,' DATE FROM THAT TIME."

Harvey had promised Magladery "a full professorship, etc... but he never fulfilled that promise and Dr. Magladery finished his tenure as associate professor, as did Frank Ford."

What was it like, back in those days? "Few of the photos of Dr. Magladery's residents from about 1946 or 1947 until 1969 are available, having been lost when the Department of Neurology moved into the Meyer Building." So we can't see the young faces of the residents – who all began their training at City Hospitals, "except David Clark," said Moses, "who refused to go there." But we can imagine: The Neurology Division's office was on Osler 3. The faculty was small: Magladery, Robert Teasdall, who had an electrophysiology laboratory down the hall; Charles Luttrell, who did neurovirology as well as some pediatric neurology; Clark, "who was a pediatric neurologist and neuro-pathologist and did some adult neurology," said Moses; Thomas Preziosi and Ford. "Frank Ford had nothing to do with the Division, however... he and Dr. Magladery did not speak with each other and Dr. Ford did not participate in any teaching in the department except to sit in on the clinics from time to time."

At Baltimore City Hospitals (later, Francis Scott Key Medical Center, and now Johns Hopkins Bayview Medical Center), the neurology division had a ward on the second floor of the B "or Chronic Building, where there were chronic neurological patients with classical examples of neurological disease, various strokes, syphilis, chorea, degenerative changes, demyelinating disease, various muscular dystrophies, etc." One floor down, "one room was set aside as the residents' headquarters, and there Dr. Magladery did some of his important work on the spinal cord reflexes." This was back in the days when residents actually lived in or very close to the hospital, and "single residents had the choice of occupying rooms on the top two floors."

Weekly Rounds, held on Thursday mornings, "began with a review of all the important charts in the department," read by various residents and critiqued around a conference table, "followed by Grand Rounds, which were highly clinically oriented." Thursday afternoons,

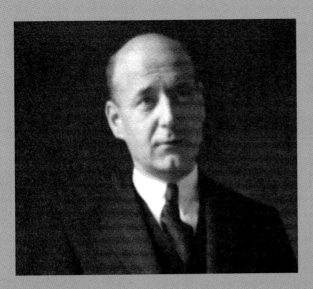 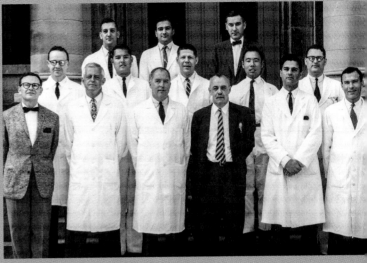

FRANK FORD (LEFT) **AND JOHN MAGLADERY'S DIVISION OF NEUROLOGY, 1963-64** (RIGHT)
Frank Ford and John Magladery: "both intelligent, estimable men, kindly and concerned for patients, Hospital and colleagues, good friends and sturdy enemies. Beyond an interest in the nervous system, they had really nothing in common." **Division of Neurology, 1963-64** *Front Row:* John Menkes, Robert Teasdall, John Magladery, David Clark, Thomas Preziosi, Howard Moses. *Second Row:* Michael McQuillen, Robert Jay Whaley, Ted Chonister, Masao Honda, Leslie Weiner. *Back Row:* Leo Coleman, Thomas Lamassa, William McLean.

Magladery made his rounds at City Hospitals. Magladery designed the neurology outpatient clinic at Hopkins, on the second floor of the Carnegie Building, "in a unique fashion," Moses continued. "Examining rooms surrounded a central conference center," with curtains that could be opened so those in the conference room could see individual patients.

It is difficult to imagine this in today's highly documented and litigious medical climate, but in addition to the strained environment within Neurology itself, and between Neurology and Medicine, "there was not the warm collegiality between Neurology and Neurosurgery … as there is now," said Moses. "Drs. Magladery and Earl Walker were not on the best of terms, and Dr. Magladery was a ready critic of the surgery for intracranial aneurysms in those days. The morbidity and mortality was very high. It was not unusual for neurosurgery residents to steal patients off the neurology floors to operate on them."

Magladery wrote numerous papers, was a member of many prestigious medical societies, and among his most cherished interests at Hopkins was the Neurology Library, "which he personally set up and nurtured through the years."

A final note on Magladery, from the obituary that Moses wrote: "It is always exciting to be able to influence the lives of others, either directly or indirectly. Dr. Magladery did this in a special way, but more by example than fiat. To his residents, he was 'the boss,' and they were 'his boys.' He was a gentle man, very considerate of others, and very loyal to those who worked with him, and they in turn returned this loyalty to him. He was very much

interested in the personal welfare of his colleagues and attempted to guide them in what seemed to be the proper directions, yet he was a very private person and somewhat shy.

"He was intellectually honest and expected the same of others. He would read and reread his staff's papers until they met his standards for publication. His own papers were beautifully written in that typical English-Canadian style, not parched and dry but with a pleasing rhythm, very easy to read. He was best known for his ability to spot phonies and insincere people and would often make his thoughts about them known sooner or later. He disdained pomposity and would often make those who behaved thusly very uncomfortable. Those who knew him appreciated the fact that he was not a politician and most of his colleagues admired him for this quality. He was a classical Queen Square neurologist who performed a meticulous neurological examination with no gimmicks, a neurologist's neurologist, one to whom his residents could always come for help in unraveling a difficult neurological problem."

"The morbidity and mortality of surgery for intracranial aneurysms was very high. It was not unusual for neurosurgery residents to steal patients off the neurology floors to operate on them."

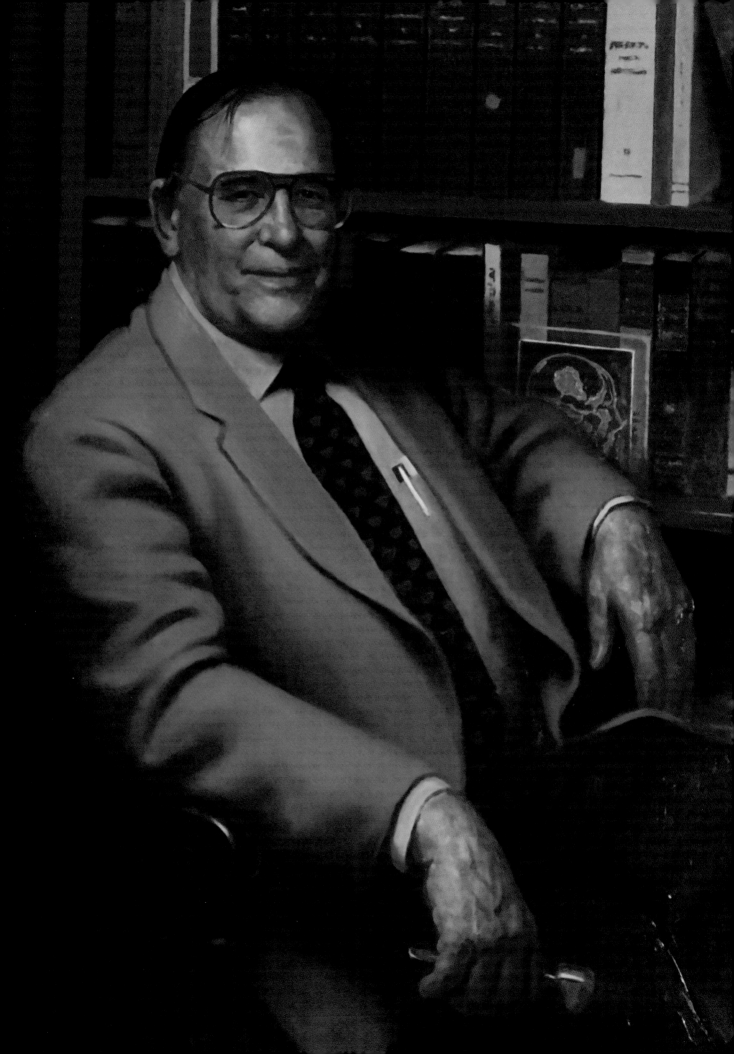

CHAPTER TWO

STARTING FROM SCRATCH

1969

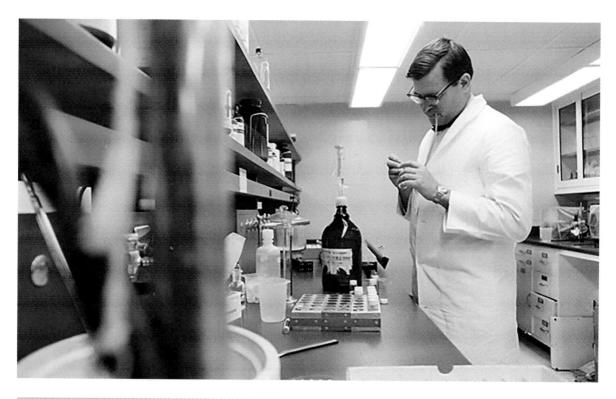

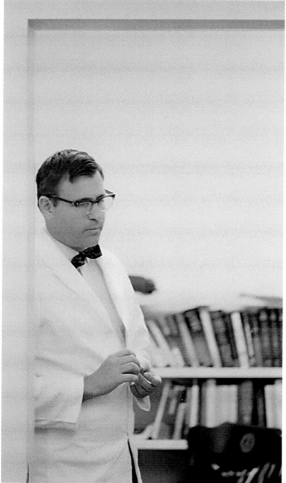

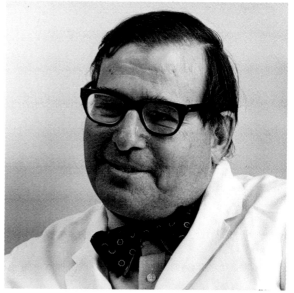

GUY MCKHANN, 1969

Guy McKhann in the early days. Some academics thought "the time for building new departments had passed, that the NIH was running out of money, and that building a new department couldn't be done. Guy, with his indomitable enthusiasm, proved them wrong."

It is one thing to get funding, as Dean Thomas B. Turner did, and to establish two brand-new professorships – and with this feat, to create a Department of Neurology.

It is quite another thing to figure out what that department should do, and be. This is the task that faced Guy McKhann in January of 1969, when he left Stanford and came to Baltimore to be the first Director of the Department of Neurology.

Fortunately, McKhann had plenty of time to think about it: When he first got to Baltimore, and for the rest of the school year, "I left my family out in California and I'd go back every other weekend or so," he says. During that time, he lived in Reed Hall, right across Broadway from the Hospital, in a small apartment with a tiny kitchen. "I would talk to people about the Department in that kitchen – plan and talk about what we might do. A lot of my talks were with Dick," neurologist Richard Johnson, an internationally renowned expert on infections of the nervous system. "First of all to convince him to come here, and then about how we might do things."

This was a fairly similar living arrangement to the one he'd had in 1957, when McKhann came to Hopkins for a year as a pediatric resident – except "in those days, I lived up by the top of the Dome, and I would go weeks without ever leaving the Hospital. Residency was a 24/7 job, to say the least, and furthermore, there was no place to go, because there was nothing around Hopkins. There was one Italian restaurant we went to, and that was about it. I didn't have a car, so I didn't see much of the rest of the city at all."

Back then, and later as a department chairman, McKhann had come to Hopkins in large part because of Robert Cooke, head of the Department of Pediatrics. Cooke had been on the faculty at Yale, where McKhann had gone to medical school, "and I worked in his lab," says McKhann. "So when he came to Hopkins, he called me up and said, 'I'd like you to come down here as a resident.' I said, 'Bob, I don't want to go into pediatrics. My father was a professor of pediatrics. My mother was a professor of pediatrics. That's not a good thing for me to do!' He said, 'Just come for one year.' So I did come down here, and I was a resident, and I had a very interesting time, actually. I didn't know any pediatrics, which probably helped me." After that year, McKhann went to Massachusetts General Hospital to train in pediatric neurology with Philip Dodge, then to the NIH, where he spent two years studying cerebral metabolism with Don Tower, and then to Stanford, where he was director of pediatric neurology. "My first job was as head of pediatric neurology at Stanford, and then I began doing more adult neurology. I was there seven years."

Cooke, who with Vernon Mountcastle (see Chapter 1) was on the search committee, "had wanted to re-develop child neurology at Hopkins," wrote Hopkins neurologist John Freeman in his book, *Looking Back: A Career in Child Neurology*, "but none of the potential candidates would come without a department of adult neurology. Therefore, Cooke also pushed hard for its creation and for Guy McKhann."

The choice had come down to McKhann and Dick Johnson, says McKhann, "and Vernon Mountcastle apparently decided, 'Let's get 'em both. So they got some money for two professorships: $12,000 for me and about the same amount for Dick. So I came to essentially run the Department and be the inside person, and Dick could do his thing (neurovirology — see Chapter 5) on the outside."

Hopkins was not alone in lacking a Department of Neurology; in the late 1960s, "there were a few departments, but not very many," says McKhann. "Ray Adams had a department at Mass General,

"As Guy pointed out, 'At that time, Baltimore was sort of a dump, made worse by the recent riots. The waterfront consisted of broken-down factories, and there was almost no reason for anyone to go downtown at night or on week-ends. Having come from sunny California, I was concerned about whether I would be able to recruit anybody. However, in a few years no one seemed to want to leave.'"

Derek Denny-Brown had one at Boston City, Houston Merritt at Columbia, Russell DeJong at Michigan." One reason why there were so few departments was "that professors in medicine didn't want to have one, and that was certainly true here" (see Chapter 1). "Strong departments in medicine didn't want to see neurology splitting off. Interestingly enough, it was the same thing they went through about 10 years later with oncology." The same issue: medicine didn't want oncology splitting off, "and in retrospect, from the medicine point of view, they were probably right. Because look what Oncology has done. Look what Neurology has done." The independence of both Neurology and Oncology inevitably siphoned off good people from the pool of internal medicine, and also diminished its scope, which would not have happened "if they had stayed within the framework of medicine."

Even though Dean Thomas Turner had secured two professorships – McKhann was the John F. Kennedy Professor and Johnson was the Dwight D. Eisenhower Professor – these were not endowed chairs. The funds to support these chairs came each year from the United Cerebral Palsy Foundation." Freeman listed some of the challenges facing this new department: "As Guy pointed out, 'At that time, Baltimore was sort of a dump, made worse by the recent riots. The waterfront consisted of broken-down factories, and there was almost no reason for anyone to go downtown at night or on weekends. Having come from sunny California, I was concerned about whether I would be able to recruit anybody. However, in a few years no one seemed to want to leave.' It was Guy's charisma and his 'build it and the money will come' philosophy which enabled the meteoric rise in the national stature of this new department. Others said that the time for building new departments had passed, that the NIH was running out of money, and that building a new department couldn't be done. Guy, with his indomitable enthusiasm, proved them wrong."

Although McKhann had to create the Department from scratch, he didn't start with an empty slate, nor without any help at all: There were four remaining members of the old Division of Neurology: John Magladery, Robert Teasdall, Charlie Luttrell, and Tom Preziosi, and Howard Moses as part-time faculty (see side story). This group soon more than doubled in size with the addition of McKhann, Johnson, Freeman (McKhann's junior associate in pediatric neurology at Stanford, who was recruited to start the child neurology program at Hopkins), Dan Drachman, whom Freeman described as "a rising star in the neuro-muscular firmament," who came from Harvard (Boston City Hospital, the NIH and Tufts), and Bob Herndon, an expert in electron microscopy of the central nervous system.

There was some attrition of the longtime Hopkins folk: Magladery had health problems and retired, Teasdall became head of the neurology department at Henry Ford Hospital in Detroit, Luttrell became head of neurology in Seattle, and only Tom Preziosi stayed on at Hopkins.

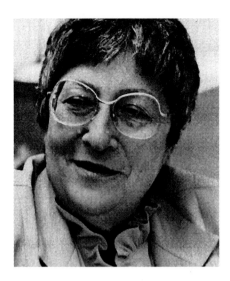

SHIRLEY SOHMER
The adult neurology ward, created on the second floor of the old Brady Building, consisted of a few cubicles curtained off from one another. It was run by Shirley Sohmer, a fantastic nurse and nursing leader, who put together a crew of neurologically trained nurses.

But soon, this "small but stellar faculty," as Freeman described it, was joined by "a spectacular group of new residents." Indeed, says McKhann, "we were very fortunate in the people we were able to attract right at the beginning." These included Bill Logan and Gary Goldstein, both from Stanford, Mark Molliver, from the anatomy department at Hopkins, and Alan Percy, who all became residents in pediatric neurology. In adult neurology: Les Weiner, who was already a resident in the Hopkins program, followed by Jack Griffin, Larry Davis, and David Zee.

"I think the thing that attracted them," says McKhann, "was that we were starting a new department, and we had no constraints on what we were going to do. And that it wasn't going to be a monolithic department. Most departments prior to that had been built around a chairman who essentially dictated what the department was going to be."

The kitchen table conferences, which had worked so well in McKhann's small Reed Hall apartment, continued even after he and his family had moved into a house. "Faculty meetings were held around Guy's kitchen table," recalled Freeman. "We were all about the same age (35-37), and a very close-knit group. The neurology department offices were located on the 12th floor of the Blalock Building. The adult neurology ward was created on the second floor of the old Brady Building, and consisted of a few cubicles curtained off from one another and run by Shirley Sohmer, a fantastic nurse and nursing leader, who put together a crew of neurologically trained nurses."

It may or may not surprise the faculty and residents who were there at the beginning to hear McKhann say that "there wasn't any real master plan. My basic philosophy was to get the brightest people we could find and stay the hell out of their way, and let them do their thing, let them build up their parts of the program. And that's what we did. Dick built up neurovirology, Dan built up neuromuscular disease, particularly his work on myasthenia gravis. Jack Griffin became interested in peripheral nerve disease, and then built up one of the best groups ever. Dave Zee got interested in vestibular function, and built up his program quite independently."

Despite that lack of a detailed plan – or more likely, *because* of the lack of micromanagement from the top – the small Department thrived. "From the start, the goal of the Department was to train academic neurologists," said Freeman, "individuals who would advance the field and then train others." McKhann's leadership style, Freeman continued, "was non-autocratic and very supportive of new ideas and directions. Guy's advice was uniformly helpful as he allowed and encouraged each of us to pursue our own directions. The faculty was cohesive and helpful to each other. It was a wonderful time to be in a wonderful department."

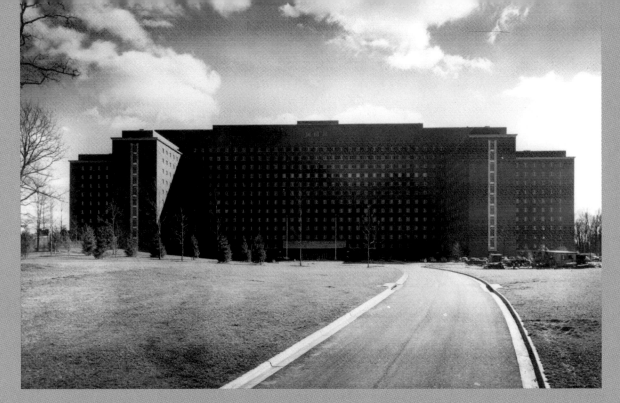

THE CLINICAL CENTER AT NIH, 1960, also known as Building 10. What the NINDS accomplished, McKhann wrote, "was the introduction of neuroscience to neurology." The research that
happened there in the 1950s and 1960s shaped the field of neurology – and, as a downstream effect, also helped reshape the fields of medicine and psychiatry. *Credit: National Institutes of Health*

The Formative Fifties and Sixties

How the NIH Changed Neurology

In 1951, not only were independent departments of neurology mostly unheard of: there was also a dearth of scientific research into diseases such as multiple sclerosis, myasthenia gravis, cerebral palsy, muscular dystrophy, Parkinsonism, and epilepsy.

But this would soon change, dramatically – because this was the year the National Institutes of Health (NIH) established the National Institute of Neurological Disorders and Stroke (NINDS, originally the National Institute of Neurological Disorders and Blindness). Under its first director, Pearce Bailey Jr., this new institute funded intramural research programs and in 1953, it hired G. Milton Shy to be its Intramural Clinical Director.

Not too long afterward, in 1957, Guy McKhann arrived at the NIH as a clinical associate in neurochemistry. McKhann wrote about his decades of working with the NIH in a chapter for the 2004 book, *Mind, Brain, Body, and Behavior: Foundations of Neuroscience and Behavioral Research at the National Institutes of Health*.

What the NINDS accomplished, McKhann wrote, "was the introduction of neuroscience to neurology." The research that happened there in the 1950s and 1960s shaped the field of neurology – and, as a downstream effect, also helped reshape the fields of medicine and

psychiatry. "It is rather ironic that we fought so hard to separate ourselves from psychiatry... and yet now neurology and psychiatry are very much coming back together again. We describe cognitive neuroscience as a joint field. We talk jointly about approaches to disease ... We have also made an interesting liaison again with internal medicine. We now have fields we call neurovirology, neuro-oncology or neuro-cardiology, so ... neurology is returning to internal medicine, but it is now on our own terms."

The NINDS served as an incubator for academic physician-scientists, McKhann wrote.

"IT WAS A VERY RICH ENVIRONMENT" FOR A GROUP OF BRIGHT PEOPLE RIGHT OUT OF MEDICAL SCHOOL OR RESIDENCY "WHO CAME HERE WITH ALMOST NO RESEARCH EXPERIENCE. IT IS A TRIBUTE TO COLLEAGUES LIKE LOUIS SOKOLOFF OR (DONALD) TOWER THAT THEY WOULD PUT UP WITH SOMEONE LIKE ME."

The intramural research program brought to neurology the ability to focus on long-term problems, "in areas that would probably have been impossible to fund within the medical school framework." Take, for example, the work of Roscoe O. Brady on metabolic disorders. "He would talk about enzyme therapy and genetic manipulation. In the 1950s, we had to deal with family history. We had simple genetic patterns: dominant, recessive, x-linked. But our major lead-in was the pathology, and the pathology was almost showing accumulation of some material. Brady was working on disorders of glycolipids: Tay Sachs disease, Gaucher disease, and other diseases of lipid metabolism. First the accumulation as identified, then the enzymes involved, and later they were used for diagnosis. That was a pattern that really started at the NIH with Brady and he carried the research forward: in the mid-1970s, by bringing other techniques in enzyme therapy, and now in the 2000s, by looking at risk-factor genetics, transgenics. That is not so much looking at enzymes anymore but at what proteins are abnormal in these disorders."

The same process happened in Alzheimer's, McKhann continued. "When I first began in neurology, it was considered a very rare disease; it was considered a pre-senile dementia. It had about the same frequency as Creutzfeldt-Jacob disease, and if a neurologist saw one or two cases in his practice, that would be a lot. In the 1960s, we did not think the disease existed.... What changed all this was the work of the group at the Albert Einstein College of Medicine who recognized that the pathology of what was considered pre-senile dementia and what we were calling senility or hardening of the arteries was essentially the same." In the 1970s, "we went back to exactly the same steps that Brady had gone through... the accumulation of a particular compound, the mechanism by which that compound was being metabolized, the enzymes involved, how they might be used for diagnosis, and how they might be used for therapy."

IN COGNITIVE NEUROSCIENCE IN THE 1950S, "WE WERE NOT DOING MUCH BETTER THAN PAUL BROCA HAD DONE IN THE NINETEENTH CENTURY. WE TALKED ABOUT LESIONS IN DISEASE AND POSTMORTEM, AND THAT WAS OUR APPROACH TO THE ASSOCIATION OF BEHAVIOR AND NEUROLOGICAL LESIONS. PATIENTS WERE EXAMINED, SOME YEARS LATER THEY DIED, AND THEN THE BRAINS WERE LOOKED AT."

At the same time, "there were a lot of people in the field of theories of cognition who did not know very much about the brain at all. These fields were brought together, not by clinicians, but by people like Mortimer Mishkin, who could look at systems in primate brains and say, 'These are how some systems work.' The challenge to us as clinicians was, how do we get from that kind of primate physiology to human physiology?"

The leap has come through the advent of imaging: "lesion location, functional imaging and, it is to be hoped, functional correlations."

There were no cellular therapies in the 1950s, either. In fact, back then "if a person had gone to an NIH study section... and said, 'I think we would like to transplant some cells into the brain,' not only would the application have been rejected, but the person would have been locked up, as well." When cellular therapy began in the 1970s, "no one paid too much attention to it." Now, great hope lies in the promise of stem cells and other cellular therapies.

The beauty of the NINDS and NIMH intramural research programs is that "they allow people to do research that would be very difficult to do in the medical school environment." However, McKhann wrote, "I do have some suggestions for change: Anyone who has run a neurology department is aware of the fact that you cannot do everything. You have to focus and identify what the strengths of your department are going to be," and the NIH must do the same thing. "When I was here in the 1950s, the NIH was unique." The research, in those days, "very much focused on epilepsy, and there were not many other epilepsy-oriented programs then. But over time, epilepsy programs sprang up all over the country, so one could now argue whether the NIH has a unique role to play in epilepsy or not. If it does, one ought to rethink how it would be different from the programs for which it was essentially a model."

Another issue to be faced, McKhann wrote, is the problem of maintaining flexibility with scientific staff. "Every medical school faces this problem – aging faculty, tenure problems – yet still wants this atmosphere of bright young people. Forty years ago, we were all in our late twenties or early thirties. That was what made this a really great place. It is very important that (this) group of young people be established and maintained. It is hard to do.

"Many people who came to the NIH in the 1950s did not know what the NIH was. They did not know much about research, and they did not know much about what their laboratories were doing. I would argue that, sadly, to some extent, this is still a problem and that one of the NIH's challenges is to get out and tell the young people what a great opportunity it can offer."

Decades before phrases like "tearing down silos" or "knocking down ivory towers" popped into academic language, McKhann was doing just that.

BUILDING MANY BRIDGES

Under McKhann's leadership, neurology took collaboration to unprecedented levels at Hopkins. Decades before phrases like "tearing down silos" or "knocking down ivory towers" popped into academic language, McKhann was doing just that.

Although, colleagues may note, he wasn't accomplishing this in faculty meetings: "I sure wasn't," he agrees. "In those days, every month, we had a meeting of the departmental chairs in the medical school, and the same people with a few others would meet *the very next day* with the hospital side. **WE HAD THESE TWO LONG MEETINGS EVERY DAMN MONTH THAT COVERED THE SAME MATERIAL! SO I JUST STOPPED GOING TO THE HOSPITAL MEETING, AND IT REACHED A POINT WHERE I FINALLY CAME TO ONE, AND ONE OF MY COLLEAGUES SAID, 'I KNEW THE HOSPITAL WAS IN TROUBLE, BUT WHEN YOU COME TO ONE OF THESE MEETINGS, IT MUST BE REALLY BAD!'** Fortunately, I recruited (Hamilton) Chip Moses. Chip had been a resident with us, and he was interested in administration. He actually went on to be a big muckety muck in the hospital and then in other areas. Chip really handled a lot of that stuff for me. He liked doing it; I didn't."

What McKhann *did* like doing, however, was building the Department in ways that made sense, and one of the smartest and best things he did was to get Neurology and Neurosurgery working together. "Don Long and I were, and are, close friends," says McKhann, who helped recruit Long from Minnesota in 1973 to be the first director of the new Department of Neurosurgery at Hopkins. "We had a single administrator. We met once a week, Wednesday mornings at 7:30. We would discuss problems that were coming up, what we could do together or independently. That was very helpful, because Neurosurgery didn't go in one direction and we in another. We made a big point of working together."

McKhann made sure both departments were situated close together, as well, so faculty and residents could talk to each other and feel like part of the same team. This was a far cry from the days when Magladery and A. Earl Walker were in charge of neurology and neurosurgery, respectively, didn't get along very well, and it was not uncommon for neurosurgery residents to borrow neurology patients from their hospital beds to operate on them (see Chapter 1).

When McKhann first arrived, however, "we were scattered all over the place."

Years after Mac Harvey retired as director of the Department of Medicine, he wrote books about Hopkins history. In one of them, *A Model of Its Kind, Vol. 1*, Harvey described the rather dismal research and clinical situations McKhann had to work with: "Space for the department turned out to be a patchwork arrangement," Harvey wrote. "Offices, clinical activities, and research laboratories were scattered through several buildings, wherever

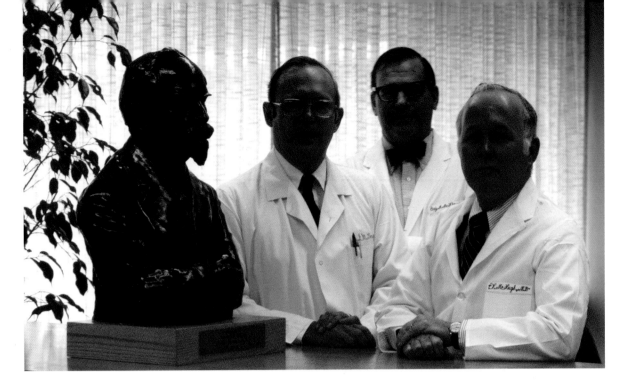

BETTER TOGETHER
From left, Donlin Long, Director of Neurosurgery, Guy McKhann, Director of Neurology, and Paul McHugh, Director of Psychiatry, with the bust of Adolf Meyer. *"One of Guy's ideas was to build a department of clinical neurosciences to link the neurology, neurosurgery and psychiatry departments more closely together, since they all had to do with the brain and clearly were overlapping spheres."*

rooms or beds were available. Neurology's first offices were situated outside Osler 3 – in space given up by the Department of Medicine – and laboratory space was made available by Joel Elkes, director of the Department of Psychiatry, who relinquished half a floor in the Traylor Building. McKhann remembers his shock at seeing the original location for neurology patients, Brady 2. Having come from a relatively new hospital at Stanford, he had not realized that such primitive wards still existed. Brady 2 was soon remodeled to become the new department's first clinical base."

McKhann helped move the process along in his own way, as well: "I had an unusual role in the medical school: I was head of the building committee." He figured that just charging in and trying to improve his own department's accommodations was not the best tactical approach. Thus, he decided: "We've got to take care of Medicine and Surgery, get them what they want," and "that worked out very well. Prior to that time, Medicine had a building, and Surgery had a building. What we did was change things so they were horizontal – so that cardiology and cardiac surgery would be on the same floor. All of that came about, and that satisfied them. So then I could turn to what I wanted to get done – which was, essentially, to build up Neurology."

Putting Neurology and Neurosurgery in close proximity was "very important," he continues. "First of all, we saw each other all the time, and Don and I were very focused on things working together." These two departments were soon linked with a third: Psychiatry. "One of Guy's ideas was to build a department of clinical neurosciences," wrote John Freeman, "to link the neurology, neurosurgery and psychiatry departments more closely together, since they all had to do with the brain and clearly were overlapping spheres. Although at the time we couldn't put the adult programs in one location (that would happen later), we were able to join the pediatric neurology and pediatric neurosurgery patients on the same floor as child psychiatry inpatients in the relatively new Children's Medical & Surgical Center. Guy and Dick Johnson subsequently recruited Paul McHugh to be chair of psychiatry. Paul was a neurologist who had been a contemporary of both Guy's and Dick Johnson's at Harvard, then trained in psychiatry."

This triumvirate of Neurology, Neurosurgery and Psychiatry – the departments and their patients, as well – would, in 1982, be housed all together, in the eight-story Meyer Building.

What happened in Neurology over the next 50 years is the subject of this book, so just keep reading. McKhann served as director of Neurology until 1988, when he stepped down and was succeeded by Richard Johnson. He then started something new – the Mind/Brain Research Institute, now the Zanvyl Krieger Mind/Brain Institute. "I moved my base from the medical school to Homewood to start it. This was an idea of Vernon Mountcastle's – essentially studying higher brain function in an organized way – so Vernon and I set up this institute." Mountcastle, who was also stepping down as director of Physiology, moved to the Homewood campus, too. Their institute is devoted to understanding how neural activity in the brain translates to thoughts and feelings – perception, memory, knowledge, decision, and action, and will doubtless be the subject of its own history book someday.

For the last 25 years, McKhann has been the scientific advisor to the Dana Foundation, a private philanthropic organization that supports brain research in the U.S. and Europe. Among many honors, he also was elected president of the American Neurological Association – an organization that, "when I first started in neurology, was a very sleepy place," he recalls. "They had a single meeting, and all the old guys who were members sat in the first couple rows and the rest of us sat in the back, and it was anticipated that we wouldn't cause any trouble. Somebody would give a talk, these old guys would make a few comments, and they'd move on to another subject. It was very uninspiring. Gradually, that changed." McKhann – as he puts it, "not a very good meeting attender," used to go to these meetings "for a day, and then go home." So he was somewhat surprised when an old friend, Pennsylvania neurologist Art Asbury, Chairman of the Membership Committee, called to tell him he'd just been voted President-Elect. "He said, 'I want to make it clear it has nothing to do with your attendance or contributions up 'til now.'"

In a recent interview with Justin McArthur, Director of the Department of Neurology since 2008 (when he took over from Jack Griffin), McKhann was asked if he had any advice to neurologists who are new to administrative or leadership roles. He did: "First of all, you have to have some idea what you want to get done – but you can't be impatient. It takes a while. So you may have all these ideas of what you want to do, but don't rush, because it also takes you a while to learn who your friends are – people you can count on to help, and you need that in any institution – and who your enemies are. Next, find the brightest people you can to work with you and to help you – they're there, and you can find them all over the place; you never know when someone is moveable.

"When I first went into neurology, people said to me, 'What do you want to do that for? All you can do is describe things; you can't do anything.' Well, that certainly isn't true anymore."

"This is a very exciting time in neurology. When I first went into neurology, people said to me, 'What do you want to do that for? All you can do is describe things; you can't do anything.' Well, that certainly isn't true anymore. Neurology is more and more becoming a treatment field, and it's going to become even more so. We have some big imponderables like Alzheimer's disease, but people have ideas about how to treat it. And we will. We're going to come up with answers. So all of a sudden, we're going to have more and more areas where treatment is going to be a very important part of what we do.

"If I were a young guy, I'd go into neurology. This is such an exciting time, and the tools that we have are changing so much."

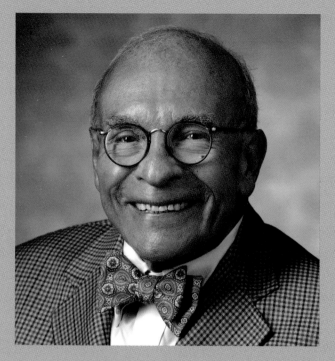

Master Clinician

When Howard Moses went into private practice, Mac Harvey denied him admitting privileges at Hopkins. Guy McKhann not only changed that; he made Moses – a skilled diagnostician and excellent teacher – an assistant professor.

Howard Moses, a 1954 graduate of the University of Illinois Medical School, got drafted, chose the Navy, went to submarine school, earned his dolphins (insignia pin), finished his service in December 1957 and a few weeks later came to Hopkins to begin his residency in neurology.

He was the only neurologist out of his medical school class. "Neurology was not a very popular specialty," he says. In fact, Moses was not officially a neurology resident "because A. McGehee (Mac) Harvey said any internist can learn neurology, so there was no reason for it to be a separate department." Instead, the residents in various medical subspecialties were Osler fellows.

There was some neurological research happening: Dick Johns and David Grob, both internists, studied myasthenia gravis, although "at that time they didn't know it was an immune-related disease. In addition to a small herd of spasm-prone Barbary goats, kept by Harvey on the roof of the School of Hygiene, there was a pasture with sheep at the corner of Wolfe and Monument, used for "various assays," says Moses. "Charlie Luttrell, a pediatric neurologist, did work on myoclonus in cats. Jack Magladery had a lab in the Chronic Building at City Hospital; in that building, too, were "one small room that had electrophysiology equipment, and another on the third floor. There wasn't that much."

A resident was always assigned to neuropathology, Moses continues, "and that was done at the City Morgue, at the foot of President Street, part of the Pumping Station of the City of Baltimore." These neuropathology cases were led by Richard Lindenberg, who came to the U.S. from Germany. "Every Tuesday night, residents, neuropathologists and surgeons would all troop down to the Pumping Station to do the brain cutting. All the brains from all the mental hospitals in the state, all the trauma cases, and brains with various neurological conditions were cut. It was a fabulous experience."

Pediatric neurologist David Clark, "an interesting character in a department that was full of characters," also was a neuropathologist and "did brain cutting at Hopkins, not the city morgue." Clark was an excellent clinician, Moses recalls, and also led rounds one night a week "of all the interesting patients in the hospital. Afterwards, we'd go to a local bar, George's, and have beer. Once a week, we would climb into Dave's old jalopy and go out to Crownsville and see all the neuropsychiatric patients."

Moses writes "When I was interviewed for the residency, David Hubel was the co-chief resident under Magladery. Collaborating with Torsten Wiesel, Hubel went on to win the Nobel Prize in 1981 for insights into the workings of visual cortex." Moses finished his residency in 1961 and was board-certified in neurology in 1963. Despite the attempts of Magladery and others to get him going in research work in various labs, what he enjoyed most was "my one day a week working in the clinic. I decided I wanted to go into private practice, because I only wanted to diagnose and treat people with neurological disease." He also wanted to teach neurology to medical students and house officers.

"DAVE CLARK TOLD ME, 'YOU'RE NOT GOING TO BE ABLE TO MAKE A LIVING IN BALTIMORE, AND YOU'RE NOT GOING TO BE ABLE TO DO ANYTHING AT HOPKINS. YOU'D BETTER GO OUT OF TOWN."

Nonetheless, on July 1, 1965, he set up shop across the street from the Hospital, in the Medical Arts Building. "I shared offices with Frank Schuster, pediatric neurologist, whom I had taught when he was a resident. In that same building, at the corner of Cathedral and Reed Street, Frank Ford also had his offices, which he shared with Josiah Moore, so that was the place to be. I had a business plan: I wanted to bring the highest quality of academic neurology to the Baltimore community. There wasn't anything" – no neurologists available for consulting at most of the hospitals in the area.

As Clark had predicted, Mac Harvey denied Moses admitting privileges at Hopkins, "So I applied for privileges at every hospital I could find,"all the way down to Anne Arundel, up to Harford County, and throughout Baltimore and Baltimore County. He wound up seeing many of his local patients at St. Agnes and Sinai hospitals. Still, he wanted to teach. "I went to Hopkins at least one day a week to run the clinic, pro bono." But if he wanted to admit a patient at Hopkins, he had to do it "through Bob Teasdall or some other neurologist."

When Guy McKhann arrived in 1969, Moses met with him. "He said, 'What do you want?' I said, 'I want admitting privileges and I want to be an assistant professor.' He said, 'Okay, not a problem.'" And just like that, the gate was lifted. Moses could admit patients to Hopkins and do as much teaching as he liked. For many years, he was recognized in *Baltimore* magazine as a top neurologist, and he is one of only a few part-time faculty to have been awarded the coveted School of Medicine Professor's Award for Teaching Excellence.

Justin McArthur, Director of the Department of Neurology, enjoys watching Moses every week at Neurology Grand Rounds. "Residents have come to recognize that within a minute or two of presenting the case, he's got the diagnosis."

His secret? Because Moses learned how to diagnose patients when imaging capabilities were very limited, "I really focus on the pattern of symptoms. For instance, a discussion about a young child presented today, with proximal weakness, signs of numbness, some peripheral neuropathy as well: I said, 'It's got to be a polyradicular neuropathy.'"

His advice to neurology residents today: "You cannot learn medicine by looking at a computer screen. This is not like how to repair a watch or fix a diesel engine. One must know how to sit down with a patient, or the family, who may or may not be fluent, and how to take a careful history and how to narrow down the problem. How to ask the right questions: that's number one. Number two is how to examine a patient, how to lay your hands on a patient, how to separate psychosomatic from true organic neurological findings, how to elicit reflexes, how to respect their privacy, their space, not to insult them. You must learn how to examine by examining live patients. You must do it that way." Moses adds that he was fortunate to have trained in an era of outstanding clinicians: "Ben Baker, John Eager Howard, Lewis Krauss, Bob Mason. To watch them examine a sick patient – that's the only way you're going to learn medicine."

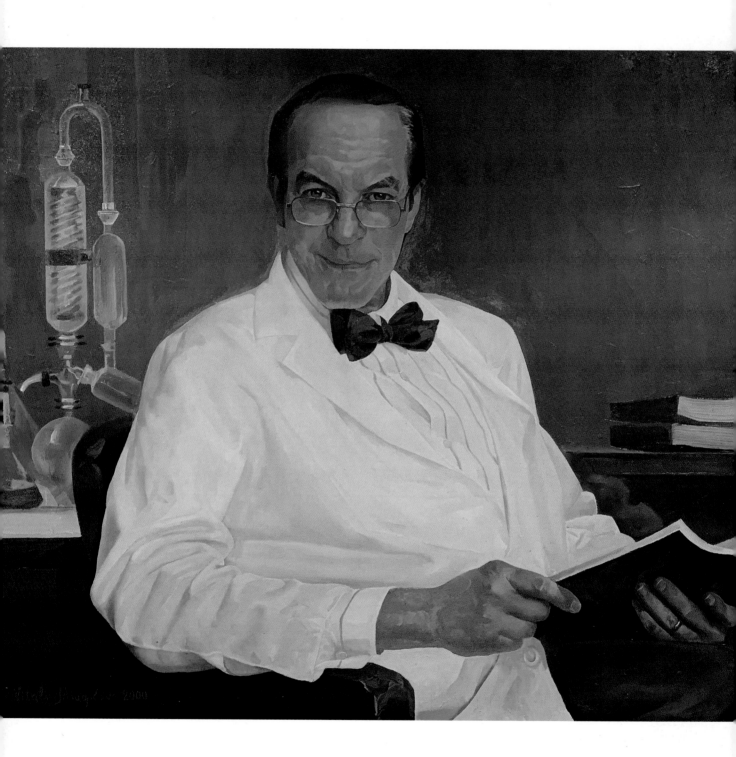

CHAPTER THREE

THE DANIEL B. DRACHMAN NEUROMUSCULAR DIVISION

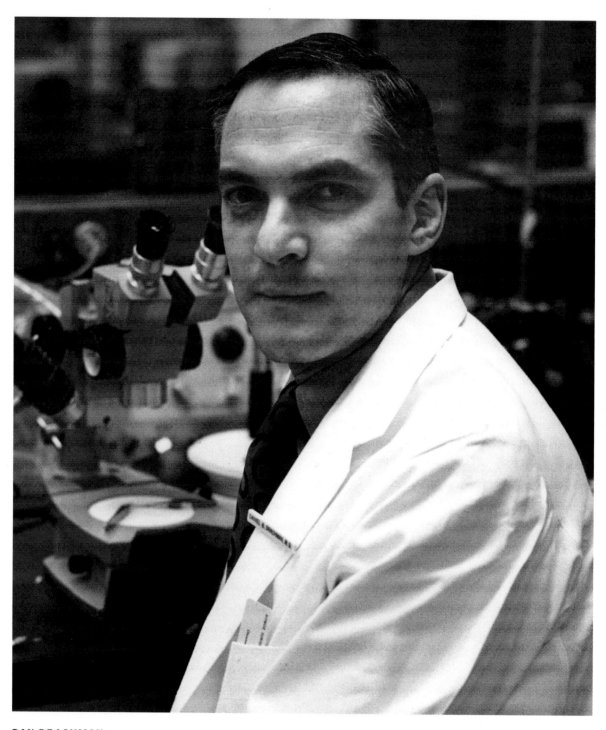

DAN DRACHMAN

Drachman has earned international acclaim for his groundbreaking work: he brought neuroembryology, neurophysiology, neuropathology, and neuroimmunology to the study of neuromuscular illnesses.

"I figured, 'Oh, my God, I signed on for neuropathology, and the neuropathologist has left!' But it all worked out for the best."

At the writing of this book, the Neuromuscular Division includes 14 faculty members. In 1969, there was one.

Today, "well over 50 clinician-scientists and basic researchers have trained in the Daniel B. Drachman Neuromuscular Division" and established Neuromuscular units spanning the globe, says the Division's current director, Ahmet Höke, M.D., Ph.D. "Virtually all the early Neuromuscular Fellows have done well in academic institutions," he continues: Marjorie Seybold was Professor of Neurology at the University of California-San Diego; Ed Myer was Professor of Pediatrics at the Medical College of Virginia; Jack Griffin became interested in Neuropathies and developed the Johns Hopkins Hospital Neuropathy lab as well as becoming Chair of Neurology at Hopkins. Klaus Toyka (see side story) became Professor and Chairman of the University of Wurzberg, Germany; Alan Pestronk, Professor of Neurology and Chief of the Neuromuscular Unit at Washington University School of Medicine in St. Louis; Ronald Haller, Professor of Neurology, University of Texas Health Center, Dallas; and Elise Stanley, Director of the Division of Neurosciences, Toronto.

But we're getting ahead of ourselves – talking about later additions to a great building, if you will, without discussing how well the foundation was laid.

It wouldn't be right to tell the story of the Neuromuscular Division without starting with the man in whose honor it is named: Daniel B. Drachman, M.D.

Dan Drachman knew from an early age that he wanted to be a doctor. He and his twin brother, David, both went to Columbia University and then to New York University Medical School. "I interned in Boston at Beth Israel, and my brother at Duke," he says. "David had one rare weekend off. He came up to Boston, and he and I talked about what we were going to do. Here we were in internal medicine, which we loved. He and I said, 'Look, we cannot learn all of internal medicine. We can learn all of neurology.' That weekend, we decided to go into neurology. So we both applied to the Harvard schools. I got into the Boston City, he at the Mass General. We spent the next three years there and then went to the National Institutes of Health."

Both became distinguished neurologists. David Drachman, who died in 2016, was the founding chair and professor of the Department of Neurology at the University of Massachusetts Medical School from 1977 to 2002, and earned international acclaim for his groundbreaking work on understanding dementia, Alzheimer's disease and related disorders; the neurology of aging; and the diagnosis and treatment of dizziness.

Dan Drachman has earned international acclaim for his own groundbreaking work, on neuromuscular diseases. Just as Guy McKhann brought neuroscience to the study of neurological illnesses, Drachman brought neuroembryology, neurophysiology, neuropathology, and neuroimmunology to the study of neuromuscular illnesses.

"My first two years of training at Harvard were clinical. I decided to take a third year and do neuropathology." Then Joe Foley, the neuropathologist, took a job at Seton Hall in New Jersey. "I figured, 'Oh, my God, I signed on for neuropathology, and the neuropathologist has left! But it all worked out for the best. Dr. Foley felt extraordinarily guilty because he had 100 cases of slides that were yet to be studied microscopically. He would come every week and go over the trove of neuropathological material. Derek Denny-Brown also felt a need to make up for the departure of Dr. Foley and he, too, taught me neuropathology. So I learned neuropathology from these two superb teachers, as well as Betty Banker and Oscar Marin."

Drachman's early mentors in neurology had special interests in neuromuscular diseases, as well. "In particular," Drachman recalls, "Betty Banker, the neuropathologist at Boston Children's Hospital, had a special interest in arthrogryposis multiplex congenita (AMC), a congenital disorder with widespread joint deformities. She had published on the subject, but the pathogenesis of AMC was still obscure."

Drachman wondered exactly what caused the joint deformities in AMC: was it something that did or didn't happen *in utero*? His opportunity to explore this question came in March 1960, when Boston was being pummeled by a terrible snowstorm. An infant with AMC died soon after birth. Drachman spent 24 hours doing a very thorough autopsy, dissecting muscles and peripheral nerves from all the limbs with abnormal joints, and removing the spinal cord and brain. He fixed the muscles and nerves in Zenker's solution. "On the following day," he recalls, "I realized that the Zenker's solution needed to be washed off in order to avoid wrecking the tissues. Although the snow in the Boston area was nearly three feet high, I hiked from Cambridge, where I lived, to Children's Hospital in Brookline and changed the fixative solution. Since that was before HIPAA, I was able to telephone the deceased infant's mother to ask her about the pregnancy. She told me that this infant had barely flicked its fingers, in contrast to her two older children who had done somersaults *in utero*."

It turned out that during this pregnancy, the woman's older children had developed German measles (rubella). She discussed the potential risk with her obstetrician, who asked whether she had ever had rubella. She said yes, and he told her not to worry. The mother probably never had rubella: "When I carried out microscopic examination of all the tissues," Drachman continues, "I discovered that all the muscles around each of the abnormal fixed joints were atrophied, and the spinal motor neurons were markedly reduced, with those remaining showing severe damage and inflammation – as would be expected if there had been a viral infection. I published the case report with the hypothesis that movement was critical for prenatal joint development, which led to my later experimental study at the NIH on the subject."

Like Guy McKhann (see Chapter 2), Drachman went to the NIH, where he worked with G. Milton Shy, "one of the few neurologists (at that time) who emphasized the importance of applying modern science to neurology." He discussed this case with Shy, and they concluded that the lack of movement did lead to the abnormality of the joints – that joints, "like old-fashioned car motors, require movement for development. Without that, they don't develop properly. It requires mechanical movement to develop joints."

During this pregnancy, the woman's older children had developed German measles (rubella). She discussed the potential risk with her obstetrician, who asked whether she had ever had rubella. She said yes, and he told her not to worry.

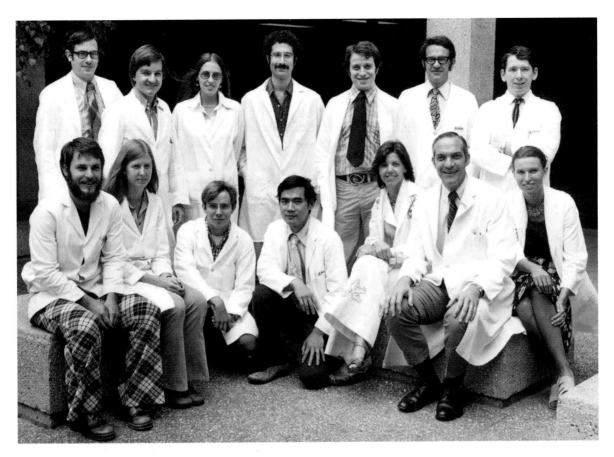

THE NEUROMUSCULAR UNIT, 1976
Drachman taught fellows and residents how to do EMGs and interpret muscle and nerve biopsies. He also got approval and accreditation for a clinical Neuropathology and Neuroimmunology Lab.

Learning From Chickens

Also at the NIH was a neuroembryologist named Alfred ("Chris") Coulombre. "He taught me about chick embryo neuroembrology," says Drachman. "The chick embryo was ideal because it is confined within an egg, which in some ways is like a uterus." Drachman developed a method of paralyzing chick embryos using a homemade micro-catheter to infuse tiny amounts of curare (a paralyzing toxin that comes from a South American plant) into the egg. "The key was to be able to maintain a very slow, continuous infusion," he notes. "This required doing an IV in the tiny chorioallantoic vein," which is just 300 microns wide.

"I infused curare, paralyzed the embryos, and they came out with two changes: not only were the joints abnormal, but the muscles were severely atrophied, as though the nerve had been cut." Drachman proved that movement prior to birth was essential for joint development, and that the absence of movement led to joint deformities including clubfoot, the most common congenital birth defect.

These findings led to many years of research on the role of neurotransmission. "What curare does is prevent the access of the neurotransmitter acetylcholine from motor nerves so that it doesn't reach the muscle's receptors." That's what paralyzes the muscles. Drachman hypothesized that interfering with synaptic activity had resulted in atrophy of the downstream muscle cells, causing trans-synaptic atrophy. To prove this, he carried out a series of experiments with other synaptic transmission-blocking agents – succinylcholine, decamethonium, hemicholinium, and eventually, *botulinum toxin*. "These produced the same types of abnormalities of joints and muscles and established the principle that the synaptic effect of the nerve is 'trophic,' and 'atrophy' results from the lack of synaptic activity."

Botulinum toxin. **Botox? The same injected substance that keeps Hollywood stars wrinkle-free?** Yes, but we'll come back to that in a bit.

Drachman left the NIH and returned to Boston, to do basic research and clinical neurology at Tufts New England Medical Center. He heard about the new Neurology department starting at Hopkins, and that Guy McKhann was going to be the Chair. Drachman called McKhann, who was still at Stanford. "Guy said, 'Why don't you come out and we'll talk?' So I went out there." During the interview visit, he flew a kite on the campus. "I think the neurology folks out there were impressed about some guy who would fly a kite while he was there for a job interview." Whether or not it was the kite, McKhann liked what he saw, and hired Drachman. In turn, "I was persuaded to come to Hopkins after talking to Guy. Guy is and always was an extraordinary leader. The thing about Guy is that whether or not he did what you wanted, he heard what you said. People who really listen are valuable."

"Guy said, 'Why don't you come out and we'll talk?' So I went out there." During the interview visit at Stanford, Drachman flew a kite on the campus. He got the job.

Drachman saw plenty of room for opportunity at Hopkins: "There was only minimal interest in neuromuscular disease at JHU when I came in 1969 – in spite of interest in myasthenia by Alfred Blalock, Richard Johns, Mac Harvey, and Michael McQuillen. The Muscular Dystrophy clinic met rarely, as part of Medicine, and had just a few patients."

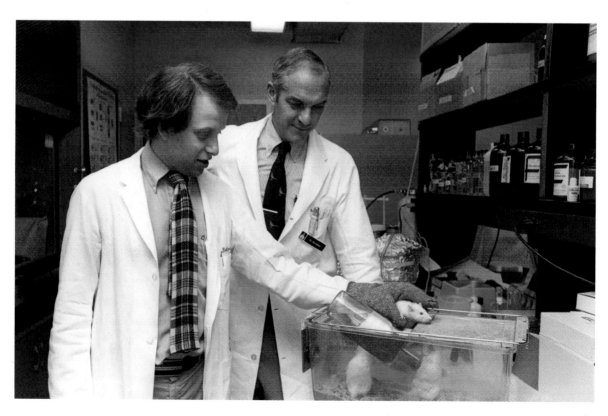

DAN DRACHMAN AND ALAN PESTRONK carrying out one of many preclinical studies of the neuromuscular system.

One of his first official functions was to found a Neuromuscular Clinic – at first, in the Kennedy Building; years later, then-Chairman Jack Griffin would rename this the "Daniel B. Drachman Neuromuscular Unit." A lack of equipment was no deterrent for Drachman; he was a fan of a do-it-yourself approach. "There was no commercially available EMG (electromyography) machine when I first came here," he recalls. "But there was a rack of electronic stuff over at the Kennedy Institute, and they weren't using it. I asked if I could have it, and they were glad to give it to me in Neurology. So I put it together as a serviceable EMG machine with a cathode follower, a cathode ray oscilloscope, a Polaroid camera, and a Grass stimulator. I then worked with the TECA company to develop their first professional EMG machine, and was rewarded by getting one free. I've always programmed electronics, and I soldered the parts together; I did a lot of electronic work with other studies on the trophic influence." His first Neuromuscular Fellow was Armando Filomeno, whom Dick Johnson had met in Peru. The Women's Board contributed funds to buy a cryostat, and Drachman hired a histochemistry technician with funds from the Muscular Dystrophy Association. Drachman taught Filomeno, and the fellows and residents who would follow over the years, how to do EMGs and interpret muscle and nerve biopsies. He also got Maryland State and Federal CLIA approval and accreditation for a clinical Neuropathology and Neuroimmunology Lab. "We don't need to do our own immunology anymore," he notes, "as it's available commercially." But for years, not only did Drachman do his own immunology tests; he taught the Neuromuscular fellows how to do them, as well. "The Histochemistry Lab, now under the direction of Andrea Corse, is the successor to the Neuropathology lab."

The lab that Drachman established "serves patients and provides important muscle, nerve, and immunological materials for research," says Höke. "Under the leadership of Ralph Kuncl then Andrea Corse, the Neuromuscular Pathology lab has grown and continues to play an important role in the care of our patients, research, and training of Neuromuscular fellows."

BREAKTHROUGH IN DUCHENNE MUSCULAR DYSTROPHY

Through serendipity, Drachman made a breakthrough in treatment for Duchenne Muscular Dystrophy (DMD). "I had two patients, both middle-aged, who had either an inflammatory myopathy or maybe a dystrophy. I didn't know which it was." He decided to treat them with adrenal corticosteroids, and he measured the leakage of the enzyme creatine kinase (CK) from their muscles. "The CK went down by about a third," although the patients did not improve clinically. Drachman wondered whether the steroids made the muscles less leaky. "So I thought, 'Let's try it in a disease where we have been told that steroids don't make patients better.' I tried it on 14 of my patients

For years, not only did Drachman do his own immunology tests; he taught the Neuromuscular fellows how to do them, as well.

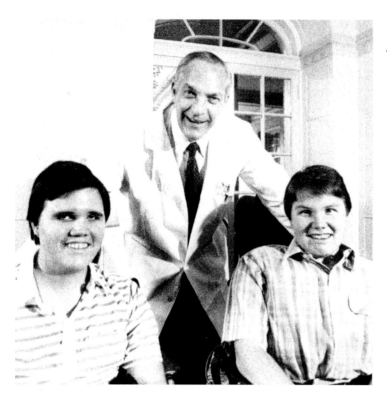

*Every year at meetings,
"I would see my friends
from the MDA and say,
'Try steroids. They help.'"
But no one did. In fact,
Merritt's Neurology text-
book "emphatically said
that steroids are not helpful
in muscular dystrophies."*

**DRACHMAN AND TWO
OF HIS DMD PATIENTS.**
After his study, published
in the *Lancet*, he
kept treating the boys
because "their parents
wouldn't let me stop."

with DMD (which only affects males), thinking that if the steroids don't help, maybe they'll at least lower the CK leakage." In those days, Drachman notes, "it was a lot easier to get people to agree to do research."

At the end of six months, the patients had become objectively stronger, and the CK levels in their blood – as in his earlier two patients – had been reduced by about a third. He published this finding in the *Lancet*, and he kept treating the boys – because "their parents wouldn't let me stop." Back then, he continues, the Muscular Dystrophy Association "would try virtually anything to treat Duchenne dystrophy," but "everything they tried failed." Every year at meetings, "I would see my friends from the MDA and say, 'Try steroids. They help.'" But no one did. In fact, Merritt's *Classical Neurology* textbook "emphatically said that steroids are not helpful in muscular dystrophies."

Drachman persisted in treating his DMD patients with corticosteroids, and continued to have encouraging results: "I had shown that kids stayed out of wheelchairs for three or four years longer, and they were better off," with measurable clinical benefit in their strength. "So my colleagues from MDA said, 'We've run out of agents to try. Let's set up a study and prove Drachman's wrong.' They did a one-year study, and to their amazement, they found that it did indeed help, although the benefit is limited." By then, Drachman had accumulated 15 years' worth of follow-up data, which he published, and "that's how it became the standard of care for treating kids with Duchenne dystrophy." Initially, we used prednisone, but soon switched to a less toxic, related drug, deflazacort, which is now widely used."

Klaus Toyka: My 44-Year Connection With Hopkins Neurology

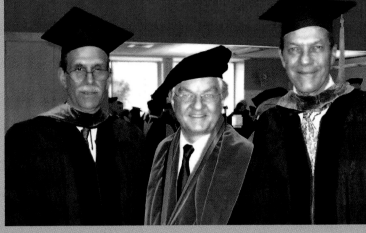

From left: David Zee, Klaus Toyka, and Dan Drachman.

Klaus Toyka, M.D., has been connected with Hopkins Neurology for 44 years – first as a Neuromuscular fellow in 1974, and today as an adjunct faculty member.

Toyka hit the ground running at Hopkins: "The principal postdoc working on myasthenia had to leave on short notice for family reasons, and so I stumbled into two running research projects at the same time. With some experience in pharmacology and chemistry, I had very little knowledge about immunology, pathology and electrophysiology. Nor did I know how to handle experimental mice." He got plenty of instruction from Drachman and others in the lab – Luke Kao, Alan Pestronk, Jack Griffin, and Ken Fischbeck. "Moreover, Dan taught me all about networking with other researchers with expertise," including Diane Griffin, Jerry Winkelstein, and George Santos.

Also, "I had to learn how to do muscle biopsies, EMGs, and all the pathology procedures, after focused instructions. This was the hard way, one would say – 12 up to 14 work hours per day including midnight neuromuscular ward rounds." But it was good, and the pace was rapid.

"It was only two months (before) Dr. Drachman published the first paper with me in *Lancet*, and only five months until we obtained the breakthrough results in the passive transfer of myasthenia gravis from man to mouse using patient IgG antibodies to acetylcholine receptors. The first account was accepted in *Science* in 1975, just before being presented to the scientific community as a totally unexpected yet conclusive discovery. More work included the role of additional pathogenic mechanisms, of the complement system and the modes of the receptor-antibody interaction, all published in the *New England Journal of Medicine*. These papers became citation classics. We all realized that this would have immediate consequences for the emergency treatment of myasthenic crisis, but we failed being the very first to actually do it. In any case, we had become the experimental initiators of an effective short-term treatment in the first established antibody-mediated neuro-receptor disorder."

After his fellowship, Toyka returned to Germany and continued studying the disease mechanisms of myasthenia. "A few years later Reinhard Hohlfeld in my Dusseldorf lab isolated and characterized the first human neuro-receptor-specific, T-helper lymphocytes that were the main regulators of B-cell derived plasma cells and their auto-antibody production. This work we published in *Nature*. Then we attempted to passively transfer human monoclonal antibodies from patients with multiple myeloma and paraproteinemic neuropathy to mice, with Uwe Besinger as the principal investigator and Archinto Anzil as the neuropathology expert. Using the paradigms developed in the myasthenia studies, we were successful in inducing a mouse neuropathy; this was published in *Science*."

Toyka returned to Hopkins for "several enjoyable sabbaticals" working with Jack Griffin, and playing chamber music – he is a violinist – with Drachman, an accomplished clarinet player. "Jack and our group worked successfully on the pathogenic interaction of IgG ganglioside antibodies derived from patients with GBS and with chronic inflammatory demyelinating neuropathy." Later, Toyka and colleagues discovered that autoantibodies to amphiphysin and to glutamic acid decarboxylase 65 may induce the typical signs of the stiff-person syndrome on passive transfer to the rat. This was published in *Lancet*.

Looking back over the four decades, "it is clear that my research career was shaped during the pioneering years at Hopkins. More importantly, these years were followed by a continuing exchange of ideas how to structure research, how to educate junior researchers, and how to keep work successful – and enjoyable – for every member of the team. My friends and colleagues were always important clinical advisors, including Guy McKhann, followed by Dick Johnson, Jack Griffin and Justin McArthur. The clinical structures at Hopkins also became a template for my later work as a chairman and as the Dean and Vice Dean of the Würzburg University Medical School. When Dick Johnson spent his two sabbaticals in the Würzburg Virology Department, we often discussed the similarities and differences of the education between Hopkins Medicine and the Würzburg Medical School, founded in 1582. We agreed it was a great success that the superb pre-WW II Neurology education in Germany could be re-established with help from U.S. institutions such as Johns Hopkins.

*"I should have
patented that,
and I would be
billions of dollars
ahead!" But
back then, most
academic scientists
didn't patent their
discoveries.*

DRACHMAN DISCOVERS THERAPEUTIC POTENTIAL OF BOTOX; DOESN'T MAKE BILLIONS

Now, back to botox: In his studies of various neuromuscular blocking agents, Drachman used botulinum toxin to study the role of acetylcholine transmission in maintaining the motor nerve's "trophic" function on skeletal muscle, at first in chick embryos, and later in single muscles in rats. In this, as with the other agents, "I was interested in what the nerve does to prevent atrophy. Also, the nerve muscle synapse is the most readily available synapse – so the principles from that model are also relevant to virtually all synapses within the nervous system."

Drachman's work with botulinum toxin paved the way for its subsequent widespread clinical therapeutic use. Where did he even get botox – a potential biological weapon – to study? "From Ed Schantz at Fort Detrick," a U.S. Army Medical Command base in Frederick, Maryland. "Ed was anything but an evil poisoner! He was the gentlest, nicest guy you could imagine." In those more innocent days before Homeland Security, "Ed would send me vials of enough botulinum to poison all of Baltimore through the mail!" In the chicken embryos, once again, the action of botulinum made it look as if the nerves had been cut: "They were virtually meatless chickens, because there was so much atrophy. Then at a meeting on embryology at Hopkins, I met a colleague from Australia. Professor P.D.F. Murray, who was the world's expert on the head and neck bones and joints of the chicken embryo." They made plans to meet the next year in England, "after I sent him a batch of botulinum-poisoned chicken embryos" for study. Dr. Murray and his wife took a boat to meet Drachman in London. Unfortunately, "he died on the boat. His wife gave me all the chicken embryo slides that he had prepared. I then learned everything about the head and neck joints of the chick embryo, and published a long paper about the role of movement in the development of bones and joints. Then I thought it would be important to try it in a mammal."

Drachman figured out how to dilute botox enough to affect one muscle of a rat, without killing the rat. "That's how botox really got discovered: Alan Scott, an ophthalmologist in San Francisco, wanted to use it for strabismus, so he called me up, and asked me how to do it." Drachman didn't think this was a very good idea, but he told Scott how. "I should have patented that, and I would be billions of dollars ahead!" But back then, most academic scientists didn't patent their discoveries. However, "I do get written credit for having devised this."

As Drachman predicted, botox didn't work very well in strabismus. "But it did work very well for many other problems, such as dystonia." He discovered this when his friend, the renowned classical pianist, Leon Fleisher, developed dystonia of his right fourth and fifth fingers. Drachman arranged for Fleisher to get local injections. "He's played hundreds of concerts since then," and even made an album called "Two Hands." In 2006, Fleisher's story was made

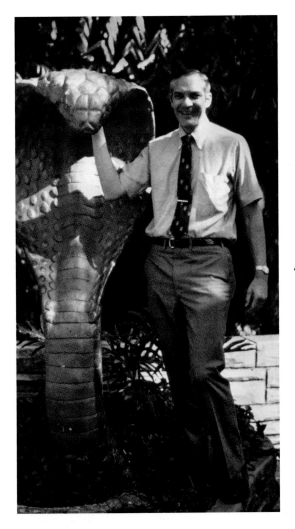

AT THE MIAMI SERPENTARIUM
Venom from certain dangerous snakes (not this one) binds to acetylcholine receptors at neuromuscular junctions, a discovery that helped Drachman and Doug Fambrough learn about these receptors in patients with MG.

into an Oscar-nominated documentary, and Daniel B. Drachman is listed as one of the stars of that movie. He spent many years working on botulinum toxin, and organized a meeting at the New York Academy of Sciences on its use. "That eventually led me to myasthenia gravis."

ANTIBODIES AND MYASTHENIA GRAVIS

It would be difficult to limit Dan Drachman to one particular area of his specialty, because his interests are many. That said, Drachman "has been a seminal figure in the history of myasthenia gravis (MG)," notes Höke. "He identified the acetylcholine receptor deficit in MG; this was the first receptor disorder described. He then elucidated the role of autoantibodies in the pathogenesis of autoimmune MG, and developed treatments as well as diagnostic tools based on these discoveries."

All of this took many years. "Since MG was thought to involve the nerve muscle junction, I wondered to what extent this was similar to what I was seeing in the chicken embryos and rats," says Drachman. Then two Taiwanese scientists, Drs. Chang and Li, discovered that venom from a dangerous snake called the Many-Banded Krait binds *specifically and irreversibly* to the acetylcholine receptors at neuromuscular junctions. With Hopkins biochemist Doug Fambrough, Drachman tested the number of acetylcholine receptors in motor point biopsies of a series of patients with MG. "Lo and behold, we discovered that there were far too few receptors at the myasthenic neuromuscular junctions."

In a groundbreaking paper published in 1975 in *Science*, he demonstrated that "if you purified immunoglobulin from people with myasthenia, and transferred it into mice, they would develop typical features of MG." This was the first passive transfer model, and "it really proved that myasthenia was an antibody-mediated autoimmune disease." In complex studies in muscle cultures and animals, Drachman showed that "there are three different mechanisms by which the antibodies cause disease. First, the antibodies cross-link the receptors. When they are cross-linked, they are endocytosed – pulled into the muscle cells and degraded – and there are fewer of them. Second, we showed that the antibodies could also block the receptors. More important, in association with complement, the antibodies damage the receptors." This led to the idea that either reducing the antibodies, or removing them by plasma exchange, could help.

In genetically engineered mice, Drachman was able to turn off this single acetylcholine receptor-antibody response. "I wanted to develop a method to eliminate the abnormal autoimmune cells without damaging the remainder of the immune system" he says. This approach has wide-ranging implications for other

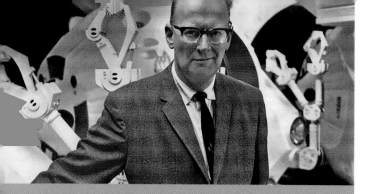

Arthur C. Clarke had been told that he had ALS. Fortunately, Drachman found that this diagnosis was wrong. *"I said, "You don't have ALS. You've got post-polio syndrome.' He said, 'Thank goodness, I will live to 2001!'"* He died in 2008.

Lessons from Shostakovich and Clarke

One day, Dan Drachman got a call from the NIH. The legendary Russian pianist and composer, Dmitri Shostakovich, had been diagnosed with ALS. "He went to the NIH to be examined, and they said, 'Come see him.' So Guy and I went there."

After spending several hours with Shostakovich, they confirmed that he had ALS – "but he had a most unusual story," says Drachman. "He had been playing the piano and conducting, and he turned and couldn't move his left hand. So, at that point, I asked for a CT scan" (MRIs didn't exist yet). It turned out that Shostakovich had injured his spinal cord. "There is a group of patients who probably develop ALS following some sort of cord injury." For Shostakovich, sadly, this turned out to be the case.

Another day, and Drachman got another call, "from someone in D.C., who said, 'Would you be willing to see Arthur C. Clarke?' In those days, we were allowed to admit people for diagnosis." Clarke arrived, and Drachman carried out a very thorough physical exam. "I spent a long time with him. Some of the astronauts came to visit him while he was here." Clarke had this story to tell: "He said, 'Several years ago, I was going upstairs. I bumped my head. Then I was in bed with a fever for weeks, and I've been weaker since.' I said, 'Well, this sounds like post-polio syndrome.' I did diagnostic studies, found that he had severe paraspinal muscle atrophy, obtained an EMG and a muscle biopsy, and a CT scan.

At the end of the week, Clarke was ready to go home. "We had an exit interview. He said, 'There are two things I didn't tell you. Number one, before I saw you, I saw your friend in London, (neurologist) John Newsom-Davis.' And number two, John told me that I had ALS.' I said, "You don't have ALS. You've got post-polio syndrome.' He said, 'Thank goodness, I will live to 2001!'" He died in 2008.

autoimmune diseases, as well. The result of this research was a seminal 2012 article in the *Journal of Neuroimmunology*: "Specific Immunotherapy of Experimental Myasthenia Gravis *in vitro* and in vivo: The Guided Missile Strategy." This was, he says, "probably the most intricate, detailed, and complex paper I ever did. It took 10 years to develop, and it worked phenomenally. But it hasn't yet been tried in humans." Drachman hopes it will be, one day. "Present treatment of MG depends on suppressing the immune system, more or less, as a whole. Ideally, we should suppress only those cells that are involved in making the pathogenic antibodies. To achieve that, we developed genetically engineered 'guided missiles' capable of seeking and destroying only the specific T cells that provide help to the B cells that actually produce the pathogenic antibodies in MG. We modified the dendritic cells to present the antigen to the T cells, together with a warhead capable of killing those cells." In cultures and in mice, this worked spectacularly, and "our strategy dramatically demonstrated proof of principle: the highly specific "guided missiles" drastically reduced the number of pathogenic T cells and virtually eliminated the pathogenic myasthenia antibodies without affecting antibodies to anything else, only antibodies to acetylcholine receptor."

Another approach he developed – targeting potential therapeutic agents to motor neurons, by means of the binding domain of botulinum toxin – has not yet been tried in humans, either. Drachman believes this strategy has potential as a treatment for amyotrophic lateral sclerosis (ALS), as well. And in still other landmark MG research, in collaboration with Bryan Traynor at the NIH, Drachman organized and conducted a genome-wide association study of more than 1,000 MG patients. They found three genes related to susceptibility to MG, and this discovery is leading to a new therapeutic approach.

WORK IN ALS

Drachman also spent years working on ALS. He had the freedom, back in the day, to study what he wanted to – something he regrets that young physician-scientists don't often have. "The field has changed," he says. "When I began, I could do anything. If I wanted to do micro-electrode recordings, I did them. If I wanted to do immunology, I was able to do it. These days, the complications involved in doing research are drastically different: funding, approval of procedures, and the complexity of the latest science. The way I learned genetics," in the late 1980s, "was, I had a postdoctoral fellow, Bing Zhi Yang, who came to work with me. He knew genetics. I didn't. So I said, 'Look, I'm going to take a sabbatical in my lab. You teach me genetics.' He did," and Drachman applied what he learned to his research on MG as well as ALS. In ALS, nobody knows what causes the terrible damage to motor neurons. "The motor neurons are badly affected; they die," says Drachman. But he believes that if some protective agent could be introduced directly into these neurons, they could be saved.

"What can get into motor neurons? Tetanus toxin, but we're all immunized against it; that's no good. Polio virus, but that's dangerous. Botulinum toxin binds to gangliosides," complex lipids on the terminals of motor neurons, "and then it enters. There's a Trojan horse part and a toxic part of the botulinum toxin molecule. I managed in this work to purify the Trojan horse part (the toxin's heavy chain end) and fuse it to avidin." Streptavidin is a protein purified from the bacterium, *Streptomyces avidinii*, and it really likes biotin; in fact, it sticks to it like molecular Krazy glue. In a feat of delicate and complex genetic engineering, Drachman purified the binding part of the molecule of botulinum – this is the Trojan horse that tricks the motor neuron into letting it in – and bound it to streptavidin, so that it can deliver a tiny payload capable of rescuing the motor neuron.

"The goal is to biotinylate a virus that would then carry a cell-saving substance to the motor neurons. The trick is to target it precisely to the motor neurons, and this worked phenomenally" in cultures. Unfortunately, that strategy has yet to be tested in animals or humans.

Over the years, says Höke, the Neuromuscular Division has continued "a strong track record of research to unravel the mysteries of ALS and other motor neuron diseases started by Ralph Kuncl and Jeffrey Rothstein; later joined by Nicholas Maragakis, Brett Morrison, Tom Crawford and Lyle Ostrow." These later advances in ALS are discussed Chapter 13.

BIKING ACROSS AMERICA

With his wife, Jephta, Drachman also promoted the cause of ALS awareness and raised $40,000 for research by sheer sweat equity: in 1990, they rode their bikes across the U.S. – a distance of 4,605 miles – from Baltimore to Seattle.

The trip, which took three months, was partially sponsored by the Baltimore Relief Society, a group of young, idealistic businessmen who wanted to give back. "When we did it, the country was so different from now," he comments, "a much more idealistic and optimistic place."

It wasn't just a spur-of-the-moment, "Hey, let's ride our bicycles across the country!" decision. Drachman, a lifelong bike rider, had been interested in taking a longer trip. Jephta suggested riding across the country. "I said, 'It's a big country.' My wife convinced me by saying, 'Well, if you don't do it now, the next wheeled vehicle you use will be a wheelchair.'" That was in November 1989. Taking advice from neuropathologist Don Price, they started cross-training – swimming, biking, running – to build up their strength and endurance. They had two bicycles custom-built by an English bike maker who lived in Reisterstown.

On May 5, 1990, "we started out from our driveway," recalls Drachman. "I kept thinking of the old Chinese proverb, 'Every journey of 1,000 miles begins with a single step.'" They had bought a carrier van, and "hired a young couple from Towson State University – who later got married! – to meet them every morning and evening. "My pre-condition was no camping. I wanted a bed and a shower every night. Jephta's condition was that her mother needed her to call every night; there were no cell phones then. So that's what we did." In those days before GPS, they followed maps all the way to Seattle.

"It was a remarkable life experience."

One more favorite memory from Drachman's time as head of the Neuromuscular Division: "We have an orchard. Every year, when the apples ripened, I would invite the entire Neuromuscular group and many of the other neurologists" to an apple-picking picnic. "We've got about 30 trees, and most years we had tons of apples. We had volleyball and hamburgers, wonderful cookies and brownies, and terrific hot dogs." After the picnic, "I would take about 40 crates of apples up to Biglerville, Pennsylvania, to be made into cider. It was the best cider ever." For more, see side story.

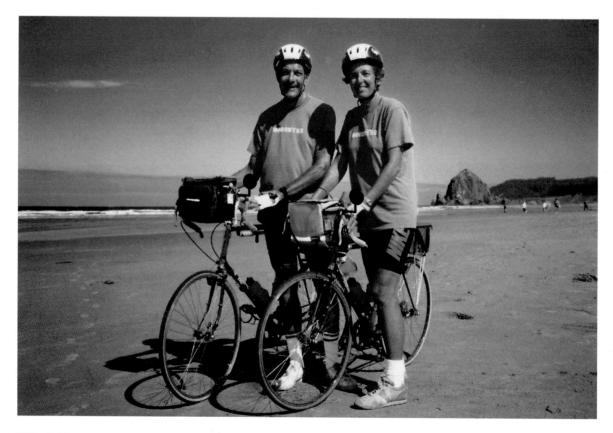

THE FINISH LINE
Dan and Jephta Drachman in Seattle, 4,605 miles from their driveway, the starting point of their mammoth bike trip across the country to raise money and awareness for ALS.

Our Apple Pick

When we first moved to the Baltimore area, we bought a big old house in the Green Spring Valley. We chose it mainly because of two beautiful Copper Beech trees, which later succumbed to a mysterious blight, but importantly, there was also an apple orchard.

Although the trees were old, they yielded delicious fruit, which turned out to be Stayman, Winesap, York Imperial, and some Jonathan apples. We planted more of the same, totaling nearly 30 apple trees in the orchard.

We soon realized that our Residents, Fellows and Neurology Staff would enjoy the apples, and every year we invited them to come on the weekend when the apples were going to be ripe; initially, it was the last weekend of October. More recently, it has been two weeks earlier.

We bought the best hot dogs and hamburgers from Lenny's Deli. My wife, Jephta, made hundreds of delicious sandwich cookies, and two varieties of brownies. We prepared hot cocoa and lemonade, and thawed many gallons of cider that had been frozen from the previous year's crop. The Residents, Fellows, and Staff came with their families. To pick the apples, they either climbed the trees or ladders that we provided, or used the apple-picking long poles with baskets on their ends. They ate dozens of hot dogs and hamburgers, hundreds of cookies and brownies, and took home all the apples they could possibly use. I hitched a big orange wagon to my Kubota tractor, and gave tractor rides to all the kids. I drove them around to see my wife's wonderful metal sculptures (giraffe, manta ray, prehistoric farm animal, hippo, etc). I often told stories about the mythical Indians who lived and made fires on the property. At the end of the day, I would drive the tractor around and collect as many as 50 or more crates of apples that had been picked.

Several days later, we would take the remaining apples to be made into cider. At first, we used an old-fashioned cider mill run by Roger Mann in Westminster, until he left (and went to Florida, where he pressed oranges for orange juice). Since then, we have taken the apples to Benderville, Pennsylvania (just beyond Gettysburg), to the Kime Cider Press, where Rick Kime presses and pasteurizes the cider. Usually we make about 70 gallons of the world's best cider.

Many of the Residents and their families remember every year's "Apple Pick," which they and we always loved. — Dan Drachman

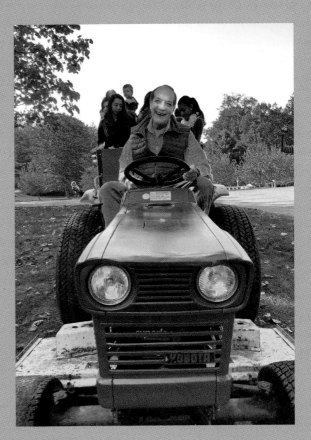

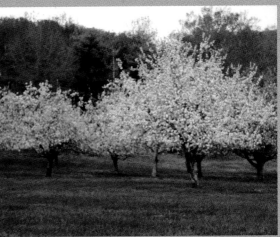

THE DRACHMANS' ORCHARD
Drachman hitched a big orange wagon to his Kubota tractor, and drove all the kids around to see Jephta's "wonderful metal sculptures -- giraffe, manta ray, prehistoric farm animal, hippo, etc." Here are a few of his nearly 30 apple trees.

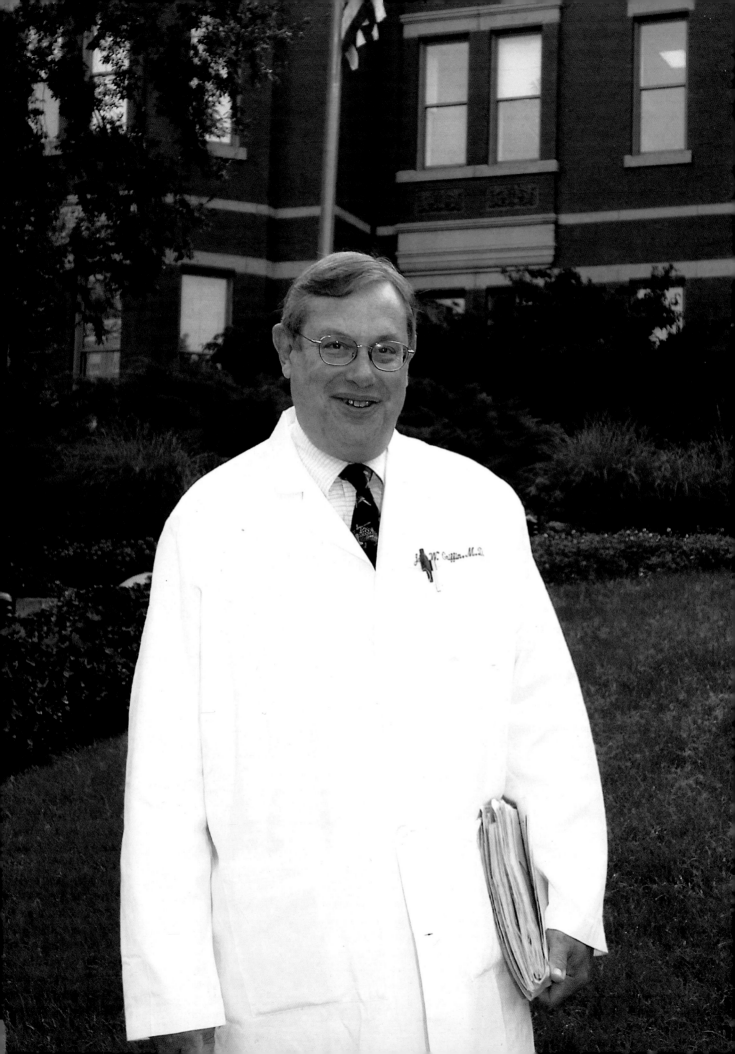

CHAPTER FOUR

THE PERIPHERAL NEUROPATHY GROUP

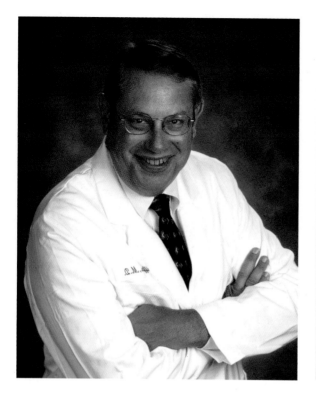

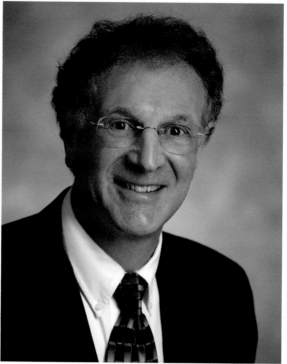

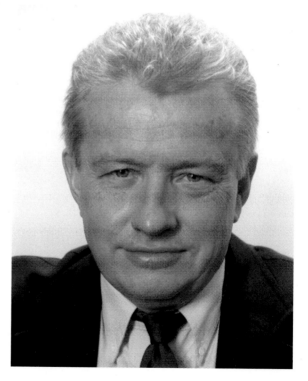

PIONEERING TRIO

Clockwise from top left: Jack Griffin, Paul Hoffman, and Don Price. Together, in a *Science* paper, they showed that exposure to IDPN selectively impairs slow axonal transport. Then they showed that axon caliber is controlled by the transport of neurofilaments.

Building on the Department's strong neuromuscular foundation, Jack Griffin developed a peripheral nerve center at Johns Hopkins that would become world-renowned. Early on, Griffin – who joked that Hopkins was his "nervana" – concentrated on axonal transport mechanisms. With neuropathologist Don Price and neuro-ophthalmologist Paul Hoffman, he demonstrated the role of neurofilament transport in axonal development and regeneration.

In a *Science* paper published in 1978, the trio showed that exposure to IDPN (beta,beta'-iminodipropionitrile) selectively impairs slow axonal transport. Then, using the IDPN model, they showed that axon caliber is controlled by the transport of neurofilaments. "This observation," reflects Ahmet Höke, M.D., Ph.D., Director of the Neuromuscular Division, "has importance not only for understanding the development of the peripheral nervous system, but for understanding nerve regeneration and the pathogenesis of certain peripheral neuropathies, as well."

GUILLAIN-BARRÉ SYNDROME (GBS) AND THE CHINA COLLABORATION

Today, 30 years later, we are still learning from the results of a remarkable research project that was sparked from an observation made by Guy McKhann. Here's how the China GBS collaboration began:

Plasmapheresis as a treatment for Guillain-Barré Syndrome (GBS) was pioneered by McKhann in the 1980s, when he was caring for a small number of patients with a rare, chronic form of the disease. Unlike more common forms of GBS, where patients tend to recover and then go on with their lives, "these patients don't do that," McKhann says. "They very slowly get worse and they stay worse. If they get better, it's very gradual. I had two or three of these folks; I didn't know what to do with them. I said, 'Let's see what happens if we plasmapherese them.' We did. The first patient got up and walked. It was amazing. But then after a while, he'd get worse again, so we'd have to re-plasmapherese him." McKhann published the results from a small series of patients. Then, with three residents – Robert Fisher, William Mobley, and Fred Server – he decided to evaluate plasmapheresis in the normal form of GBS. They set up a controlled trial involving about a dozen institutions.

Puzzlingly, the plasmapheresis trial went better than expected for some patients, and worse than expected for others. "About halfway through the trial," McKhann recalls, "the group from Canada said, 'We want to drop out of the trial. It's just not working.' About the same time, I got a call from the people at Mass General. They said, 'We don't have to run a trial anymore. The damn technique works every time.'"

How could this be? McKhann invited researchers from both institutions to Baltimore, and said, "'We've got a problem, team. It doesn't work for you, and it works for you. So what's the difference?' Well, it didn't take long to figure out what the difference was: The group in Boston was seeing these patients right away. The group in Montreal was treating patients who had been to four or five other hospitals. By the time they got to plasmapheresis, it was quite late. So it was very clear that *when* you get treated was very important."

A Different Kind of GBS

Then, in 1986, McKhann went to China. He had intended to go with his father, Charles Freemont McKhann, a retired professor of Pediatrics at Case Western Reserve, to visit Zhu Fu Tang. Professor Zhu had learned Western pediatrics with Guy's father at Boston Children's Hospital in the 1930s and since had become known as the "father of modern Chinese pediatrics." Guy's father was not able to make the trip, so instead, McKhann brought Dick Johnson and David Zee. At the Beijing Children's Hospital, the team talked with Zhu and his colleagues about the Hopkins experience with plasmapheresis in GBS. "Zhu Fu Tang said, 'would you like to see some of our patients?' So I went up to the ward, where there were all these little kids paralyzed. I said, 'I didn't think you still had this much polio.' They said, 'that's not polio; it's the Guillain-Barré syndrome. We have it every summer.' Well, in the United States, we don't see a lot of kids with GBS, and it certainly isn't seasonal. I thought, 'this is strange.' So I put a research group together: Jack Griffin, myself, Art Asbury, from Penn, Dave Cornblath, and Tony Ho, a Hopkins medical student, who could translate Chinese."

McKhann's observation – that what was happening to children every summer was, neurologically speaking, a different kettle of fish – turned into a landmark study of GBS. The initial research group was soon joined by Irv Nachamkin at Penn, who studied *Campylobacter jejuni*, and Dr. Li (who had been a visiting scientist in Griffin's lab).

Asbury vividly remembers Cornblath "tightly grasping his portable EMG machine throughout China." Cornblath's efforts were worth the trouble: his EMG tests provided the first evidence that this illness was not due to demyelination. Cornblath's work revealed that these forms of GBS involved primary axonal damage; this discovery expanded electrodiagnostic criteria for GBS to include axonal damage. Griffin and Asbury, from autopsy tissue, identified "Wallerian-like degeneration of motor axons and, in a few instances, sensory axons." The research team identified two variants of neuropathy that were related to infection with *Campylobacter jejuni*: AMAN (acute motor axonal neuropathy) and AMSAN (acute motor and sensory axonal neuropathy).

This international collaboration proved "one of the most compelling examples of the power of interdisciplinary research to integrate knowledge, observation and skills to advance scientific understanding of human disease," says Asbury. In fact, he notes, one teaching hospital in Hebei put up a sign that said, "Research is the Future of Medicine."

Among the many insights the scientists gleaned from studying the patients in China, notes Höke, is better understanding of the autoimmune pathogenesis. Since the Chinese GBS was shown to result from an immune response to infection with *Campylobacter jejuni*, it contributed to the 'molecular mimicry' hypothesis to explain this archetypical autoimmune disease." In 1994, Kazim Sheikh, a postdoctoral fellow in Jack Griffin's group, showed that gangliosides on *Campylobacter jejuni* were critical in initiating the autoimmune response, and developed mouse models that lacked the enzyme essential for synthesizing complex gangliosides. Now at the University of Texas in Houston, Sheikh has continued to make important contributions to understanding the molecular mechanisms of GBS.

One teaching hospital in Hebei put up a sign that said, "Research is the Future of Medicine."

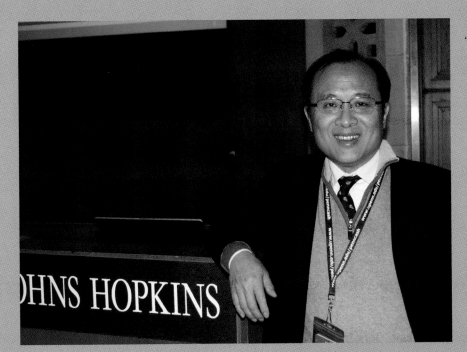

TONY HO

"There were so many children, they had to commandeer other wards to accommodate them all."

Children and Chickens

"TONY HO IS A GOOD EXAMPLE OF THE ABILITY OF GUY MCKHANN AND JACK GRIFFIN TO IDENTIFY TALENT, MENTOR, AND LAUNCH YOUNG PEOPLE TO DO INDEPENDENT RESEARCH," SAYS ART ASBURY. "AS A MEDICAL STUDENT, TONY HO HAD NO SPECIAL INTEREST IN NEUROLOGY. BUT GUY AND JACK 'DRAFTED' HIM INTO THE CHINA GBS EXPERIENCE, WHICH CHANGED ALL THAT."

Ho's part in the China research started in 1989, when "Guy secured some funding from the Rockefeller Foundation to go to China. We visited Professor Zhu Fu Tang at Beijing Children's Hospital; he was about 90 years old. He led us to a ward full of children on respirators."

Ho will never forget his first view of that ward: "What was shocking was that it was not only one ward; there were so many children, they had to commandeer other wards to accommodate them all.

"The histories were all very similar: most of them came from the countryside. Typically, the first symptom was unsteadiness and falling, followed by symmetrical bilateral leg weakness. The disease then might skip to the cranial nerves, with facial weakness and swallowing difficulties, and then progress to breathing difficulties. The last phase would be bilateral weakness of the arms. Many children eventually developed respiratory paralysis that required ventilation. Upon examination, we found that despite the severe paralysis, almost all the children had intact sensation.

Another curious observation was that many of the children had very severe neck stiffness. We could literally lift them off the bed like a board. Naturally, we inquired about the CSF results and all of them had the typical albuminocytologic dissociation of GBS."

It was especially striking, Ho notes, for Westerners to learn that many of the children were being kept alive by their parents, who were squeezing manual respirator bags: "I would later find out that since the hospitals did not have enough respirators to go around and the respirators they had were very rudimentary (all of them were constant-speed air pumps), these children were manually respirated by their families 24/7 until their respiration improved," Ho says. "Amazingly, despite this and the open-air windows of the wards, the complication, infection, and mortality rates of these patients were extremely low. Although they were untrained, the family members were able to take care of their loved ones with quality no less than what was found in the West."

Ho, who is now Executive Vice President and head of Research and Development at CRISPR Therapeutics in Cambridge, Massachusetts, started out in China as a guide and translator. On return trips as a neurologist, he saw patients, performed nerve conduction studies, and taught local physicians how to culture *Campylobacter*. From autopsy tissue studies, Ho, Griffin, Asbury, and others identified the presence of IgG and complement activation bound to the axolemma of motor fibers.

Continued next page >

Continued from page 47 >

WHY IN THE SUMMER?

Professor Zhu Fu Tang said that he hardly ever saw this type of paralysis until about 30 years ago; then it happened almost every summer: "hundreds of kids would turn up with paralysis," says Ho. "Guy immediately started asking, 'What happened 30 years ago? Why in the summer?' Professor Zhu Fu Tang said he did not know." McKhann kept asking every day. "To my surprise, Professor Zhu all of a sudden opened up. Many times, he said, the children would come in after the rain," after they had been drinking unboiled water. "They almost never saw children under one year old. These clues eventually led us to link this disease to a waterborne bacterial connection. Later, I asked Guy why he kept asking the same question over and over again. He smiled and said, 'I just wanted to jiggle his memory.'"

After the first trip to China, "Guy said, 'Let's go see Albert.'" And with Ho, he drove to Albert Sabin's home in Washington, D.C. Sabin, famous for his work on poliovirus, "opened the door and, before we could even start to say why we were there, he handed us a research paper and said, 'I saw those children from Beijing, too, and this is what they have,'" recalls Ho. The paper, by Sabin and his Mexican colleague, Michael Ramos-Alvarez, had been written in 1969 and was entitled, "Paralytic Syndromes Associated with Non-inflammatory Cytoplasmic or Nuclear Neuronopathy."

THE LINK TO CHICKENS

Based on reports of the association of the organism *Campylobacter* with GBS from Australia by Kaldor and Speed, they found that many of the Chinese patients had elevated anti-*Campylobacter* antibody titers. In 1992, Ho spent the summer at Shijiazhuang. One day, he says, "a 14-year-old girl came in with advancing disease. After feeding the chickens, she fell ill and became paralyzed. We sent a team to her village to examine these chickens and took stool cultures from them. The pictures were striking: all these sick chickens had heads drooped to one side. The nerve pathology showed the typical axonal damage we had seen in humans. We were able to isolate *C. jejuni* from this girl and these chickens.

"Dr. Li bought some live chickens from the market and fed them the *C. jejuni*. In the first batch of 33, all got diarrhea and half became weak. In the second, one-fourth developed paralysis. These weak chickens had pathology in their sciatic nerves similar to AMAN patients. An animal model of *Campylobacter*-associated AMAN had been developed!

"The chickens were housed next to six monkeys that had been in the animal facility for almost 10 years. Four monkeys came down with diarrhea, followed by paralysis! The first paralyzed monkey was cultured positive for *C. jejuni*. By the fifth day, he was quite sick. The subsequent autopsy showed minor changes in the ventral roots. Monkey #2 also came down with paralysis but slowly, over one to two months. His teased fibers showed extensive axonal damage consistent with AMAN."

The animal model and subsequent pathology studies confirmed the relationship between *Campylobacter* and the Chinese GBS. Clearly, an immune response to a ganglioside on the organism triggered an autoimmune disease, leading to paralysis.

Ho says that today's excitement in the medical community about the gut microbiome, and how bugs in the gut can modulate immune attacks against cancer, is satisfying to see. But "little do they know: neurologists learned about the power of gut bacteria and their ability to incite disease almost two decades earlier," in China.

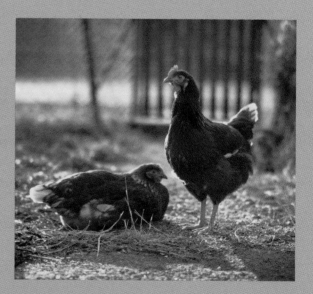

The discovery that chickens had *C. jejuni* led Ho and Li to develop an animal model of *Campylobacter*-associated AMAN.

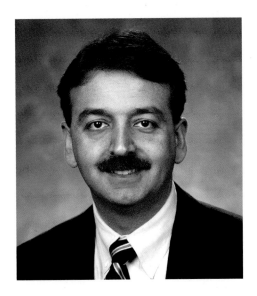

"Jack invited me to come back to Hopkins and join the faculty," an offer that Höke accepted without asking about what his salary or startup package would be. "I just trusted Jack. "

AHMET HÖKE
Höke developed models of HIV-associated sensory neuropathy, a major complication not only of HIV, but of the early drugs to treat it. Today, he is working to prevent chemotherapy-induced peripheral neuropathy.

"I Never Looked Back"

Ahmet Höke joined the Neurology residency program in 1994, after completing his doctoral work with Jerry Silver at Case Western Reserve University on central nervous system regeneration. Soon after his arrival, Jack Griffin "persuaded me to do research on the potential of unmyelinated peripheral nerve axons to undergo myelination," Höke recalls. With the help of "industrial quantities" of GDNF (Glial Derived neurotrophic factor) from Amgen, Höke was able to show that unmyelinated axons in an intact nerve can be induced to myelinate when they are given appropriate signals through the Schwann cells. Through this work, Höke says, "I got hooked on peripheral nerve research." After completing his residency, as a condition of their J-1 visas, Höke and his wife were obliged to return to Canada. "Jack suggested that I go to Calgary to work with the respected peripheral nerve researchers, Tom Feasby and Doug Zochodne." Höke wasn't there long. In 1999, at the American Academy of Neurology's annual meeting, "Jack invited me to come back to Hopkins and join the faculty"– an offer that Höke accepted without asking about what his salary or startup package would be. "I just trusted Jack," says Höke. "This was the environment and allure of Hopkins. I never looked back."

When he returned to Hopkins, Höke pursued a line of research that tapped into the Department's extensive resources and environment available for HIV research. He developed *in vitro* and *in vivo* models of HIV-associated sensory neuropathy – a major neurological complication not only of HIV itself, but of many of the early drugs to treat it. Today, Höke's research involves the neuropathy that happens after treatment with chemotherapy drugs. "Chemotherapy-induced peripheral neuropathy (CIPN) is the ideal clinical target for development of neuroprotective drugs," Höke says, "because one can intervene before the injury to the nervous system occurs." With this goal, he began a drug development program and has identified ethoxyquin as a potential therapy to prevent CIPN. "Currently, preclinical development of novel ethoxyquin analogues are under way."

Jack Griffin brought together Höke and Thomas Brushart, M.D., Chief of Hand Surgery, to work on Schwann cell heterogeneity and the role of Schwann cells in peripheral nerve regeneration. Together, Brushart and Höke have changed the concept of Schwann cells beyond just the "glue" of the peripheral nervous system to specialized, axon-supportive cells. In exciting collaborative work with colleagues in Biomedical Engineering and Plastic Surgery, Höke has developed the first biodegradable peripheral nerve conduits made of electrospun nanofibers as a potential replacement for nerve grafts.

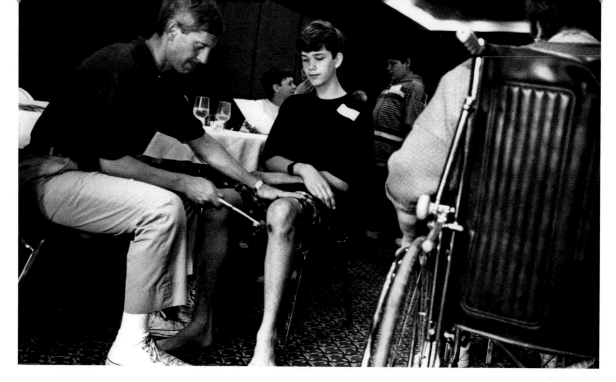

DAVID CORNBLATH Cornblath is director of the EMG Laboratory, a vital part of the Peripheral Nerve Group's strong clinical service. The Peripheral Nerve Clinic, established by Jack Griffin and Cornblath, sees thousands of patients annually.

THE PERIPHERAL NERVE GROUP GROWS

Mohamad Farah, a Ph.D., scientist, was Jack Griffin's last postdoctoral fellow. During his fellowship, Farah worked on understanding the role of BACE1 (beta-secretase 1) inhibition in improving nerve regeneration. When he established his own laboratory, he went on to explore the molecular mechanisms by which this happens, and also BACE1 inhibition's therapeutic implications in various forms of peripheral neuropathies. **Charlotte Sumner**, a previous Neuromuscular fellow who was completing her research fellowship at the NIH with Kurt Fischbeck, was Griffin's last recruit to the Peripheral Nerve Group. Peripheral nerve research is in Sumner's genes: she is the daughter of Austin Sumner, a preeminent neuromuscular neurologist and peripheral nerve expert. In her fellowship years at Hopkins, Sumner had helped identify a defective gene, TRPV4, as the cause of a form of Charcot Marie Tooth (CMT) disease. After she joined the Neuromuscular Division, she went on to develop mouse models and tools to explain how TRPV4 affects axon biology and how mutations in TRPV4 cause neuropathy. Sumner also has made significant contributions to understanding the pathogenesis and treatment of spinal muscular atrophy (SMA; see Chapter 9). Specifically, she demonstrated that SMA is a *developmental* disease – in which the peripheral nerves do not form appropriately – as well as a *degenerative* disease.

Recent recruits to the Peripheral Nerve Group include **Brett Morrison, Thomas Lloyd, Lyle Ostrow, Ricardo Roda, Mohamad Khoshnoodi, Lindsey Hayes**, and **Brett McCray**. Morrison and Lloyd, working together with Jeffrey Rothstein, study ALS and also peripheral neuropathy. Morrison explores how metabolic support of axons is maintained in normal and disease states, and how this affects nerve regeneration. Lloyd straddles the scientific worlds of CMT, ALS and IBM (inclusion body myopathy) with elegant work using the fruit fly as a disease model. Ostrow's main focus is on ALS and developing biorepositories for the disease; he also sees patients with inflammatory neuropathies. Roda studies the role of mitochondrial dysfunction in myopathies and neuropathies. Khoshnoodi works with Michael Polydefkis, who runs the Johns Hopkins Cutaneous Nerve Laboratory, to explore the role of distal axonal degeneration in peripheral neuropathies. Hayes and McCray, current K08 awardees, are working with their mentors to explore the mechanisms of neurodegeneration in ALS and CMT.

CLINICAL PERIPHERAL NERVE GROUP

In addition to its robust program of basic research, the Peripheral Nerve Group maintains a very strong clinical service. Initially established by Jack Griffin and David Cornblath, Director of the EMG Laboratory, the Peripheral Nerve Clinic now boasts more than 10 faculty members who see thousands of patients annually. In recent years, further subspecialty clinics have been established, including the GBS/CIDP Clinic, CMT Clinic and Diabetic Neuropathy Clinic. The Hopkins Peripheral Nerve Clinic's physicians are the largest contributors to the multicenter Peripheral Neuropathy Research Registry, a national cohort study – the largest of its kind – of idiopathic peripheral neuropathy patients. This academic collaboration, established and initially funded by a patient of Höke's, promises to be an invaluable resource for many future research projects, one that will yield genomic insights into neuropathies and lead to the discovery of new biomarkers.

CUTANEOUS NERVE LABORATORY

The Peripheral Nerve Group at Hopkins could not have functioned without the leadership of Michael Polydefkis and the Johns Hopkins Cutaneous Nerve Laboratory. Established in 1993 by Justin McArthur and Jack Griffin with the goal of developing a simpler, better way to identify small nerve fibers in the skin that are frequently affected in some types of peripheral neuropathies, the Cutaneous Nerve Laboratory was the first CLIA-certified lab to use epidermal nerve fiber analysis as a diagnostic tool. Ever since, it has been at the forefront of assessing the diagnostic and prognostic value of skin biopsies in neurological disease.

Polydefkis, who completed his residency and fellowship at Hopkins, is its Director. Under his leadership, the Cutaneous Nerve Lab serves as an invaluable clinical and research resource. Polydefkis is a pioneer in this emerging field: he has developed two experimental models for human peripheral nerve regeneration – both the first of their kind. These capsaicin-denervation and excisional-denervation models are powerful tools that help us examine the potential regenerative capacity of new drugs. Using these models, Polydefkis has shown that cutaneous nerve regeneration is impaired in diabetic and HIV patients with neuropathy. He also was the first to show the utility of skin biopsies in diagnosing amyloidosis.

A common theme among the peripheral nerve experts at Hopkins is that, like Polydefkis, almost all of them have completed at least part of their training here. "This is a testament to the intellectual environment that keeps young, promising neurologists at Hopkins and nurtures their academic careers," says Höke. It is an established tradition in the Department. Jack Griffin once said:

"As a chair, I need three faculty members to do the clinical workload of one full-time clinician, so that each one can have the time to devote to research and academic pursuits."

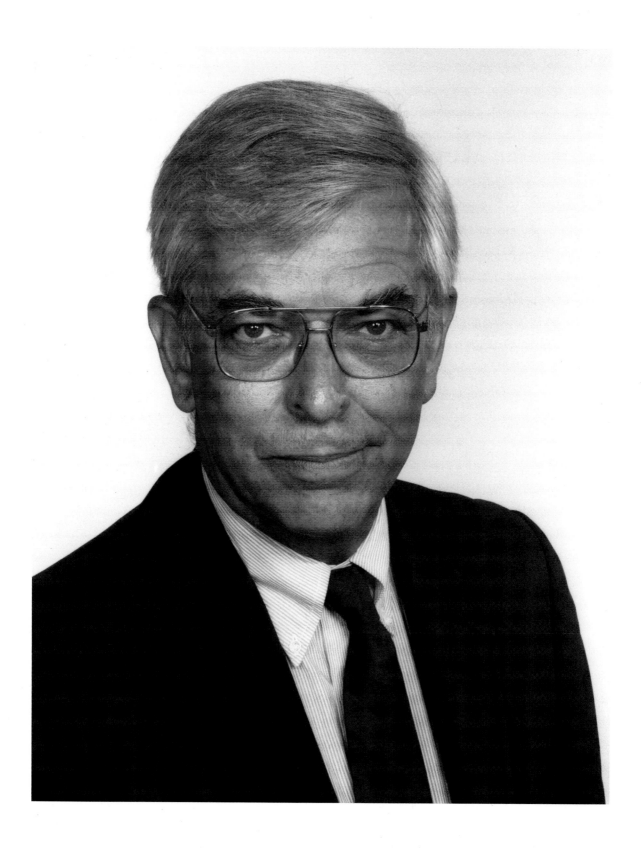

CHAPTER FIVE

THE NEUROVIROLOGY GROUP

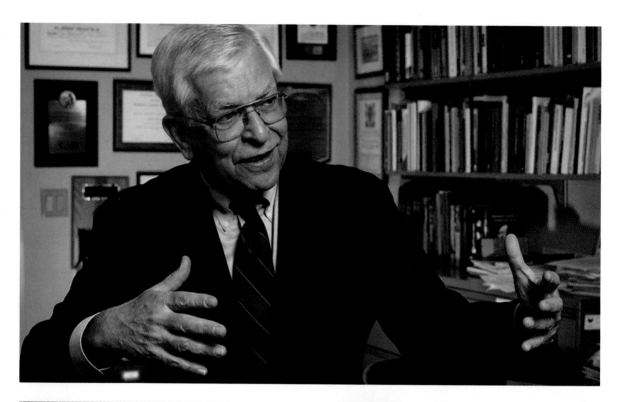

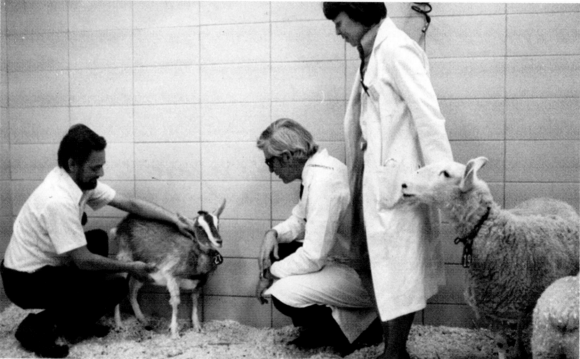

Above: Dick Johnson's "sharp wit and relaxed demeanor belied a mind of intense acuity, and his kind, approachable manner ensured that he would never be short of mentees."

Below: Bill Narayan, left, studied bluetongue, a virus transmitted to ruminants like goats and sheep by insects. Johnson is in the middle, with Diane Griffin at right.

Previous spread: Fresh out of his residency at Stanford, Johnson joined the Walter Reed Army Institute of Research as a clinical pathologist. He had expertise in neither research nor virology; in fact, he recalled, "I had never done any research, and there was no field that I knew less well than virology." But he quickly started learning about both.

Richard Johnson, Father of Neurovirology

Dick Johnson brought to Hopkins expertise in neurology, pathology and virology, and here he combined them to forge an entirely new field: Neurovirology.

Like many people throughout the history of Hopkins Medicine, Johnson happened to be at the right place – whether that was Russia, Peru, Papua New Guinea, Thailand, or Baltimore – at the right time. He traveled to "all corners of the globe," wrote Hopkins neurologist Nicoline Schiess, M.D., M.P.H.. This caused some colleagues "to believe that he spent as much time in the air as he did in his office;" in fact, she said, they dubbed him the "Pan Am Professor." Johnson loved working in exotic locations. When he was abroad, his correspondence to colleagues toiling away back at Hopkins began with a gleeful "Dear Shut-Ins" or something similar, recalls immunologist Diane Griffin, M.D., Ph.D., who came to Johnson's lab in 1969 as a postdoctoral fellow.

Johnson had another unofficial title, as well: "the Father of Neurovirology." He "was often at the epicenter of many of the innovative medical breakthroughs in neurovirology," Schiess wrote. Abroad and at home, "his sharp wit and relaxed demeanor belied a mind of intense acuity, and his kind, approachable manner ensured that he would never be short of mentees."

Many of his fellows went on to become leaders in the field. For instance: **Diane Griffin** became chair of the Department of Molecular Microbiology and Immunology at the Johns Hopkins Bloomberg School of Public Health, and currently is Vice President of the National Academy of Sciences; **Henry McFarland** became Chief of the Neuroimmunology Branch of NINDS; **Bill Narayan** became Distinguished Professor and Director of the Marion Merrell Dow Laboratory of Viral Pathogenesis at the University of Kansas. **John "Jack" Penney** went to Harvard where, among other achievements, his work led to the cloning of the gene that causes Huntington's disease. **Howard Lipton** joined the faculty in Microbiology and Immunology at the University of Illinois College of Medicine at Chicago. **Ray Roos** became Chair of the Department of Neurology at the University of Chicago and is an internationally recognized authority on the relationship between viral infection and neurological disease; **Janice Clements** became Director of the Department of Molecular and Comparative Pathobiology at Hopkins; **Jerry Wolinsky** was interim Chair of the Department of Neurology at the McGovern Medical School, University of Texas. **Bob Herndon**, now at the University of Mississippi, was Director of the Center for Brain Research at the University of Rochester. **Don Gilden** was Chairman of the Department of Neurology at the University of Colorado for nearly 25 years.

"The Slow Virologists"

Dick Johnson earned his M.D. at the University of Colorado School of Medicine in 1956, did his residency in internal medicine at Stanford, and then joined the Walter Reed Army Institute of Research as a clinical pathologist. He had expertise in neither research nor virology back then. In fact, he recalled, "I had never done any research, and there was no field that I knew less well than virology." But he quickly started learning about both when he was promoted to Assistant Chief of the Department of Virus Diseases; after his military service, Johnson wanted to learn even more. He did another residency, in neurology, at Massachusetts General Hospital, a clinical fellowship in neuropathology at Harvard, and spent a year as a teaching fellow at the Medical School of King's College, Newcastle-upon-Tyne, England. During these years, he became particularly interested in slow virus infections.

"At the American Embassy, there was a small marquee. The top billing listed Marlene Dietrich, the second the Harlem Globetrotters, and there we were, the third listed... 'The Slow Virologists.'"

"His expertise was established at a critical time in the field," wrote Schiess, "preparing him for the multiple opportunities that arose. The concept of slow virus infections was just becoming popular, and because of his expertise ... his participation in this emerging field was sought by fellow practitioners around the world."

Johnson joined the U.S. Public Health Service in 1962, and soon afterward was appointed to be part of an elite team of U.S. scientists to visit Russia; USSR researchers announced they had reproduced Amyotrophic Lateral Sclerosis (ALS) in monkeys after injecting them with fluid from the spinal cords of people who had died of the disease. The Russians said that the "virus-like agent discovered has been passaged twice in monkeys without consequent attenuation." Johnson later recalled the U.S. delegation's inauspicious arrival in Moscow: "At the American Embassy, outside the office handling upcoming cultural exchanges, there was a small marquee. The top billing listed Marlene Dietrich, the second the Harlem Globetrotters, and there we were, the third listed... 'The Slow Virologists.'" No one ever managed to replicate the ALS-producing "virus-like agent," and the U.S.-Russian collaboration was cut short by escalating political tension – particularly, the U.S.'s Operation Rolling Thunder in Vietnam. Johnson returned to his post in Canberra, Australia, where he was working as an Honorary Fellow in microbiology at Australian National University.

KURU

In 1964, Johnson's mentor, the noted Australian virologist, Frank Fenner, asked him to go to Papua New Guinea. His mission: to examine people stricken with Kuru, a rare, degenerative, incurable neurological disorder that turned out to be caused by a cannibalistic ritual (eating the brains of dead people). The disease had been described a few years previously by Carlton Gajdusek and Vincent Zigas; in 1976, Gajdusek would receive the Nobel Prize for his work. Johnson was the second neurologist ever to examine these patients, and later, he examined the first chimpanzee to develop clinical signs of the disease after being inoculated with brain extracts from a human patient. "At the time," Schiess noted, "no one knew that these original descriptions and subsequent scientific discoveries were the starting point for an entirely new type of infectious agents called prions – the cause for more well-known diseases such as Bovine Spongiform Encephalopathy," or Mad Cow Disease. That same year, Johnson joined the faculty at Case Western Reserve, where he worked until he came to Hopkins in 1969 as the Dwight D. Eisenhower Professor of Neurology, a position he would hold for the rest of his life.

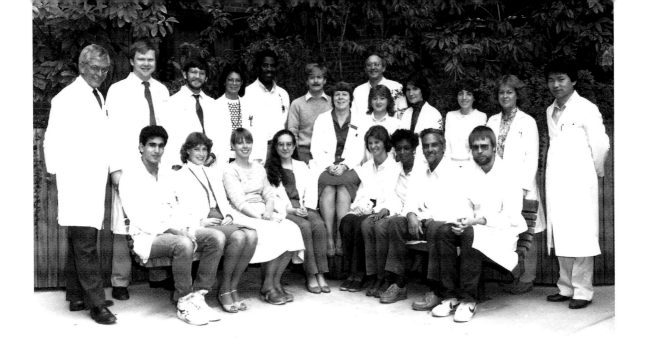

JOHNSON'S NEUROVIROLOGY GROUP

Johnson formed the Neurovirology Group soon after his arrival. "It was a great rookie team of enthusiastic young investigators, who each brought and shared diverse talents. Research was never more fun than during those early years."

THE NEUROVIROLOGY GROUP

Johnson formed the Hopkins Neurovirology Group soon after his arrival. The very first members were Opendra (Bill) Narayan, Ph.D., a veterinary virologist originally from British Guiana; Leslie Weiner, M.D., fresh out of his fellowship in neurology and epidemiology at Hopkins; and Robert Herndon, M.D., recruited from Stanford, who ran the electron microscopy laboratory. Soon came postdoctoral fellows Diane Griffin and Larry Davis; graduate student, Bill Flor, who had come with Herndon from Stanford and was working on his thesis; and Howard Lipton, who joined after service in Vietnam and a neurology residency. "It was a very collegial group, and Dick was an outstanding leader," says Herndon.

It was also a very young group, recalls Weiner: "The oldest person was Dick Johnson, who was 37. Guy was 36; Dan (Drachman) was 36. John (Freeman) was 35. Bob Herndon was 36. I was 31, so I was the junior person. They were friendly. They were caring. Dick Johnson and I and Herndon and Diane Griffin, we spent a lot of time laughing. It was just wonderful." Many in Johnson's lab and in McKhann's lab next door had young kids, all around the same age, Weiner adds: "Guy had five children. Dick had four children. Bob Herndon had three or four children. I had four."

Johnson, in an appreciation of Narayan in the *Journal of Neurovirology*, wrote in 2008: "It was a great rookie team of enthusiastic young investigators, who each brought and shared diverse talents. Research was never more fun than during those early years. Although the lab was small, we usually had bag lunches crowded around a coffee table in my office; we discussed new data but also shared personal stories. Bill's tales of 'house calls' in frigid, windswept Manitoba (where he had a large animal veterinary practice before getting his Ph.D.) were memorable. His story of driving his VW Beetle with an incompetent heater out 100 miles in subzero temperatures to deliver a heifer in the middle of the night was chilling, and very funny."

Diane Griffin describes the group as "very familial. There weren't that many people on the faculty. There weren't that many people in Dick's laboratory. It was an exciting time, it was a new Department of Neurology." Johnson was "easy to be around," she adds. "He was interesting, full of stories, partly based on his travels; and infrequently upset... He would take things in stride; this was particularly notable when you traveled with him. I worked with him in Peru (on that country's measles outbreaks; see below), so we traveled together a fair amount. No amount of inconvenience or impending disaster really bothered him that much." He was also a good writer. "I learned so much about scientific writing and writing clearly and with simple sentences. He was an inveterate editor of manuscripts before they went out." Like McKhann, Johnson was a great teacher as well, she adds. "They were both intellectually curious, always thinking and asking questions, and had breadth that was beyond just the science."

Johnson's approach "was that you needed a pathologist, you needed immunologists, you needed virologists, you needed neurologists, you needed neuroscience people, and eventually you needed molecular biologists."

Johnson believed in tackling something so complex as as a virus-induced disease from many sides. Says Griffin: "his approach was that you needed a pathologist, you needed immunologists, you needed virologists, you needed neurologists, you needed neuroscience people, and eventually you needed molecular biologists, but at that point we didn't really have that aspect of virology. Where he really got his variety of specialties was from postdoctoral fellows like me, an immunologist," with antibody expertise; "Bill (Flor), and Henry McFarland," who had expertise in cellular immunology.

Janice Clements, Ph.D., came to Johnson's lab in 1975 as a postdoctoral fellow and joined the faculty in 1978. "Dick recruited me because I came from molecular biology and genetics. I knew how to clone. I knew how to biochemically isolate proteins. He saw that as an opportunity for the rest of his people, and that's what was great about Dick. He saw you as an asset, as somebody who had these resources – not somebody who is different and doesn't fit in, but that you would bring that expertise to his group."

In 1975, when Clements arrived, "we could all fit into Dick's office; there were eight or nine of us. Every Monday morning, he would talk to every one of us about what we were doing. You never missed that meeting. On Friday afternoon, we had a research seminar, and that was a clever way of keeping us there Monday through Friday and even on the weekends. Saturdays, when we dropped in, he loved to be there because that was the time he could catch up and find out what was going on, not only in science but your home and what you were doing, and who you were dating, and what was happening. He was the science mentor, but you also felt like he was part of your family."

In those first few years, says Griffin, "everybody had their own virus, which would be "impossible now. Now you really have to specialize more." Narayan studied bluetongue, transmitted to ruminants by insects; Clements studied lentiviruses, and Griffin worked on the Sindbis virus, a mosquito-borne alphavirus that causes encephalitis in mice. "Dick had started working on that virus, and brought it from Australia."

The Sindbis virus primarily infects neurons, and "one of the questions my lab asked early using this model system was, what's going on with the immune response? We had strains where the mice get sick for a few days, and then they recover," says Griffin. How, indeed, could the immune system get rid of a virus in a neuron without killing it? "The answer was antibody." It took many years to figure this out, but Griffin and her lab did, in work published in *Scientific American* in 1992. "It turns out that the antibody is made against a surface protein on the virus, "which also happens to be expressed on the surface of the infected cell. So the antibody actually binds to the surface of the cell and then signals. We're still trying to figure out what it actually does. It's inducing changes in the cell that restrict virus replication so the virus can no longer grow and produce more virus."

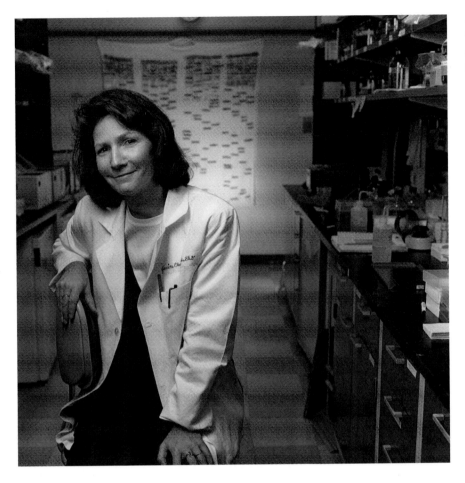

JANICE CLEMENTS
Clements came to Johnson's lab in 1975 as a postdoctoral fellow. Back then, "we could all fit into Dick's office. Every Monday morning, he would talk to every one of us about what we were doing. You never missed that meeting... He was the science mentor, but you also felt like he was part of your family."

THE SV40 MYSTERY

In the early 1970s, says Bob Herndon, "one of our first major accomplishments was the isolation of a virus from a case of progressive multifocal leukoencephalopathy (PML)." But to everyone's surprise, "the virus isolated was SV40, not JC virus!" This discovery – that fragments of the simian virus 40 were in the brains of patients – was so unexpected that no one was quite sure what to do about it.

"That was almost the end of my career," recalls Les Weiner. "We had a patient who was diagnosed with PML by biopsy. People recognized that it was a virus," but no one could isolate it. After much work and many meetings, they concluded that the SV40 virus was real, but was a contaminant – not the cause of PML. Weiner left Hopkins, at age 39, to become founding chair of the Department of Neurology at the University of Southern California in 1974, but he stayed in touch with his Hopkins colleagues: "Guy, Dick, Dan, Bob Herndon, we would get together at meetings. They'd come to my house. When Dick was in Los Angeles, he would stay with us. Guy loved my house, because it was full of red – red carpet, red drapes – and he said it looked like a brothel! It still looks the same way."

In those first few years, says Griffin, "everybody had their own virus, which would be "impossible now. Now you really have to specialize more."

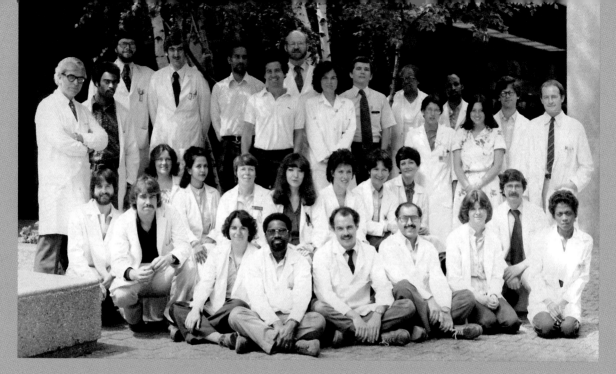

The Neurovirology Group-- in this picture, way too big for everyone to sit around a table in Johnson's office.

A Rich Environment

THE NEUROVIROLOGY GROUP STUDIED MANY VIRUSES, AND THE SCIENTISTS WHO TRAINED WITH JOHNSON MADE IMPORTANT CONTRIBUTIONS TO THE FIELD. HERE ARE JUST A FEW EXAMPLES:

The mouse hepatitis virus causes a demyelinating disease in mice. Bob Herndon studied it with Les Weiner, and "using autoradiography with tritiated thymidine we were able to demonstrate both regeneration of oligodendroglia and remyelination," says Herndon. "Both of which, according to the dogma of the period, were not supposed to happen. We also demonstrated some recurrent demyelination in these animals."

Dick Johnson had demonstrated that mumps ependymitis in hamsters could cause closure of the aqueduct with hydrocephalus. "Larry Davis collected spinal fluid from several patients with mumps and headache," continues Herndon, "and by using electron microscopy, we were able to demonstrate infected ependymal cells in the spinal fluid" – confirming the suspicion that, in rare cases, the same denuding of the cerebral aqueduct that occurred in hamsters could also occur with mumps infection in humans, resulting in hydrocephalus.

Mary Lou Oster-Granite, M.D., Ph.D., joined Johnson's laboratory in 1970 as a graduate student from the anatomy department, and began work on a parvovirus called PRE308 in newborn hamsters. "Parvoviruses are very small, single-stranded DNA viruses which do not have any DNA polymerase," explains Herndon.

Thus, "they can only replicate in dividing cells. The PRE308 virus has a predilection for the external germinal layer of the cerebellum; when cats are infected *in utero*, it causes destruction of the external germinal layer with cerebellar malformation." Oster-Granite and Herndon collaborated with neuroscientist Anne Young, who later became Chief of Neurology at Massachusetts General Hospital, to establish that glutamate was the neurotransmitter of cerebellar granule cells. Oster-Granite completed her thesis and went on to become a section head in Child Neurology at NIH.

Larry Davis worked on viral infections of the inner ear and has remained a world authority in that area. He is now Professor of Neurology at the University of New Mexico in Albuquerque and Chair of Neurology at the Albuquerque Veterans Medical Center. John Greenlee began work on PML and carried out a search for PML markers in human tumors. While at Hopkins, he began his studies on paraneoplastic cerebellar degeneration. He also has studied K-virus extensively. He is currently a Professor of Neurology at the University of Utah medical school and has published extensively on paraneoplastic syndromes and K-virus. Others who spent time in the Neurovirology Group include Jan Mullinix, M.D., Jeff Swarz, Ph.D., Maria Mazlo, a pathologist from Budapest, Hungary, John Kasckow, M.D., Ph.D., Professor of Psychiatry at the University of Pittsburgh. Says Herndon: "The Neurovirology Laboratory was a marvelous experience for those of us lucky enough to participate in its development."

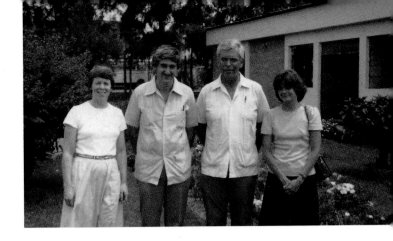

THE PERU TEAM *From left:* Diane Griffin, Robert Hirsch, Dick Johnson, and Susan Cook. Johnson's work in Peru grew into a decade-long collaboration between Peruvian and American scientists and an anti-measles program funded by the NIH. It also resulted in several papers, including two published in the *New England Journal of Medicine.*

MEASLES IN PERU

In 1971, Johnson was invited to spend three months teaching in Lima, Peru. "I accepted enthusiastically," he recalled. He was going to a country with a big problem: yearly measles outbreaks that were incapacitating, wrote Schiess. "The disease was so prevalent that one of the main hospitals in Lima reserved an entire pediatric ward from January to March to accommodate the large number of patients affected by the virus. Recognizing that the high birth rate, lack of effective vaccines, seasonal variation, and annual migration patterns offered an unusual chance to study the disease, Johnson jumped at the opportunity to conduct research at the Universidad Peruana Cayetano Heredia in Lima." Johnson's lab at Hopkins had developed measles assays, which his team in Peru used to study the outbreaks. "Much of the research from this work became, and still is, applicable to current measles outbreaks in the U.S. due to anti-vaccine choices among some communities," noted Schiess.

Johnson's work in Peru grew into a decade-long collaboration between Peruvian and American scientists and an anti-measles program funded by the National Institutes of Health. This also resulted in several scientific papers, including two published in the *New England Journal of Medicine.* For his contribution to controlling measles in Peru, Johnson was awarded the Comendador Medal by the President of Peru, the Charcot Prize from the International Federation of Multiple Sclerosis Societies, and an Honorary Professorship in the Peruvian University.

NOT HTLV, BUT HIV

One of Johnson's smartest decisions was setting Janice Clements to work on lentiviruses, which are retroviruses: they turn RNA into DNA. "I had been working on the lentiviruses, because they cause this slow, remitting and relapsing disease which is like Multiple Sclerosis. It was a central nervous system (CNS) infection that caused inflammation, and then it would go down." Clements had found the molecular basis for this activity while working in Johnson's lab: "The virus changed in response to the immune response to the virus," she explains. "The virus would infect cells, and the immune response would react against that virus, and the virus would then evolve, within one host, to be resistant to that antibody. So we actually understood how it created this remitting and relapsing disease – we understood that, but we also showed that it was not like any other retrovirus."

Scientists initially thought the HIV virus that caused AIDS was a cancer-causing virus. But this virus did not cause cancer; the Kaposi's sarcoma seen in many AIDS patients happened as a result of immunosuppression; it was not caused by the oncogenic effects of the virus itself. "The biology was different," Clements says. "When you looked at the other aspects of HIV, it killed T cells, it caused immune inactivation. It caused CNS disease. It caused multi-organ disease. That fit a lentivirus."

The two scientists who found the virus, Luc Montagnier in France and Robert Gallo at the National Cancer Institute, "knew it was a retrovirus," says Clements. "They knew it was a human retrovirus, because it came from people, and the only other known human retrovirus at the time was the HTLV-1

Scientists initially thought the virus that caused AIDS was a cancer-causing virus. But the Kaposi's sarcoma seen in many AIDS patients happened as a result of immuno-suppression; it was not caused by the oncogenic effects of a virus itself.

virus, which was oncogenic. So they assumed it was in that family, and that's why Gallo called it HTLV-3."

Clements, with Bill Narayan, Gallo, and Matt Gonda, a virologist at the National Cancer Research Facility in Frederick, proved that HTLV-3 was actually a lentivirus "that infects the host and causes a slow, progressive infection of immune cells," Clements says. "That's the other thing: lentiviruses infected immune cells but didn't transform them. HIV infected immune cells and killed them." Gallo and Narayan were first and last authors on this paper, but "we (Clements and Gonda) did the work. I didn't care; I cared about the science, and we were so excited when we saw the results that said, 'Absolutely, visna virus and HIV are much closer than HTLV-1 and the HIV virus.' It was one of those times when you go, 'Yes!'"

Clements and colleagues then discovered the mechanism for HIV infection in the brain: the virus could enter and infect brain cells without the need to use CD4, a specific receptor molecule on the surface of white blood cells and most immune cells that viruses can latch onto. "We showed that the viruses that were in the brain could get into those cells without CD4. The CD4-independence was important, because it explained infection in cells in the brain, like microglial cells, perivascular macrophages, and astrocytes."

In 1988, with a $5.6 million grant from the National Institute of Neurological and Communicative Disorders and Stroke, Hopkins established a research

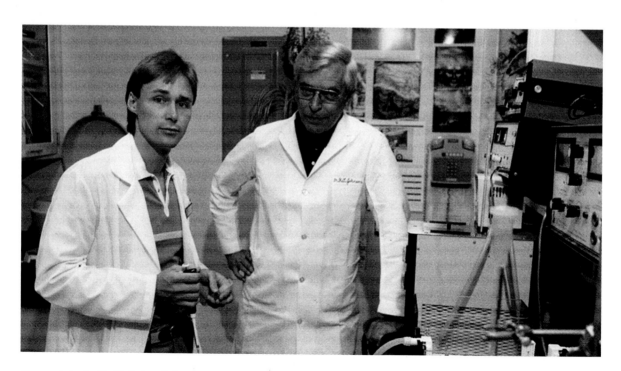

Research by Justin McArthur, left, and Johnson showed that HIV invades brain cells early in the course of AIDS. In 1988, Hopkins established a research center to examine HIV's effects in the brain, spinal cord, and nervous system.

center to examine the complications of HIV in the brain, spinal cord, and nervous system. Research by McArthur and Johnson had shown that HIV invades brain cells early in the course of AIDS, and David Cornblath, M.D., Jack Griffin, M.D,. and McArthur had found that many patients with HIV experience severe pain, numbness or weakness in one or more limbs, indicating that the virus also invades the peripheral nervous system. Another important study, by McArthur and Ola Selnes, Ph.D., reversed a University of California-San Diego study and showed that most healthy men with HIV have normal brain function – a finding that had important implications for employment policies, in an era when discrimination against people with the virus was common (see side story).

So little was known then about the neurological effects of HIV, and Hopkins neurologists were at the forefront of the investigation: Cornblath and McArthur studied the symptoms and characteristics of peripheral neurological complications; Johnson looked at genetic and cellular changes in myelin and also studied brain tissue in areas of the brain affected by other forms of dementia. Diane Griffin investigated the immune system's response in the nervous system, and Clements and her team later went on to explore how the HIV virus affects the latent immune system – specifically, the macrophages. "When the virus went latent because of anti-retroviruses," drugs that treat AIDS effectively, "people focused on the T cell; they ignored the macrophage. They didn't think it was important any longer." But that may not be the case; in collaboration with Bob Siliciano, Clements proved that the macrophage in the brain and other tissues is a latent reservoir for SIV (simian immunodeficiency virus), and they now are working on HIV.

Compassion and HIV

To anyone who didn't live through the early days of HIV, back when it was known as the HTLV-3 virus, it may be hard to imagine the prejudice, isolation, and callousness caused by fear and misunderstanding, which those first affected by this virus had to endure.

Justin McArthur, M.B.B.S., M.P.H., Director of Neurology, was an Osler medical resident in 1981, when the first reports came out describing an odd phenomenon: a rare form of pneumonia and Kaposi's sarcoma in a few young homosexual men. It was a tiny ripple that would become a tidal wave. By 1984, when McArthur was a resident in Medicine at Hopkins, human immunodeficiency virus (HIV) was known to be the cause of the acquired immunodeficiency syndrome (AIDS), and Hopkins was lucky enough to have John Bartlett, M.D., at the helm of the Division of Infectious Diseases. McArthur worked closely with Bartlett to care for these patients in the clinic and as inpatients.

In the early 1980s, in addition to having a terrible disease that nobody knew how to treat, patients suffered from the huge stigma attached to AIDS.

IT IS NO EXAGGERATION TO SAY THERE WAS PUBLIC HYSTERIA ABOUT THE VIRUS – FEAR THAT IT COULD BE "CAUGHT" FROM A TOILET SEAT, OR FROM TOUCHING SOMEONE WHO HAD IT. COMMUNITIES, HOSPITALS, AND EVEN CEMETERIES SHUNNED AIDS PATIENTS. THEY WERE PARIAHS; NOBODY WANTED THEM.

Hopkins did. Bartlett told his colleagues a story of a woman who was in tears as she came to see him in the clinic: When he asked what was wrong, she told him that when she had signed in to register at the Hospital, the admitting clerk asked her to put the pen down – and then had gotten a Kleenex, picked up the pen and dropped it in the trash can. "You know how that made me feel?" the woman asked.

In 1984, Johns Hopkins Hospital opened the AIDS inpatient service; it was one of only two in the country; the other was at San Francisco General Hospital. In those days, before the universal red bags and safety precautions for use and disposal of needles, some health care professionals did acquire the HIV virus from needle sticks. It took doctors and nurses with courage as well as compassion to care for these patients in the early days of the HIV epidemic, and Hopkins had them.

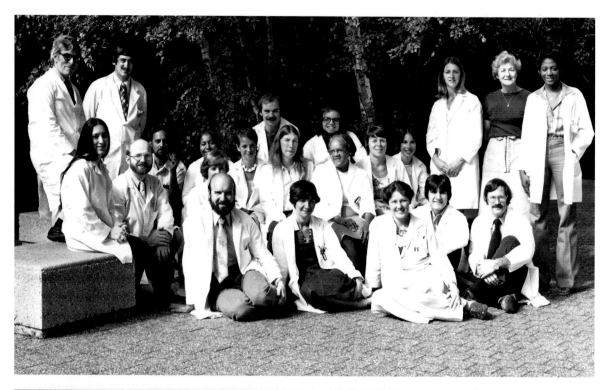

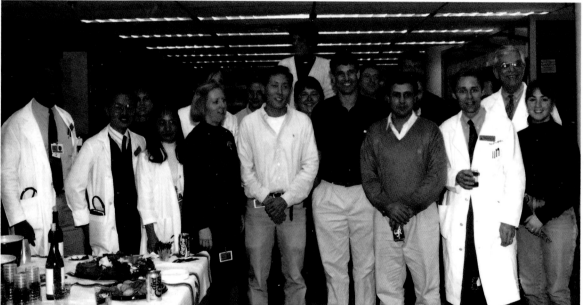

JOHNSON'S NEUROVIROLOGY GROUP

Dick Johnson influenced "literally hundreds, if not thousands, of medical students, undergraduates, and postdoctoral fellows through his charismatic, spellbinding lectures, and through direct mentoring. Many people considered him a 'mentor's mentor,' because of his insight, perseverance, and enthusiasm for his trainees."

Japanese Encephalitis in Thailand

In Thailand, Johnson learned such important skills as "avoiding cobras while wading through floodwaters."

In 1984, at the request of Major General Philip Russell, M.D., in the U.S. Army Medical Corps at Walter Reed, Johnson moved with his family to Thailand to conduct research on Japanese encephalitis. "His focus was on the cytochemistry of the virus in affected humans and monkeys," wrote Schiess. Johnson was a visiting scientist at the Armed Forces Research Institute of Medical Sciences, and a visiting professor at Mahidol University in Bangkok. "His six months in Thailand resulted in multiple publications on the inflammatory cells and immunocytochemical characteristics of Japanese encephalitis." Johnson set up a field study lab at a general hospital in the small highland town of Ching Rai, near the northernmost border of Thailand. When he got back to Hopkins, he shared some of the important skills he learned on this trip, Schiess added, "like avoiding the cobras from the nearby farm while wading through floodwaters."

"Mentor's Mentor"

Dick Johnson once said, "There are only three jobs I have had in my life that I truly loved: driving a night cab, working as a park ranger archeologist at Mesa Verde, and being a doctor."

Johnson was a skilled clinician, and patients came to see him from all over the world – particularly those with undiagnosed or unusual infections involving the nervous system. "His patients stayed with him year after year," noted Schiess. "It was not unusual to find some who had followed him for 30 years or more."

Dick Johnson died in 2015, at age 84. "The last few months of his life coincided with the emergence of the Zika virus into the Western Hemisphere," wrote Schiess. But Johnson had said for decades that the arrival of "new" neurotropic viruses was not new at all: "Over the span of his career, he observed the emergence of many so-called new viruses," including West Nile Virus and Ebola. The virologists, neurologists, immunologists, and neurovirologists investigating these viruses today are carrying on Johnson's legacy. His work "has had a tremendous impact on how viral infections are studied," says Janice Clements. "His research was novel and had a major influence on academic medicine and the treatment of virus infections of the brain."

Johnson influenced "literally hundreds, if not thousands, of medical students, undergraduates, and postdoctoral fellows through his charismatic and spellbinding lectures, and through direct mentoring," says Justin McArthur. "Many people considered him a 'mentor's mentor,' because of his insight, perseverance, and enthusiasm for his trainees."

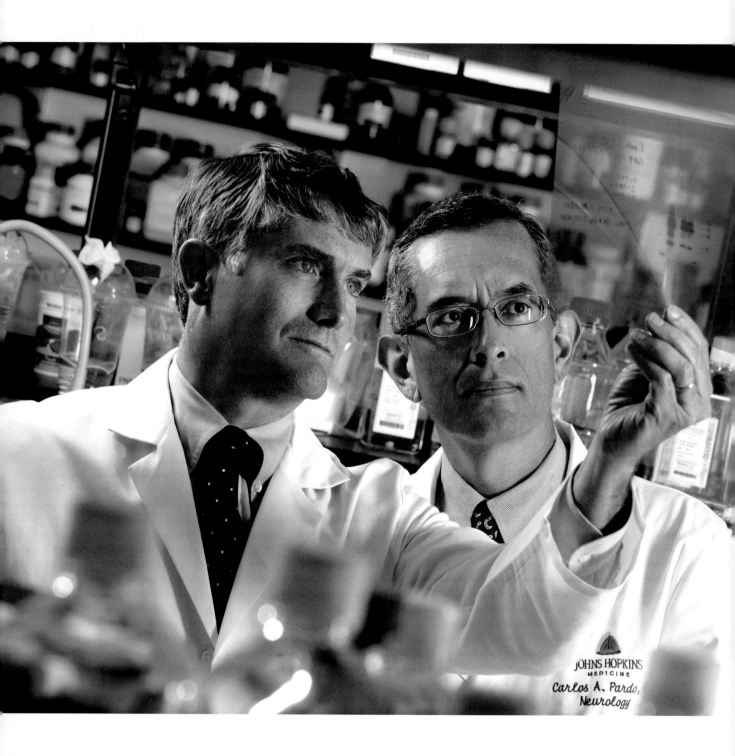

CHAPTER SIX

THE JOHNS HOPKINS MULTIPLE SCLEROSIS CENTER

At first, the Multiple Sclerosis (MS) Center was under the direction of Neurovirology, headed by Dick Johnson, based on earlier concepts of a possible infectious disease mechanism. This changed in 2003, when Peter Calabresi, M.D., a neuroimmunologist trained at the NIH, was recruited to direct the new Neuroimmunology and Neuroinfectious Disease Division.

"The expansion of Neuroimmunology was appropriate for the newer understanding of the autoimmune nature of MS," Calabresi explains, "in which disease-modifying immunotherapies were being approved for treatment." Previously, Calabresi had studied the role of interferons in the treatment of MS, showing that their therapeutic action did not depend on an *antiviral* mechanism, but rather was attributable to their effects on the *immune system*. "They profoundly affect adhesion molecules, such as VLA-4, on immune cells, and thereby block immune cell trafficking." Calabresi also had played a key role in the phase 3 trial of natalizumab, showing that the therapeutic effectiveness of this monoclonal antibody was due to its ability to block alpha-4 integrin; the successful trial resulted in FDA approval of the immunosuppressive drug for MS.

In 2005, Calabresi and colleagues Avi Nath, M.D., and Jack Griffin received a program project grant from the National Multiple Sclerosis Society. This led to productive collaborations on the mechanisms of immune-mediated neurodegeneration and the development of animal models and imaging outcome measures to facilitate clinical trials.

Nath and Calabresi explored the role of CD8 T-cell cytotoxic pathways and performed proteomic and lipidomic screens to characterize MS tissue pathology. Griffin and Calabresi used electron microscopy to show that EAE (experimental autoimmune encephalomyelitis) was actually a model of immune-mediated axonopathy, leading to studies of central neurodegeneration. Daniel Reich, M.D., Ph.D., Calabresi and Susumu Mori, Ph.D., published a series of papers demonstrating the utility of Diffusion Tensor Imaging (DTI) in MS (see Chapter 12: Neuroimaging). Later, Reich and Calabresi collaborated with Jerry Prince, Ph.D., in the Department of Biomedical Engineering, to develop post-MRI acquisition software "to quantify not only brain volumes," Calabresi says, "but cortical and subcortical grey matter nuclei, especially the thalamus," which they showed degenerates "more rapidly and reliably than white matter compartments." Reich since has developed an imaging lab at the NIH, and has become an international authority on MS imaging.

Calabresi and colleagues also examined the utility of Optical Coherence Tomography (OCT) of the retina. In collaboration with a former Hopkins fellow, Elliot Frohman, M.D., Ph.D., and a former Hopkins pre-medical student, neuro-ophthalmologist Laura Balcer, M.D., the group has published 70 papers and a textbook, putting OCT on the map as a very useful quantitative method for evaluating MS. With Shiv Saidha, M.D., then a fellow, Calabresi developed and validated a series of post-acquisition tools to quantify the retinal nerve fiber layer (axons) from the retinal ganglion cell layer (GCL). Saidha, now an associate professor, and Calabresi have the world's largest cohort of MS patients tracked with OCT for the longest period of time. They have shown that retinal neurodegeneration occurs with or without clinical episodes of optic neuritis, and that it is associated with neurodegeneration in other cerebral grey matter compartments. Thus, GCL atrophy on OCT and thalamic atrophy on 3Tesla

MRIs are now being used to measure the severity of disease in MS, to quantify the success of immunotherapies at protecting the brain, and to test putative primary CNS neuroprotective drugs. In addition, Saidha and Calabresi have found that subsets of patients, including African Americans, have more rapid retinal thinning independent of therapy. Identifying these subsets has allowed more detailed testing of genetic and metabolic risk factors.

The MS laboratory program has been actively investigating mechanisms by which the adaptive immune responses (T and B cells) activate CNS resident cells – microglia and astroglia – to mediate injury. Neurologist Carlos Pardo, M.D., has long recognized the role of microglia in neuroinflammation, and has published papers with Calabresi on effector T cells in the MS brain.

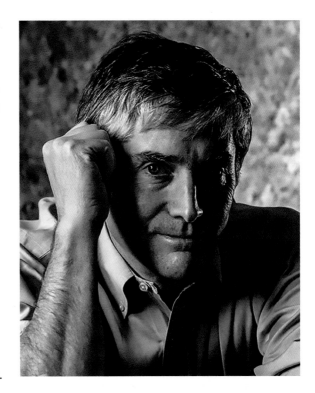

PETER CALABRESI

"The fellows trained in the Richard T. Johnson MS Program are destined to become the thought leaders of the next generation."

Previous spread:
Peter Calabresi, left, and Carlos Pardo. "From novel imaging tools and biomarkers of neurodegneration to innovative experimental therapeutics, and now the application of precision medicine," Hopkins Neurology's innovative approach has changed the way MS is treated and investigated.

REMYELINATION?

More recently, the MS team has partnered with Dwight Bergles, Ph.D., in the Neuroscience Department to examine the potential for *remyelination* in MS. Bergles, a developmental myelin biologist, and Calabresi have been studying the potential for remyelination by oligodendrocyte progenitor cells (OPCs). Their work has revealed that OPCs are abundant proliferative cells, and are the major source of remyelination in non-inflammatory demyelination. In contrast, the OPCs can be co-opted by the immune system to become mediators of inflammatory response.

In 2011, the MS Center recruited Ellen Mowry, M.D., who trained at the University of Pennsylvania and UCSF. Mowry has brought needed expertise in epidemiology and experimental therapeutics: She rapidly expanded the study of environmental risk factors and evidence-based therapeutic decision-making. Mowry showed that vitamin D deficiency was a major risk factor not only for *developing* MS, but that it was associated with more severe disease activity and worse outcomes. Mowry and Calabresi have created the Johns Hopkins Precision Medicine Center of Excellence (PMCOE; for more, see side story) that was chosen by Paul Rothman, M.D., Dean and CEO of Johns Hopkins Medicine, to be one of two lead PMCOEs for the School of Medicine. This Center has developed software to interface with the electronic medical record system, Epic, to plot patient-specific metrics on a dashboard to facilitate rapid assessment – not only of clinical outcomes, but of patient-reported outcomes and iPad acquired behavioral

"The Johns Hopkins MS Center has been at the core of virtually every major break-through in MS in the last 20 years."

tests. The MS PMCOE follows 6,000 people with MS a year, and is at the cutting edge of clinical research, with Sandra Cassard, Sc.D., and Kathryn Fitzgerald, M.D., studying environmental risk factors, cognitive and mood-related outcomes from the longitudinal cohort.

Michael Levy, M.D., Ph.D., has spearheaded the development of a neuromyelitis optica (NMO) center (see below), one of the first NMO centers in the country. Scott Newsome, D.O., directs the new Infusion Center at Green Spring Station. He also leads several investigator-initiated studies for MS therapeutics, including studies of the putative remyelinating compounds, liothyronine and anti-LINGO. Michael Kornberg, M.D., M.S., Ph.D., a recent fellowship graduate and assistant professor, studies the metabolism of immune cells with Pavan Bhargava, M.D., and Calabresi, and recently published the first report in Science of the therapeutic mechanism of dimethyl fumarate (Tecfidera), an effective drug that appears to have therapeutic effects in MS by suppressing glycolysis in immune cells.

The Johns Hopkins MS Center has recently embarked on a groundbreaking study called "Validation of Serum Neurofilament Light Chain as a Biomarker of Disease Activity in MS." As Calabresi explains, "Neurofilaments are cytoskeletal proteins which are neuron-specific and may be released following axonal damage." Increased neurofilament light chain (NfL) levels have been found in the blood and CSF in several neurological disorders with underlying neuro-axonal degeneration, including MS. "Importantly, the advent of ultrasensitive single-molecule array technology (Simoa) has enabled the measurement of low levels of NfL in blood with high accuracy and reproducibility." Serum NfL levels have been shown to be associated with clinico-radiological disease activity in MS, increased risk for conversion from CIS (clinically isolated syndrome) to MS, and have been proposed as a biomarker for monitoring response to disease-modifying therapy. Associations of baseline serum NfL and rates of change of serum NfL with long-term disability and rates of brain substructure and retinal atrophy are ongoing. "The goal is to have a commercially available assay in the next three to five years that could be used to prognosticate and monitor disease activity and response to therapies," says Calabresi.

"The Johns Hopkins MS Center has been at the core of virtually every major breakthrough in MS in the last 20 years," Calabresi points out, "from novel imaging tools and biomarkers of neurodegneration to innovative experimental therapeutics, and now the application of precision medicine. The fellows trained in the Richard T. Johnson MS Program are destined to become the thought leaders of the next generation."

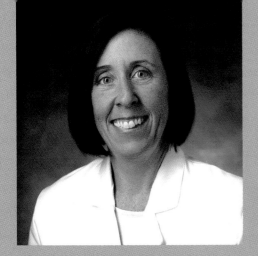

ELLEN MOWRY Mowry's research showed that vitamin D deficiency was a major risk factor not only for developing MS, but that it was associated with more severe disease activity and worse outcomes. She and Calabresi launched the MS PMCOE in 2017.

Personalizing Prognosis and Treatment: The Multiple Sclerosis PMCOE

EARLY MS IS OFTEN CHARACTERIZED BY A RELAPSING-REMITTING COURSE, THOUGHT TO BE DUE TO INFLAMMATORY DEMYELINATING EVENTS; BUT EVENTUALLY, MANY PEOPLE DEVELOP SECONDARY PROGRESSIVE MS, LIKELY DUE TO DEGENERATIVE CHANGES.

"Although relapsing-remitting MS is usually treatable, no treatment works definitively once the secondary progressive phase has begun," says Ellen Mowry. "An especially challenging issue for a newly diagnosed young person with MS is to determine whether the disease will be mild or disabling."

Calabresi and Mowry launched The Johns Hopkins MS Precision Medicine Center of Excellence (PMCOE) in April, 2017, to identify clinical, imaging, and blood biomarkers of long-term disability risk, and initiate clinical trials to identify new therapeutic strategies to prevent disability and promote repair in people with MS. The Center is designed to:

Track neurologic functional performance using iPADs at every clinic visit. All patients complete research-grade clinical performance measures and quality of life measures, which are shared with 10 MS Centers in the U.S. and Europe.

Evaluate baseline and annual non-invasive imaging of optic nerve damage caused by MS. Optical coherence tomography (OCT) measures of retinal nervous tissue loss predict brain volume and clinical outcomes 10 years later. "OCT is now being used to calculate patient-specific slopes of degeneration," says Mowry, "to identify patients with the most rapid rates of neurodegeneration."

Obtain systematic, clinic-based blood draws to identify biomarkers of prognosis and treatment response. Biomarkers that are predictive of long-term disability in MS and responses to disease-modifying therapy are needed. New data suggest that higher neurofilament light chain (NfL) levels correlate with MS disease severity and worse long-term outcomes, "but we need to evaluate such novel biomarkers in a prospective representative patient population in order to assess their true clinical applicability and generalizability," Mowry notes.

Standardize brain magnetic resonance imaging (MRI) across the Johns Hopkins Health System. "Annual brain MRI is important as a means of identifying patients who have developed new lesions, which represent new inflammatory activity that typically indicates the need to switch therapy," says Mowry. The MS PMCOE has standardized the brain imaging of MS patients undergoing clinical MRI not only within the Johns Hopkins Health System, but also within the largest network of freestanding radiology centers in the United States. "Standardization will allow for more reliable analyses of imaging studies to evaluate prognostic factors and individualize treatment plans."

Collect virtual data regarding environmental and lifestyle exposures of potential relevance to the prognosis of MS. Mowry and Kathryn Fitzgerald have launched a study to evaluate diet, exercise, and sleep health, among other exposures that appear to be related to prognosis in MS.

Translate evidence to investigator-initiated trials. MS PMCOE is conducting a randomized, controlled trial to determine whether an "early aggressive" therapy approach favorably influences the intermediate-term risk of disability: 900 people with MS will be randomized to higher-efficacy vs. first-line therapy across approximately 45 sites and followed for four years or more. Additional trials of bile acid supplementation (Pavan Bhargava), intrathecal rituximab (Bhargava, Calabresi, and Mowry), liothyronine administration (Newsome), fasting mimicker diet interventions (Fitzgerald and Mowry), intranasal insulin for cognitive impairment (Mowry and Newsome), vitamin D supplementation (Mowry), and exercise (Bhargava) are under way.

The MS PMCOE has created an outstanding clinical experience, simultaneously enhancing care of patients and creating an unparalleled research cohort, providing the opportunity to make major strides toward developing prognostic biomarkers and identifying new therapeutic targets and treatment strategies.

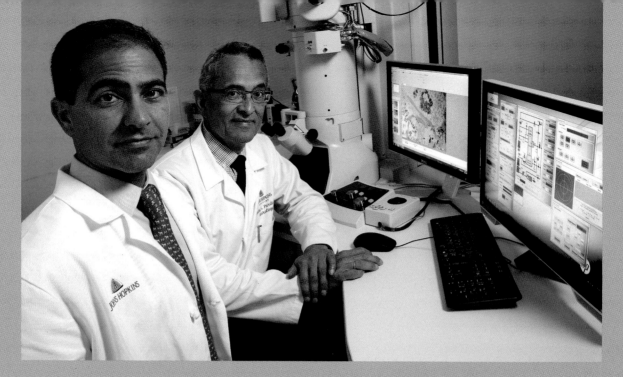

Levy, left, with Carlos Pardo, says: "We are closer than ever to finding a cure for NMO!"

"How Many MS Patients at Hopkins Actually Had Undiagnosed NMO?"

I was an on-call intern late one night at the Johns Hopkins Hospital when I met a young woman who presented with weakness and pain in her legs. This was her third admission to the Hospital in the past six months, despite her doctor's best effort to treat her for MS.

"I don't understand why these attacks keep coming," she told me, wincing in pain. "I have done everything my doctor told me to do, taken every medication he told me to take. And still, I keep getting these attacks. Something is *definitely* not right."

I stayed up with her that night trying to get to the bottom of this mystery. After scouring the medical literature, I found a study published by Vanda Lennon and Brian Weinshenker from the Mayo Clinic describing a new antibody blood test that potentially distinguishes MS from a rare disease called neuromyelitis optica (NMO). That was 2004. Back then, NMO was not on the radar at most MS centers around the country.

I SUSPECTED THAT MY PATIENT THAT NIGHT WAS SUFFERING FROM NMO, *NOT* MS, AND I SENT HER BLOOD TO THE MAYO CLINIC FOR TESTING. IT CAME BACK: POSITIVE.

One year later, Dr. Lennon discovered the target of the antibody: aquaporin-4.

This case had a profound impact on me. I wondered how many MS patients at Johns Hopkins actually had undiagnosed NMO. My mind wandered to the science around NMO, and the target of NMO, aquaporin-4. Could NMO patients have an abnormal aquaporin-4 that triggers the immune system to attack, or is aquaporin-4 just a naïve target of an aberrant immune system? For answers, I turned to Dr. Douglas Kerr, who started the Transverse Myelitis Center at Johns Hopkins and probably knew more about Transverse Myelitis and NMO than anyone else in the world! Dr. Kerr invited me to work in his lab to develop a mouse model of NMO that could help us understand what causes NMO, and provide clues for the best ways to treat it.

The other prominent person in this story at Johns Hopkins was Dr. Peter Agre, the physician-scientist who discovered the family of aquaporins and earned a Nobel Prize in Chemistry in 2003 for his work. Agre was also the first to publish the correct sequence of the aquaporin-4 (AQP4) water channel. Agre was thrilled to hear about the involvement of AQP4 in NMO, and he invited me to travel to Oslo, Norway, to attend a meeting with him about aquaporins in the brain. It was in Oslo that I learned about the AQP4 knockout mouse that would be instrumental in development of the NMO mouse model (see below!). At this conference, I met all of the major scientists in the aquaporin world, including

Vanda Lennon, the discoverer of the anti-AQP4 antibody in NMO. She kindly invited me to hang out with her and her lab at a bar that night and we stayed out until the sun finally set, close to midnight that summer in June 2008. Dr. Lennon paid the entire bill.

Upon returning home, I obtained funding from the American Academy of Neurology to profile the two different variations of aquaporin-4 found in the human brain. I found that one of them was highly expressed in areas where NMO attacks occurred – especially in the spinal cord and optic nerves. With a grant provided by the Guthy Jackson Charitable Foundation in 2009, I was hired on the faculty at Johns Hopkins to continue my work developing a mouse model of NMO. The NMO mouse proved to be more difficult to create than I originally envisioned, but with the help of the best colleagues and technicians I could find, we pressed on.

I finally had a breakthrough moment in 2012. Up to then, we were focused on the aquaporin-4 antibody. The aquaporin-4 antibody is a protein whose sole function is to bind to aquaporin-4 and trigger an immune attack. Many of us hypothesized that the antibody was harmful in NMO and caused the disease. We spent several years trying to understand how this antibody could be harmful, but in fact, it was not that harmful after all. The antibody may have contributed a little, but it was not the major player. Something else in the immune system was the cause of NMO. My breakthrough initially seemed like just another failure; I found yet more proof that the antibody was not the cause. In the course of proving that my hypothesis was wrong, I accidentally discovered that a different immune component was causing NMO— it was T-cells *reactive against aquaporin-4*.

T-cells are the thoughtful immune cells in your body: They go around and surveille for infections and cancers by communicating with each cell, and carefully consider the context of any signal.

MATURE T-CELLS ARE TRAINED TO LOOK FOR A PARTICULAR FOREIGN PROTEIN, AND WE DISCOVERED THAT T-CELLS DIRECTED TO AQUAPORIN-4 ATTACK THE OPTIC NERVES AND SPINAL CORD IN MICE, JUST LIKE IN PATIENTS WITH NMO.

It took us three more years to prove definitively that these T-cells were the cause of the disease and we published our results in 2015. Since then, two more labs in San Francisco and Germany confirmed our results.

Besides creating a mouse that develops NMO just like humans do, the more exciting news that comes from this discovery is the **potential to cure NMO.** Since we figured out exactly how to switch the immune system "on" to cause NMO, we had the capability to switch the immune system "off," permanently. We successfully patented our findings — filed December 2016 — and applied for government funding to pursue a specific treatment for NMO based on our technology. The goal is to switch the immune system "off" to aquaporin-4, and to re-educate the immune system of NMO patients so that they will stop attacking the optic nerve and spinal cord.

As a field, we have significant progress in the understanding and treatment of NMO. We now have three worldwide clinical trials ongoing to treat a rare disease. This is quite a feat! It speaks to the progress we have all made in the lab towards finding treatment targets that can help patients in the acute and preventive treatment of NMO. I am committed more than ever to achieve the goal I set out in 2004 – find the cure to NMO. In fact, I believe NMO is a proof-of-concept disease that can demonstrate how re-educating the immune system can be an effective treatment for an autoimmune disease.

We've come a long way since I met my first patient with NMO in 2004. I hope everyone reading my story feels the same hope and optimism that we are closer than ever to finding a cure to NMO!

– *Michael Levy*

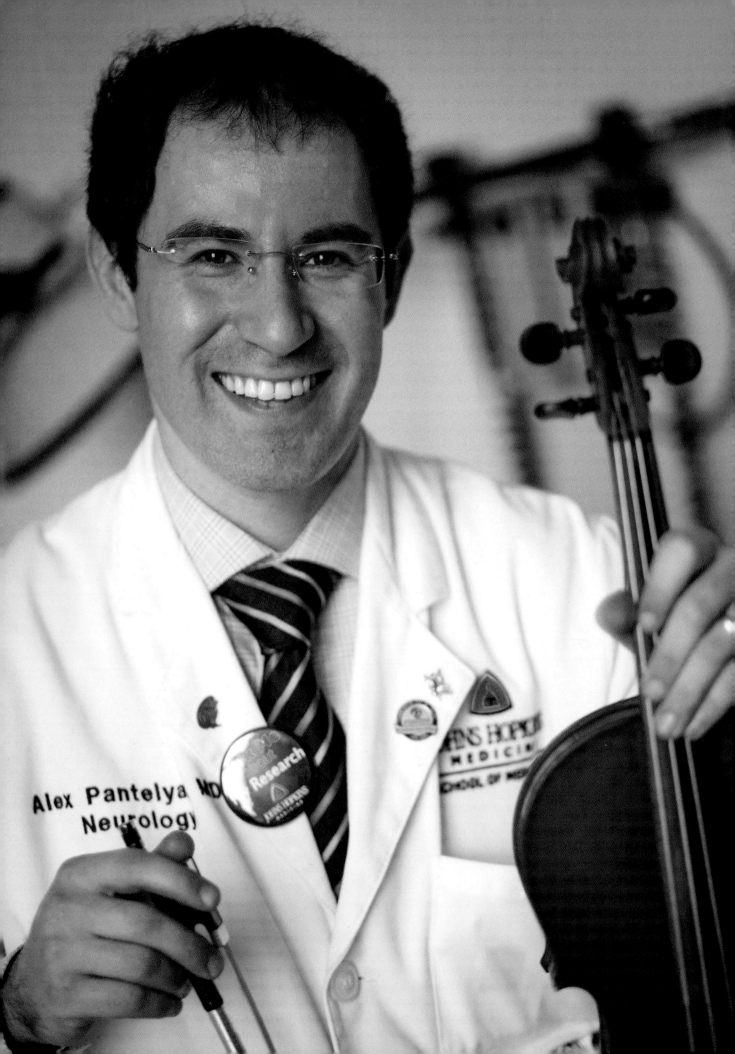

CHAPTER SEVEN.

MOVEMENT DISORDERS

PARKINSON'S DISEASE

Johns Hopkins has a long history of contributions to Parkinson's disease (PD).

Thomas Preziosi, M.D., participated in some of the early clinical trials of levodopa in patients with PD. Mahlon Delong's laboratory showed that the symptoms of PD were due in part to abnormal activity of the output nuclei of the basal ganglia, particularly overactivity of the subthalamic nuclei – and that lesioning the overactive subthalamic nuclei alleviated symptoms. Delong's pioneering work led to the use of deep brain stimulation as a treatment for PD, and in 2014, he was awarded the Lasker-DeBakey Clinical Medical Research Award (see side story) for this contribution.

THE ROLE OF NITRIC OXIDE

In the mid-1980s, Solomon Snyder's laboratory conducted pioneering work on the mechanism of action of the parkinsonism-inducing neurotoxin, MPTP, and showed that the active metabolite of MPTP, (1-methyl-4-phenylpyridinium) was taken up by dopamine neurons, selectively damaging them. Ted Dawson, M.D., Ph.D., now the Leonard and Madlyn Abramson Professor of Neurodegenerative Diseases, joined Sol Snyder's laboratory in 1990, just as research on the role of nitric oxide as an unconventional neurotransmitter was burgeoning. In 1991, Ted and Valina Dawson, Ph.D., showed that glutamate excitotoxicity was mediated by nitric oxide, which was produced by neuronal nitric oxide synthase (nNOS). This prompted the investigation of nitric oxide's role in many neurologic disorders, including Parkinson's disease. The Dawsons showed that MPTP killed dopamine neurons through activation of poly (ADP-ribose) polymerase 1 (PARP1). Knocking out *nNOS* and *PARP1* in mice prevented the loss of dopamine neurons in the MPTP model of PD.

Ted and Valina Dawson's work has revealed multiple biochemical and genetic abnormalities involved in the pathogenesis of PD, and has led to several promising therapeutic approaches.

THE ROLE OF α-SYNUCLEIN AND GENETICS OF PARKINSON'S DISEASE

PD research changed dramatically in 1997, with the discovery that mutations in the α-*synuclein* gene caused autosomal dominant PD, and that α-synuclein was the major component of Lewy bodies and neurites, the pathologic hallmark of PD (see below). Other genes also were found to cause autosomal dominant or autosomal recessive PD. In 2000, the Dawsons showed that inactivation of parkin – either due to mutations in the gene, *parkin*, or damage to parkin secondary to nitric oxide – resulted in the accumulation of two important parkin substrates (PARIS and AIMP2) in the brains of PD patients; which, in turn, contributes to the demise of dopamine neurons in PD. They found another mechanism for parkin inactivation, as well: c-Abl (the non-receptor tyrosine kinase), which leads to the accumulation of the pathogenic parkin substrates, PARIS and AIMP2. Moreover, they showed that c-Abl activation converted α-synuclein to a pathologic species, and that eliminating or blocking c-Abl reduces neurodegeneration in animal models. This work led to the current testing of c-Abl inhibitors as potential therapeutic agents for treatment of PD.

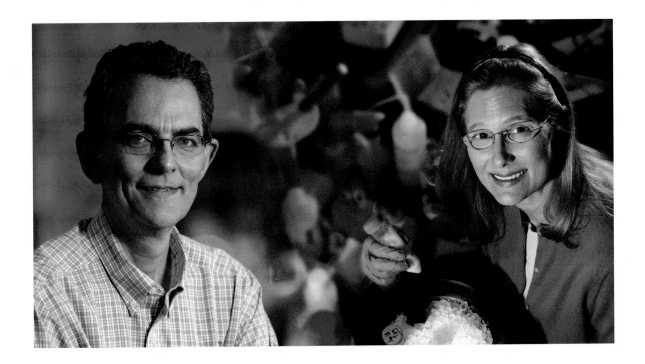

IDENTIFICATION OF LRRK2 (LEUCINE-RICH REPEAT KINASE)

The Dawsons also showed that mutations in another gene, *LRRK2*, the most common cause of autosomal dominant PD, were linked to neuronal toxicity, by substantially enhancing LRRK2's kinase activity. This work suggests that inhibitors of LRRK2 may be effective in treating PD.

PRION-LIKE SPREAD OF α-SYNUCLEIN

The Dawsons co-developed a brain-penetrant, long-acting, glucagon-like peptide-1 receptor agonist that is profoundly protective in animal models of Parkinson's disease.

Another therapeutic approach investigated by the Dawsons involves preventing the spread of α-*synuclein* from cell to cell via "LAG-3." Finally, they co-developed a brain-penetrant, long-acting, glucagon-like peptide-1 receptor (GLP1R) agonist, designated NLY01, which is profoundly protective in animal models of PD, and started a biotechnology company, Neuraly Inc., to evaluate this agent in the treatment of Parkinson's disease and other neurologic disorders.

LOOKING AHEAD

The Dawsons continue to investigate the basic underlying mechanisms of neurodegeneration in Parkinson's disease. "Our goal is to identify key nodal points that can be targeted for therapeutic intervention," says Ted Dawson. "We are dedicated to advancing the frontiers of PD research, ultimately leading to the development of agents that will modify the course of PD and related disorders."

THE DAWSONS
Ted and Valina Dawson have made great strides in understanding the basic mechanisms of neurodegeneration in Parkinson's disease, and in identifying highly promising agents to treat it.

Previous spread:
Alexander Pantelyat, who directs the Atypical Parkinsonism Center, is also co-director of the Center for Music & Medicine.

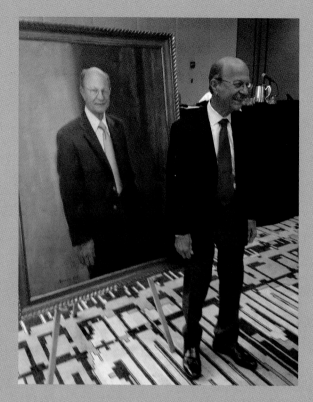

MAHLON DELONG After finishing his Neurology residency at Hopkins, Mahlon DeLong joined the faculty and continued his investigation, begun at the NIH, of the role of the basal ganglia in movement. His research led to the use of deep brain stimulation in Parkinson's disease and earned him the 2014 Lasker~DeBakey Clinical Medical Research Award.

Mahlon DeLong, Distinguished Hopkins Alumnus and Lasker Awardee

IN 2014, MAHLON DELONG SHARED THE LASKER ~ DEBAKEY CLINICAL MEDICAL RESEARCH AWARD WITH ALIM LOUIS BENABID, OF THE CLINATEC INSTITUTE IN GRENOBLE, FRANCE. THEY WERE HONORED FOR THEIR WORK THAT LED TO THE DEVELOPMENT OF DEEP BRAIN STIMULATION, WHICH HAS HELPED RELIEVE SYMPTOMS IN THOUSANDS OF PATIENTS WITH ADVANCED PARKINSON'S DISEASE.

After undergraduate studies at Stanford, Mahlon DeLong attended Harvard Medical school, and then did postgraduate training at the Harvard Medical Service of the Boston City Hospital, from 1966 to 1968. Following this residency, he went to the NIH and joined the research lab of Ed Evarts, who did single cell microelectrode recording in awake behaving non-human primates (NHP).

When Mahlon arrived at the lab, the "most desirable" areas to study (motor cortex, frontal eye fields and cerebellum) had already been assigned. He was relegated to the basal ganglia, whose role in movement was poorly understood, although their role in movement disorders, such as Parkinson's disease (PD) and Huntington's disease was widely accepted. The goal was to record electrophysiologic activity in awake behaving animals, rather than the anesthetized animals previously used for similar studies. DeLong was able to characterize the spontaneous patterns of activity in the different subnuclei of the basal ganglia; to demonstrate that individual basal ganglia neurons

were somatotopically organized (related to body parts) just as in the motor cortex and cerebellum; and to show that the basal ganglia had distinct motor and non-motor regions. The research provided novel insights into the physiology and functional organization of the basal ganglia in the intact animal, and a firm basis for his later research on the role of the basal ganglia in animal models of movement disorders, including Parkinson's disease and hemiballismus. Although he had planned to stay at the NIH for only two years, the work was so interesting and productive that he stayed for five.

NEUROLOGY RESIDENCY AND FACULTY AT JOHNS HOPKINS

After leaving the NIH to undertake a residency in Neurology at Johns Hopkins, Mahlon found that "the switch from full-time basic research to residency training was not as difficult as expected, due to the generous help and guidance by outstanding residents ahead of me, and the clinical knowledge and wisdom of Tom Preziosi, who was a model clinician and source of information." Mahlon joined the Neurology faculty after residency, and focused clinically on patients with movement disorders. With Apostoles Georgopoulos, a post-doctoral fellow, he re-explored the physiology of the basal ganglia, with different tasks, in research space provided by Vernon Mountcastle. They extended recordings to the substantia nigra and notably the subthalamic nucleus (STN), which was now recognized as an independent source of input to the basal ganglia from the precentral motor fields. As in the other subnuclei, they discovered that the STN was divided into clear motor and non-motor areas. They also demonstrated proprioceptive input, most strikingly from passive directional movements of the proximal joints. The movement-related neuronal activity was primarily related to the direction of movement, rather than the pattern of muscular activity. Neuronal activity, they found, was also related to the amplitude/velocity of limb movement. Although changes in neuronal activity occurred close to the time of EMG activation, they were not involved in initiation of movement.

Several years later, DeLong and colleagues proposed that the basal ganglia and thalamus are components of a family of largely anatomically and functionally segregated, closed-loop cortical-subcortical networks, identified as "skeletomotor," "oculomotor," "associative" and "limbic "networks. This schema is now widely accepted, with close to 8,000 citations, and readily explains the common occurrence of varied neurologic and psychiatric signs and symptoms associated with basal ganglia disturbances.

Early in the 1980s, after moving to what is now Johns Hopkins Bayview Medical Center (see chapter 19) DeLong and colleagues discovered that cholinergic neurons of the nucleus basalis of Meynert (NBM) were selectively decreased in the brains of patients with Alzheimer's disease. In collaboration with Peter Whitehead, Don Price and Joe Coyle, DeLong discovered that a reduced number of these cholinergic neurons project to the cortex; this finding had a major impact on the Alzheimer's disease field. It also led to studies that strongly suggested a role for the NBM in arousal and learning.

In 1995, Delong's group moved to laboratories in the Meyer Building, and became interested in exploring the pathophysiology of Parkinson's disease. The discovery that MPTP (a contaminant in synthetically made heroin) caused parkinsonism in young addicts, by selective uptake and destruction of dopamine neurons in the substantia nigra, resulted in a faithful primate model of Parkinson's disease. Studies by William Miller, an M.D.-Ph.D. student, revealed increased inhibitory output from the internal segment of the globus pallidus (GPi). The evolving model of circuit activity placed the STN as a key player in the signs and symptoms of this disorder; elevated excitatory (glutamatergic) drive on the output neurons of the GPi was felt to be a major factor. DeLong had shown that lesions of the STN, which caused chorea, reduced the activity of neurons in GPi. Together with Hagai Bergman and Thomas Wichmann, he showed that in the primate MPTP model, transient inactivation or lesions of the STN resulted in an almost immediate reversal of the features of Parkinsonism, including tremor, rigidity and bradykinesia.

BETTER UNDERSTANDING OF THE PATHOPHYSIOLOGY OF PARKINSON'S DISEASE AND THE SUCCESS OF DEEP BRAIN STIMULATION CONTRIBUTED GREATLY TO THE RENAISSANCE OF FUNCTIONAL SURGERY WORLDWIDE.

This finding, published in *Science* in 1990, provided a rationale and target for treating PD – but also raised the concern that it might bring back ablative procedures for PD, which had been problematic in the past. These studies, and the prior history of successful treatment of PD with pallidotomy, led the group to return to pallidotomy, but with careful microelectrode mapping of the target area in GPi. Several years later, following the discovery by Alim Benabid that chronic high-frequency stimulation of the thalamus could stop tremor just like ablation, they showed that deep brain stimulation of the STN also could reverse the features of parkinsonism in patients with PD. The STN, formerly a bit player in the basal ganglia, moved to center stage as a novel and highly effective target for deep brain stimulation. Better understanding of the pathophysiology of Parkinson's disease and the success of deep brain stimulation of the STN contributed greatly to the renaissance of functional surgery worldwide. Fred Lenz, who had experience with microelectrode recordings in the thalamus of patients undergoing thalamotomy, was recruited to begin this functional neurosurgery at Hopkins.

A number of clinical and research fellows and graduate students participated in these studies, including: *Graduate Students:* Michael Crutcher, William Miller; *Postdoctoral Fellows:* Apostoles Georgopolus, Susan Mitchell, Thomas Wichmann, Russel Richardson, Hagai Bergman, Yolanda Smith, Ikuma Hamada.; *Clinical Fellows:* Jerrold Vitek, Garret Alexander, and Jim Ash.

Because diagnosis is often complicated, the visit involves evaluations by a physical or occupational therapist, speech/language pathologist, social worker, research coordinator/educator, a Movement Disorders Fellow, and an NIH collaborator, in addition to Jee Bang and Alex Pantelyat.

ATYPICAL PARKINSONISM

Some of the signs and symptoms are identical to Parkinson's disease, but it isn't PD. What else could it be? Several similar but very different degenerative disorders fall into the category of Atypical Parkinsonism, including dementia with Lewy bodies (DLB), Multiple System Atrophy (MSA), Progressive Supranuclear Palsy (PSP), and Corticobasal syndrome/degeneration (CBS/CBD).

The Johns Hopkins Atypical Parkinsonism Center was established in 2014 at the Bayview Medical Center by Alexander Pantelyat, M.D., who was recruited from the University of Pennsylvania to serve as its Director. In 2016, the clinic grew with the addition of Jee Bang (see below), who completed her Neurology Residency training at Hopkins and spent three years at the University of California-San Francisco as a Behavioral Neurology Fellow. In 2017, the Johns Hopkins Atypical Parkinsonism Center was recognized as one of the first four CurePSP Centers of Care, and also as one of the first 25 Lewy Body Dementia Association Research Centers of Excellence.

"We have seen more than 120 patients so far," says Pantelyat Because diagnosis is often complicated, he adds, the multidisciplinary visit takes four to five hours and involves evaluations by a physical or occupational therapist, speech/language pathologist, social worker, research coordinator/educator, a Movement Disorders Fellow, an NIH collaborator (Sonja Scholz, M.D., Ph.D., of the NINDS Neurodegenerative Diseases Research Unit, Neurogenetics Branch), and two attendings: Jee Bang and Alex Pantelyat. "The average distance traveled by patients and families from their home to this clinic is greater than 120 miles," Pantelyat adds. "The goal is to have patients follow up yearly, with regular appointments in between." Data collected at each visit include multiple rating scales depending on the diagnosis and, if the patient consents, blood for whole genome sequencing at NINDS. Examinations include a two-minute walk duration, with cadence, step length, and gait velocity (baseline, with rhythmic auditory metronome cues, and repeated without cues 10 to 15 minutes later).

Several local patient-care partner support groups have been established through the Atypical Parkinsonism Center, including Atypical Parkinsonism support groups in Towson and at Sibley Hospital (in partnership with CurePSP). A Lewy Body Disease (dementia with Lewy bodies and Parkinson disease dementia)-specific support group is expected to begin in Towson in 2019, as well.

The Atypical Parkinsonism Center is dedicated to carrying out clinical and translational research for diagnosis and treatment of these disorders. Most of the work so far has been focused on PSP, with multiple current research protocols led by Pantelyat, Ted Dawson, Bang, and others.

Looking ahead, "our goals include expanding our multidisciplinary atypical parkinsonism clinic and setting up virtual visits for patients who are too impaired to travel to Johns Hopkins," says Pantelyat. "We also plan to develop clinical studies for this patient population, involving music and rhythm-based interventions (in collaboration with the Johns Hopkins Center for Music & Medicine, which Alex Pantelyat co-directs), and to expand our longitudinal biomarker studies and pharmacological studies for these diseases."

THE JOHNS HOPKINS HUNTINGTON'S DISEASE CENTER OF EXCELLENCE (HDCOE)

The Johns Hopkins Huntington's Disease (HD) Center was founded in 1980 by psychiatrists Paul McHugh, M.D., Marshal Folstein, M.D., and Susan Folstein, M.D., based on an epidemiological study of HD in Maryland. The Center represents a unique partnership between the Neurology and Psychiatry Departments. Today, Christopher Ross, M.D., Ph.D., from Psychiatry, is the Center's Director, Jee Bang is the Clinical Director, and the Huntington's Disease Center is one of the Centers of Excellence at Johns Hopkins. The HDCOE is supported by the National Institute of Neurological Disorders and Stroke, the Huntington's Disease Society of America, and other sources. In addition to conducting research on HD, the Center provides multidisciplinary clinical services, including genetic counseling and social work support, to individuals with HD and related disorders, and their families. The Center has participated in genetic studies leading to identification of the HD gene, and in clinical and imaging studies that have defined the natural history of the disease and demonstrated that "regional brain atrophy begins many years before diagnosable onset of manifest HD," says Jee Bang. The genetic defect consists of an excessive number of "triplet repeats" (more than 35 repeats of the triplet CAG in the *HTT* gene), and is inherited in an autosomal dominant fashion.

The HDCOE conducted the largest single-site clinical trial in HD, and has participated in many multicenter clinical trials, often via the Huntington Study Group. The Center continues to be a leader in basic, translational and clinical research, notes Bang. "We generated one of the most widely used transgenic mouse models of HD. We participated in the collaborative group to generate and study an induced pluripotent stem cell model of HD, and have been leaders in the study of the biochemistry of the Huntingtin protein (the *HTT* gene product)." The Center's scientists also have developed novel functional and metabolic MRI measures of changes due to the disease.

"In the HD Clinic, we see more than 150 patients every year, over one-third of whom are new patients," says Bang. Neurology, psychiatry, and genetics residents and fellows are trained in the clinic through regular rotations, and medical and undergraduate students regularly observe there. Bang and Ross lecture to medical students, residents and faculty at Hopkins, and at national and international meetings.

Treatment for HD has come a long way since the Center first opened its doors.

"Current treatment consists of symptomatic therapies for chorea and mood disorders often associated with HD, such as depression, irritability, perseverative thinking, and apathy," says Bang. Now, with new strategies for lowering the abnormal protein, huntingtin, by means of RNA interference- based reagents such as antisense oligonucleotides (ASO) or viral-vector delivered reagents, "there is real hope to alter the fundamental mechanisms of disease progression," she adds. The experience with ASO therapy for Spinal Muscular Atrophy (see Chapter 10) indicates the potential power of this approach. Antisense oligonucleotide therapies need to be delivered directly into the CNS, often via the intrathecal route. The Johns Hopkins HDCOE is the top recruiting site in the U.S. for the CSF

The Ataxia Center has flourished, providing "one-stop" service with physicians, fellows, therapists, a geneticist, as well as research and patient coordinators, all seeing the patients on the same day in the same location.

biomarker trial (HDClarity). "We anticipate being a lead site for the first-ever phase III trial of an antisense oligonucleotide drug designed for HD, initially developed by Ionis, and now sponsored by Roche/Genentech. This represents a potentially historic opportunity for disease-modifying therapy for this devastating, hereditary, neurodegenerative disease."

THE JOHNS HOPKINS ATAXIA CENTER

The Johns Hopkins Ataxia Center, begun in 2009 under the direction of Sarah Ying, M.D., grew out of a cooperation with the Chesapeake chapter of the National Ataxia Foundation and the generous philanthropic support of the Gordon and Marilyn Macklin Foundation. Its goal was to provide the best and most efficient care for people with ataxia by providing a "one-stop" experience, giving patients access on a single visit to physicians and therapists with different areas of expertise in diagnosis and management. The Ataxia Center has flourished: over the last few years under the directorship of Liana Rosenthal, it has grown dramatically in scope — with multiple physicians, fellows, students, speech and swallowing therapists, physical and occupational therapists, a geneticist, as well as research and patient coordinators, all seeing the patients on the same day in the same location. Outreach programs, a newsletter, activities for ataxia patients and their families, and support groups are all part of the ataxia program today. It truly is a model for how medical care can be delivered in the most efficient and beneficial way for our patients.

SELECTED REFERENCES

Bang J, Lobach IV, Lang AE, et al. Predicting disease progression in progressive supranuclear palsy in multicenter clinical trials. *Parkinsonism Relat Disord*. 2016;28:41-48.

Geiger JT, Ding J, Crain B, et al. Next-generation sequencing reveals substantial genetic contribution to dementia with Lewy bodies. *Neurobiol Dis*. 2016;94:55-62.

DeLong M. Lasker Award winner Mahlon DeLong. *Nat Med*. 2014 Oct;20(10):1118-20

Javitch JA, Snyder SH, Uptake of MPP(+) by dopamine neurons explains selectivity of parkinsonism-inducing neurotoxin, MPTP. *Eur J Pharmacol*. 1984 Nov 13;106(2):455-6

Brahmachari S, Ge P, Lee SH,, et al. Activation of tyrosine kinase c-Abl contributes to α-synuclein-induced neurodegeneration. *J.Clin Invest*. 2016 .126(8):2970-88.

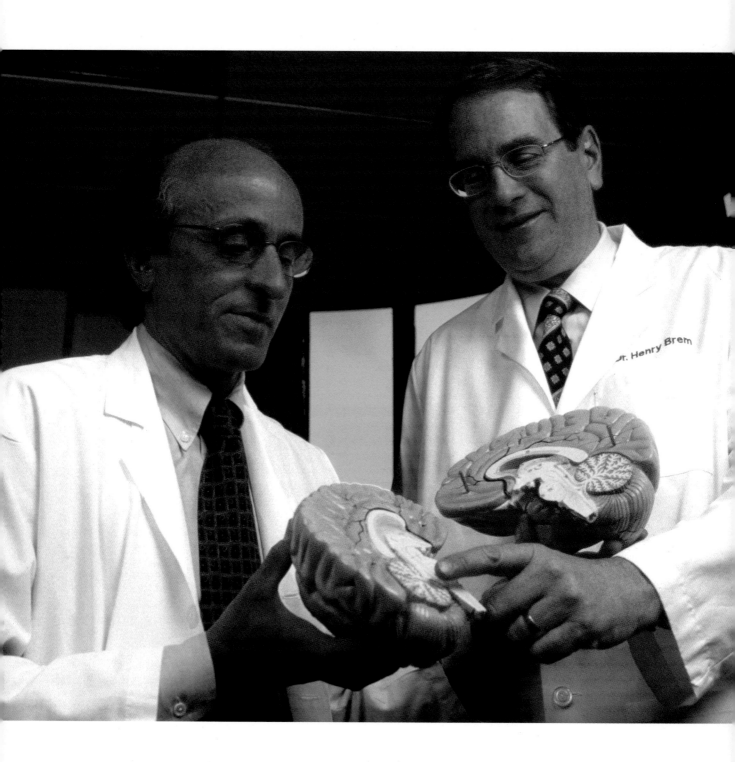

CHAPTER EIGHT

ONCOLOGY

Previous spread:
John Laterra, left,
and Henry Brem,
working to find more
effective treatments
for brain tumors,
and better ways to
deliver them.

LOCAL DRUG DELIVERY AND INTRA-TUMORAL PHARMACOKINETICS

Johns Hopkins Neuro-Oncology has long been a leader in the field of "intra-tumoral pharmacokinetics:" developing innovative methods to deliver chemotherapy directly into brain tumors.

Preclinical research in the laboratory of Henry Brem, the Harvey Cushing Professor of Neurosurgery, resulted in the development of Gliadel® chemotherapeutic wafers, implanted during surgery for treatment of glioblastoma. A successful multicenter, placebo-controlled Phase 3 clinical trial resulted in improved patient survival and FDA-approval of Gliadel in 1995. This clinical trial was a landmark in its use of a placebo-controlled study design to evaluate the efficacy of a neurosurgical procedure. While admittedly limited in efficacy as a single agent, Gliadel is also being studied for its ability to enhance the effects of immune checkpoint inhibitors and other forms of immunotherapy. Working together in preclinical and clinical trials, Hopkins Neurology, Neurosurgery and Oncology department investigators have evaluated the intra-tumoral pharmacokinetics of various treatments for gliomas – directly informing modern efforts to reduce the blood-brain barrier and enhance drug delivery to brain cancers.

DEVELOPING IMAGING BIOMARKERS FOR GLIOMAS

Using specific APT sequences, MRI can show minuscule, previously undetectable amounts – in the millimolar range – of mobile proteins and peptides.

Collaborative research between Johns Hopkins Neuro-Oncology and Neuro-Imaging (see Chapter 12) has been instrumental in developing Amide Proton Transfer (APT) magnetic resonance imaging (MRI), and in validating its diagnostic utility in brain cancer patients. This research demonstrated for the first time that using specific APT sequences, MRI can show minuscule, previously undetectable amounts – in the millimolar range – of mobile proteins and peptides. This accomplishment was pioneered by MR physicist Peter van Zijl, Ph.D. In subsequent studies, research teams led by van Zijl and John J. Laterra, M.D., Ph.D., professor of Neurology, Oncology, and Neuroscience and co-Director of the Brain Cancer Program at the Kimmel Cancer Center, used APT imaging to detect cellular proteins and peptides in rodent brain tumors, and to distinguish tumors from radiation necrosis.

Next, Jaishri Blakeley, M.D., worked with Jinyuan Zhou, Ph.D., in Radiology and several collaborators in Neurosurgery to show that APT imaging can

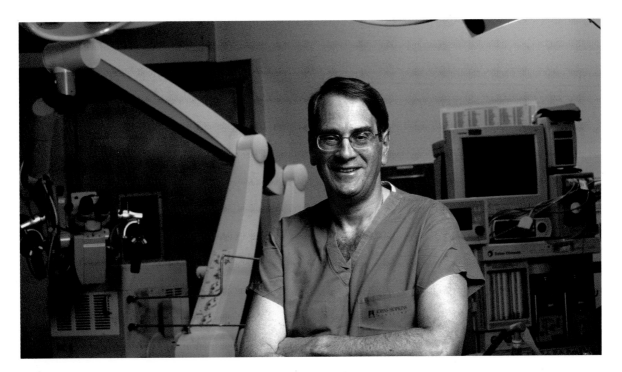

Henry Brem's innovative Gliadel wafer was a landmark in the treatment of brain tumors. Can it enhance the effects of immunotherapy? Hopkins investigators are leading research to find out.

identify optimal biopsy sites within heterogeneous malignant brain tumors. "We also found that it can distinguish recurrent brain cancer from radiation-induced brain injury in patients with brain cancer," Blakeley says. This journey of discovery from basic physics research to clinical application exemplifies the cross-disciplinary, patient-oriented research nurtured by the Division of Neuro-Oncology at Johns Hopkins.

Bacterial Therapy of Brain Tumors

Solid cancers contain regions of very low oxygen tension that enhance cancer cell survival and make tumors more drug-resistant. These hypoxic zones are unique to cancer – which also makes them excellent potential targets for treatment.

Hopkins scientists, led by molecular geneticist Bert Vogelstein, M.D., showed that the spore-forming anaerobic bacterium, *Clostridium* novyi-NT (C. *novyi*-NT) has the ability to thrive in hypoxic cancers and thereby kill tumors. Neuro-Oncology faculty member Verena Staedtke, M.D., Ph.D., translated this work to *in vivo* glioblastoma models. In animals, she showed that genetically modified C. novyi, injected intravenously, travel right to brain tumors – where they proliferate and cause tumor necrosis, *while sparing normal brain and prolonging survival.* What could make this work better? It turns out that C. *novyi* therapy and other forms of immunotherapy, such as CAR-T cell therapy (T cells modified to target tumor antigens) can be limited by systemic toxicities driven by cytokine storm. Staedtke has investigated how to prevent these toxicities: She discovered that these treatments cause cytokine-induced overproduction of catecholamines by myeloid cells – and that inhibiting catecholamine synthesis, using clinically available drugs, reverses toxicity. This work will soon be tested in patients.

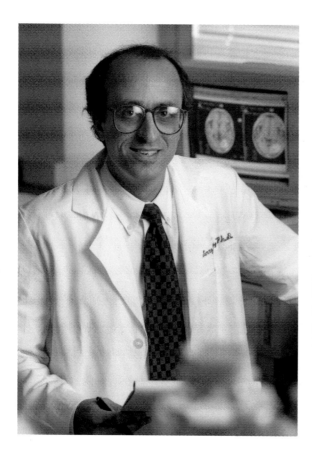

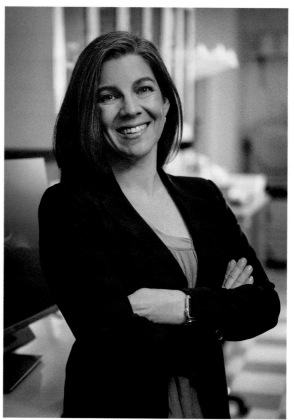

Left: John Laterra is doing innovative research in glioblastoma, using modified nanoparticles to inhibit tumor growth.

Right: Jaishri Blakeley directs the Johns Hopkins Comprehensive Neurofibromatosis Center.

TARGETING THERAPEUTIC MICRORNAS TO GLIOBLASTOMAS

Glioblastoma, like many aggressive tumors, is composed of diverse cell phenotypes; some of these are especially good at making the tumor grow and become more difficult to kill.

These cells are similar to neural stem cells and are referred to as GBM stem cells (GSCs). In pioneering research, John Laterra's laboratory has demonstrated the conversion of non-tumor-propagating GBM cells to tumor-propagating GSCs, and has found the epigenetic mechanisms responsible for this change. Oncogenic receptor tyrosine kinases stimulate GSC formation by reprogramming transcription factors that function by regulating the microRNA network. Laterra and colleagues identified microRNAs that can inhibit GSC formation, and in exciting work with Jordan Green, Ph.D., of Biomedical Engineering and the Hopkins Institute for Nano BioTechnology, Laterra has developed strategies for delivering these GSC-inhibiting miRNAs to GBM cells using nanoparticles. In preclinical studies, these modified nanoparticles have been highly promising: they have been shown to inhibit tumor growth, prolong animal survival, and enhance the response to standard-of-care radiation.

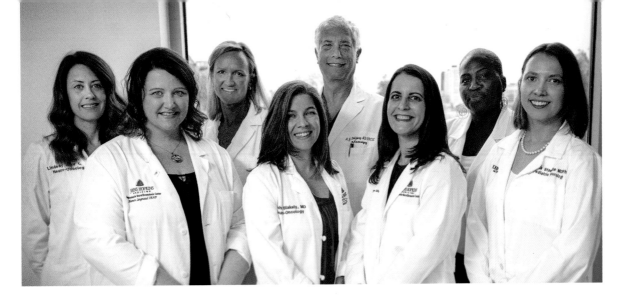

Members of the Neurofibromatosis Therapeutic Acceleration Program (NTAP), circa 2019, from left: Lindsay Blair, CRNP; Shannon Langmead, CRNP; Emily Little, RN; Jaishri Blakeley, MD; Allan Belzberg, MD; Bronwyn Slobogean, PA; Mary Brown, Verena Staedtke, MD, PhD.

THERAPEUTIC DEVELOPMENT FOR TUMORS ASSOCIATED WITH THE NEUROFIBROMATOSES

The JHCNC has become one of the world's largest clinical and research centers focused on neurofibromatosis.

The Neurofibromatoses (NF) include three rare tumor suppressor syndromes; Neurofibromatosis type 1 (NF1), type 2 (NF2) and schwannomatosis (SWN). In 2007, Jaishri Blakeley founded the Johns Hopkins Comprehensive Neurofibromatosis Center (JHCNC), and Verena Staedtke was recruited in 2016 to develop pediatric neuro-oncology and laboratory-based research in neurofibromatosis and immunotherapy. Together with Shannon Langmead, CRNP and neurosurgeon Allan Belzberg, Director of Peripheral Nerve Surgery, they direct the JHCNC – which has become one of the world's largest clinical and research centers focused on NF. Through this center, Neuro-Oncology Division members have detailed many of the clinical manifestations, long-term outcomes and imaging features of the tumors associated with NF1, NF2 and SWN. Among their important clinical therapeutic discoveries: showing that the anti-vascular agent, bevacizumab, results in sustained restoration of hearing in 36 percent of people with hearing loss related to NF2-associated vestibular schwannomas, and that the hearing and radiographic benefits gained from bevacizumab are maintained up to six months off of drug. These results are now being considered for inclusion in the NCCN Clinical Practice Guidelines as an evidence-based practice guideline for NF2.

The Neurofibromatosis Therapeutic Acceleration Program (NTAP), a philanthropically supported research program in the Division of Neuro-Oncology, was founded by Blakeley in 2012 to develop new treatments for plexiform and cutaneous neurofibromas affecting people with NF1. NTAP's research portfolio spans identifying the cell of origin and investigation of the interplay between the neoplastic Schwann cells (*NF1-/-*) and the heterozygous (*NF1+/-*) microenvironment, to participating in late-stage clinical trials showing that mitogen-activated protein kinase enzyme inhibitors (MEKi) cause reduction of plexiform neurofibroma size and resolution of tumor-associated symptoms. Such efforts have supported inclusion of the JHCNC as a Johns Hopkins School of Medicine Precision Medicine Center of Excellence. Through both of these initiatives, Neuro-Oncology Division researchers are making their data on the neurofibroma genome, proteome, methylome and response to drugs from clinical and preclinical studies *openly available to the research community*, and using these findings to create calculators to predict optimal treatment for each tumor type.

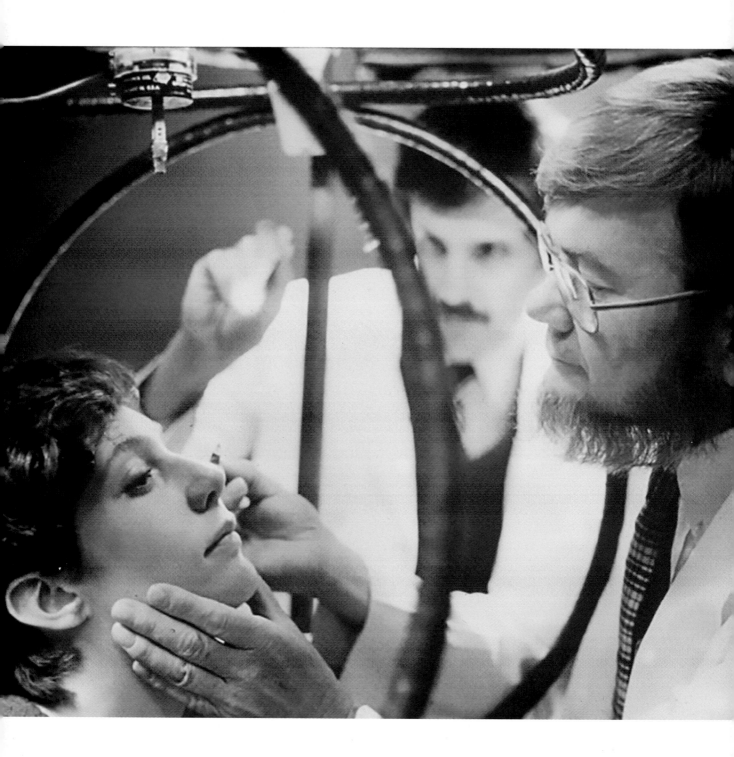

CHAPTER NINE

THE DIVISION OF NEURO-VISUAL AND VESTIBULAR DISORDERS

PREVIOUS SPREAD

The magnetic field search coil technique applied to human subjects: in this photo from the 1980s, David A. Robinson (right) inserts a small scleral annulus, developed by Han Collewijn from The Netherlands, to precisely measure eye movements, as David Zee (middle) looks on.

Beginnings

In 1971, during a noon basic science lecture to Neurology residents, David A. Robinson, Professor of Biomedical Engineering and Ophthalmology, used the medial longitudinal fasciculus (MLF) and internuclear ophthalmoplegia (INO) as an example of how to apply an engineering systems approach to understanding a clinical problem.

The clarity of Robinson's presentation inspired David Zee, a second-year neurology resident, to work with Robinson in his third-year elective time. Zee had been persuaded by Guy McKhann to pursue a Neurology residency at Hopkins, after attending Guy's evening teaching sessions for students and residents. Zee's interest in neuro-ophthalmology, kindled in a medical student summer elective at the Mayo Clinic, was strengthened during his residency by his work with a senior medical student, Neil Miller, and through exposure to Frank Walsh, one of the fathers of American neuro-ophthalmology.

During Zee's elective time, McKhann referred a patient with cerebellar dysfunction and downbeat nystagmus. With Robinson, Zee made a control systems model of this form of pathological nystagmus. Their early paper was one of the first to apply a control-systems approach (computational neuroscience) to clinical vestibular and eye movement disorders. It also emphasized developing bedside techniques for probing the function of each of the functional types of eye movements; saccades, pursuit, optokinetic, vestibular, gaze-holding, and vergence. Its final sentence read: "Eye movement abnormalities such as nystagmus can be better understood by considering them as disorders of control systems."

Origins of the Neurovestibular Unit

Robinson had invented a reliable way to record eye movements in monkeys and humans (Figure 1) and Zee wanted to use it to develop animal models of human ocular motor and vestibular disorders. He especially focused on cerebellar lesions, which ultimately allowed him to understand the pathophysiology and localizing value of many of the eye movement disorders seen in patients with cerebellar disease. Indeed, Zee says, these studies on the cerebellum made the eye movement examination invaluable for *all* patients with brainstem or cerebellar disease, "because of the precise localization of lesions indicated by many abnormal findings."

From this conceptual background came the idea of a vestibular-neurology "dizzy" clinic, "where a control-systems approach would be applied to patients with various types of vertigo and eye movement disorders," says Zee. Here, Zee's long-term research effort, using experimental lesions in trained nonhuman primates, could be applied to better understand the array of eye movement disorders seen in the clinic.

Like many burgeoning labs, the Neurovestibular Unit attracted a series of fellows from the U.S. and many parts of the world who, in turn, returned home to set up their own laboratories, bringing a quantitative systems approach to their own neuro-ophthalmology and neuro-otology clinics. John Leigh, inspired by reading the 1974 downbeat nystagmus paper, came to Hopkins in 1977 to work with both Robinson and Zee. He published papers on a number of topics, including eye movement abnormalities in unconscious patients and in Huntington's disease, during his six years at Hopkins, first as a fellow and then on the faculty. Leigh also recognized the need for an updated textbook focusing on eye movements; it had been several decades since David Cogan wrote his seminal book, *The Neurology of the Ocular Muscles*. Together, Leigh and Zee wrote the first edition of a textbook: *The Neurology of Eye Movements* (1983), now in its fifth edition.

Although it is not possible to mention the contribution made by every individual to the lab's research, some of the names of Neuro-Vestibular Lab investigators and trainees are listed in the electronic appendix of this book.

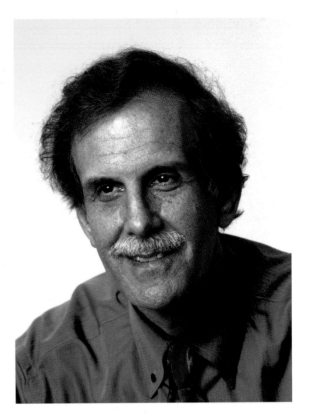

DAVID ZEE Zee's studies on the cerebellum made the eye movement exam invaluable for all patients with brainstem or cerebellar disease. This led to the idea of a vestibular-neurology "dizzy" clinic, "where a control-systems approach would be applied to patients with various types of vertigo and eye movement disorders."

INVESTIGATING HOW RAPID EYE MOVEMENTS ARE PLANNED

"The first major studies concerned abnormalities of rapid eye movements, saccades, that we use to reposition our line of sight as we scan the environment," says Zee. Working with Lance Optican at Johns Hopkins and colleagues at the NIH, Zee and Robinson studied and modeled patients with a form of dominant hereditary ataxia who showed exceedingly slow saccades. "These studies suggested a new hypothesis for how saccades were generated: the local feedback hypothesis," Zee explains, "in which the brain uses an internal model, incorporating brainstem and cerebellar circuits, to assess saccade progress and alter behavior as needed to make sure the eye arrives on target." The core of this model became, and still is, the essential concept underlying how the brain generates saccade eye movements. This model was also extended to account for saccadic oscillations: flutter and opsoclonus.

Two decades later, discovery of new cellular and molecular mechanisms of neurons in the brainstem that generated commands for saccades led to revision and improvement of the original model. Leigh and Zee, with Optican, Aasef Shaikh and Stefano Ramat, developed a new model focused on the inherent instability of brainstem circuits, which accounts for saccade oscillations. "These concepts also provided insights into a variety of tremors and dystonia affecting the limbs and head," notes Leigh, "and the elaboration of a new concept of a head-holding (integrator) mechanism. Thus, these studies of eye movements provided new insights for motor control in general."

DISCOVERING MECHANISMS AND TREATMENTS FOR NYSTAGMUS

Since the initial study on downbeat nystagmus, an abiding goal of the lab has been to understand the pathogenic mechanisms for a broad range of abnormal forms of nystagmus, looking for potential treatments. The first discoveries concerned a rare disorder, periodic alternating nystagmus, in which the direction of horizontal nystagmus reverses every two minutes or so. Robinson and Leigh developed a model for this disorder that made specific predictions, such as specifying the critical vestibular stimulus that would temporally abolish the unwanted nystagmus. "These predictions were confirmed experimentally in three affected patients," Leigh says. "The model also provided insights into successful treatment of the nystagmus with baclofen – a collaborative effort with colleagues from the United Kingdom – which was one of the first reported pharmacological 'cures' of an eye movement disorder." Since that study, the lab has had an interest in the treatment of abnormal eye movements, such as nystagmus in the syndrome of oculopalatal tremor, which arises from olivocerebellar circuits. In health, these circuits are essential for motor learning. But, in the syndrome of oculopalatal tremor, disruption of the olivocerebellar circuits causes maladaptive learning, leading to oscillations of the eyes and the cranial nerve innervated muscles derived from the branchial arches.

The first discoveries concerned a rare disorder, periodic alternating nystagmus, in which the direction of horizontal nystagmus reverses every two minutes or so.

USING EYE MOVEMENTS TO STUDY MOTOR LEARNING

Another important theme of research was how the brain adapts the vestibulo-ocular reflex (which enables clear vision during head movements) in the face of changing visual demands due to normal development and aging, or the response to disease or trauma, or even a new prescription of corrective spectacles. These studies were the beginning of what was to become a sustained research interest of the laboratory in ocular motor learning, with implications that extend to motor learning in general, such as occurs when learning a new piano piece or dance step. These studies are also fundamental to understanding how patients recover from vestibular and other disorders of movement. A series of studies also provided insights into how other eye movements – saccades, pursuit, and vergence – could adaptively modify their properties to new visual demands. Thus, the relative simplicity of eye movement control has proven advantageous in understanding basic mechanisms of motor learning and recovery from injury.

Implications of these studies extend to motor learning in general, such as occurs when learning a new piano piece or dance step.

STUDYING DEMANDS MADE ON EYE MOVEMENTS DURING NATURAL ACTIVITIES

The vestibulo-ocular reflexes include responses to linear head movements (translations) as well as head rotations. The properties of the translational vestibulo-ocular reflex had not been studied in response to head movements

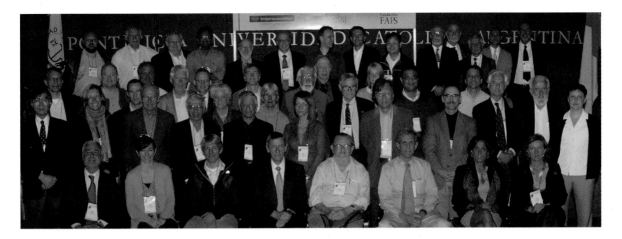

A vestibular and eye movement meeting held in 2011, in Buenos Aires, at which a dozen lab alumni presented papers.

such that occur during natural activities, such as locomotion. By applying brief, fast, head translations (rather than rotations), the translational vestibulo-ocular reflex (VOR) was shown to have quite different properties from the rotational vestibulo-ocular reflex that clinicians conventionally test. (Head rotations depend on the labyrinthine semicircular canals, whereas head translations depend on the otolithic organs). This finding led to the development with Stefano Ramat of a new "head heave" test, consisting of rapid, lateral movements of the patient's head, which was used by Daniele Nuti and Marco Mandala, David's long-standing colleagues in Siena, Italy, to detect otolithic involvement in patients with acute vestibular neuritis, and thereby evaluate prognosis. It also prompted Mark Walker, Raphael Tamargo, and colleagues to study the effect of experimental lesions of the cerebellar nodulus on the translational vestibulo-ocular reflex. These studies demonstrated the contribution of the cerebellum to the different signal processing underlying the translational and rotational vestibulo-ocular reflexes, "both of which are called on to preserve vision during the head movements that occur during our natural activities, and are pertinent to understanding why people fall," says Zee.

By applying brief, fast, head translations (rather than rotations), the translational vestibulo-ocular reflex was shown to have quite different properties from the rotational vestibulo-ocular reflex that clinicians conventionally test.

Understanding the Mechanisms for Double Vision

Ophthalmologists from the Wilmer Eye Institute have been steadfast partners in the growing focus of interest in the lab that concerned a thorny clinical problem: persistent diplopia and strabismus. This research effort included developing an animal model for trochlear nerve palsy, which was the focus of physiological experiments and collaborative anatomical studies with Joseph Demer, Jing Tian, Richard Lewis, David Guyton, and Howard Ying. These early studies were important precursors to more recent discoveries of how properties of orbital tissues and muscles, and both their afferent and efferent innervation, relate to strabismus – and how the brain attempts to adaptively realign the eyes and restore single vision when eye muscles become weak or paralyzed.

Investigating a Serendipitous Finding:
MRI Scanners Induce Nystagmus

The observation that normal subjects lying in an MRI machine report dizziness and develop sustained nystagmus led to a series of collaborative studies with colleagues from the Department

Basic discoveries made in the Hopkins lab have been applied to a broad range of clinical disorders.

of Otolaryngology-Head and Neck Surgery. The mechanism for this novel finding (motion of the endolymph in the vestibular canals, due to Lorentz magneto-hydrodynamic forces imposed by the magnetic field) was mathematically modelled, and represented a new way to stimulate the labyrinth and examine its function. Transcranial magnetic stimulation (TMS) is also being used in the laboratory by two new permanent members of the lab, Amir Kheradmand and Jorge Otero-Millan, to study normal and abnormal perception of one's sense of upright as it relates to the common, vexing, and often unexplained problem of dizziness and imbalance with which so many patients are plagued.

APPLYING FINDINGS FROM BASIC STUDIES TO CLINICAL DISORDERS AND THE EMERGENCY ROOM

Basic discoveries made in the Hopkins lab have been applied to a broad range of clinical disorders. These include the mechanism of nystagmus in internuclear ophthalmoplegia (in which the "dissociated nystagmus" reflects an adaptive response to diplopia), and the diagnostic value of abnormal saccades in Huntington's disease. New quantitative clinical vestibular tests have been developed for the dizzy patient, such as head-shaking nystagmus, optokinetic after-nystagmus, and tilt suppression of vestibular nystagmus.

Ronald Tusa and Susan Herdman, members of the lab for many years, studied the effects of experimental lesions of visual cortex on eye movements. Ron later developed one of the first animal models of congenital nystagmus. Susan became one of the founders of the burgeoning field of vestibular rehabilitation therapy.

As the lab moves forward to address key contemporary problems of modern medicine, a major clinical project is aimed at the accurate diagnosis of stroke in patients with acute vertigo seen in the emergency room setting. This research was initiated by David Newman-Toker, and involves many other colleagues in the lab, including Dan Gold, who is spearheading a telemedicine initiative.

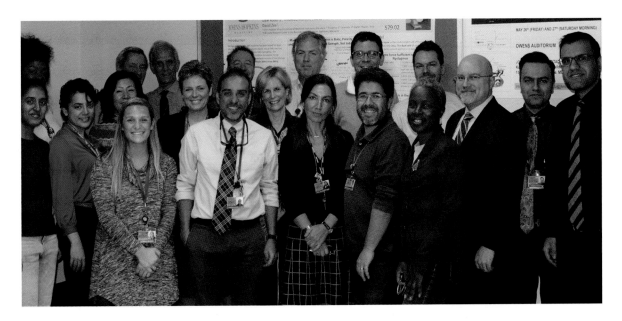

Neuro-vestibular lab members in 2018.

CONCLUSIONS AND SYNTHESIS

"Starting with little knowledge of the mechanisms of vestibular disturbance and abnormal eye movements," concludes Zee, "a sustained effort over the past half-century, drawing on the bourgeoning field of neuroscience – including neurophysiology, neuropharmacology, neuroimaging, and neurocomputation – has led to substantial progress, at an ever-accelerating rate, in understanding clinical disorders affecting balance and vision." Some of the discoveries of the Division of Neuro-Visual and Vestibular Disorders have been specific to vestibular and visual disorders, but many have generalized to a broad range of neurological disorders. "The outlook for further progress is positive, reflecting the optimism within the neurological and neuroscience communities as a whole."

Starting with little knowledge of the mechanisms of vestibular disturbance and abnormal eye movements, a sustained effort over the past half-century has led to substantial progress at an ever-accelerating rate.

SELECTED REFERENCES

Leigh, RJ, Zee, DS, *The Neurology of Eye Movements*, Fifth edition, Oxford University Press, New York, 2015.

Zee, DS, A neurologist and ataxia: Using eye movements to learn about the cerebellum, *Cerebellum and Ataxias*, 2018, PMID: 29445510

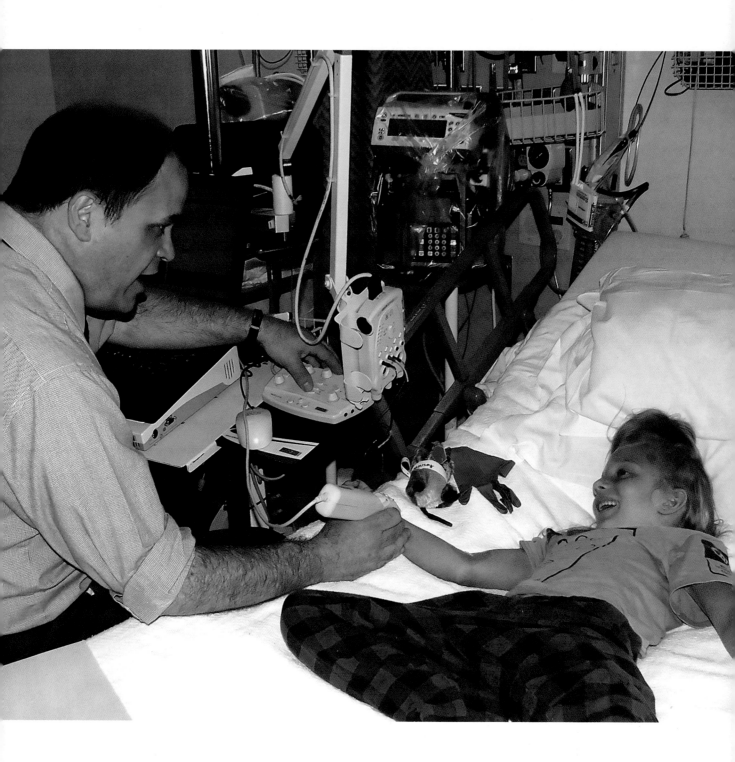

CHAPTER TEN

SPINAL MUSCULAR ATROPHY

Previous spread
THOMAS CRAWFORD
Thomas Crawford is happy to report that SMA "has shifted from one of the most hopeless of maladies to one that is treatable with novel therapies."

TRANSLATING RESEARCH INTO TREATMENT

Spinal muscular atrophy (SMA), a relatively common genetic neuromuscular disorder, was often fatal in affected infants and young children, and significantly disabling in older children and adults. But this is no longer the case: "In the last two decades, SMA has shifted from one of the most hopeless of maladies to one that is treatable with novel therapies," says neurologist Thomas Crawford, M.D.

"Babies who were once destined to die now grow and develop well. Children who would never have achieved head control can now walk."

This success required advances in multiple disciplines, notes Charlotte Sumner, M.D., "from individual patient investigations optimizing care and outcome measures to molecular genetics, animal disease modeling, neuropathology, and molecularly targeted therapeutics."

The vastly improved outlook for people with SMA is a story to which Crawford, Sumner, and other Hopkins investigators have contributed much.

FINDING A "WINDOW OF OPPORTUNITY"

In the 1970s, Jack Griffin, Linda Cork, Robert Adams, and Donald Price characterized a genetic disorder affecting Brittany Spaniel dogs that appeared similar to SMA. At that time, not much more was known about SMA beyond Werdnig's 1891 observation that identified a "spinal" cause for muscular atrophy based upon the atrophic ventral motor roots, "thus distinguishing it from genetic myopathies," says Sumner. Although the canine condition differs from human SMA by having a dominant inheritance pattern and an unknown genetic abnormality, the clinical similarities were striking. The Hopkins group showed that the early stages of muscle weakness are caused *not* by degeneration of motor neurons or their axons, but rather by hypotrophy of motor neuron soma and axons with impaired axon transport and neurofilament accumulation. Later, Martin Pinter and Hopkins Neurology-trained Mark Rich showed that these histological abnormalities are associated with impaired synaptic vesicle release at the neuromuscular junction (NMJ) in response to evoked stimulation. "Such pathological and electrophysiological abnormalities also turned out to be characteristic of genetic mouse models of human SMA and to the extent possible, patients as well," says Crawford. "This highlighted a critical 'window of opportunity' of neuronal dysfunction before degeneration" and suggested a potential point for therapeutic intervention.

In 1987, Crawford developed a pediatric neuromuscular clinic with a special focus on SMA. This enabled a number of contributions to the field, including the availability of genetic material for finding the SMA gene and identification

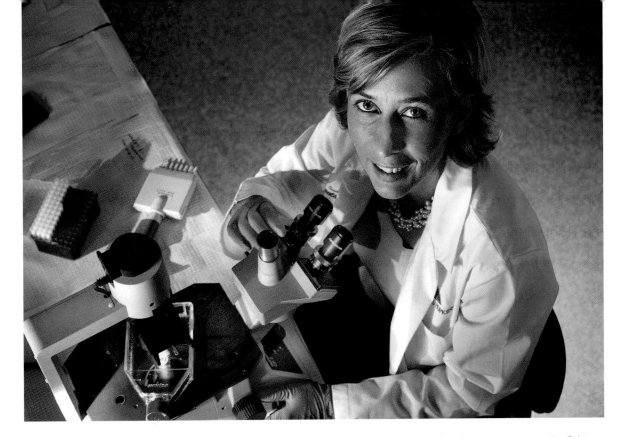

CHARLOTTE SUMNER The discovery that "neuronal dysfunction preceded neuronal loss" in humans, as in the Brittany Spaniel disease, suggested a potential point for therapeutic intervention.

of early plasma "biomarkers" of SMA. Parents of SMA patients encouraged Crawford to establish an autopsy program that evolved under Sumner's guidance to become an important resource.

During her neuromuscular fellowship at Hopkins in 2000, Sumner was influenced by the clinical exposure to SMA provided by Crawford and the neuropathological approaches championed by Jack Griffin. Identification of the SMA gene in 1995 had led to the creation of the first mouse models of SMA in 2001. "SMA is caused by homozygous mutations of the 'survival motor neuron 1' gene (*SMN1*) and retention of a partially functioning, variably spliced transcript from an adjacent *SMN2* gene that is present in variable copy number," explains Crawford. Complete absence of SMN protein would be lethal; having increased copy numbers of *SMN2* is associated with reduced disease severity. "These genetic observations led to the hypothesis that increased expression of SMN would ameliorate disease," says Sumner. During her postdoctoral fellowship at NIH with Kenneth Fischbeck and after joining the Johns Hopkins Neurology faculty in 2006, Sumner focused on understanding the underlying molecular and cellular mechanisms of SMA and on testing potential therapeutics. "It emerged that early phases of SMA disease pathogenesis in SMA mouse models were characterized by slowed development and electrophysiological dysfunction of the entire motor circuit," she says. But importantly – as in the Brittany Spaniel disease – "neuronal dysfunction preceded neuronal loss." Sumner and others studied histone deacetylase (HDAC) inhibitors that activate gene expression by promoting an open chromatin state. She found that HDAC inhibitors can increase SMN expression in cultured cells from SMA patients, while preclinical HDAC studies demonstrated the fundamental proof-of-concept insight that *increased SMN expression improves motor function and survival*. These early studies also revealed the important observation that earlier delivery was associated with enhanced efficacy – an insight that would be recapitulated in all of the successful therapy programs to come later. Although clinical trials at Hopkins and elsewhere of the FDA-approved, weak HDAC inhibitor valproic acid did not show convincing efficacy in SMA patients, much more active SMN-inducing drugs were on the horizon.

A New Generation of SMA Therapeutics

These advances in SMA genetics and understanding of the disease were happening at the same time as the rapidly evolving science of RNA splicing biology, synthetic antisense oligonucleotide development, and refinement of gene-transfer vectors. Characterization of the factors that control pre-mRNA splicing of *SMN2* led to the strategy of targeting the splice motif ISS-N1 with antisense oligonucleotides to sterically inhibit splice factors that remove exon 7. The removal of exon 7 by the splice factors would result in an inactive protein; the antisense oligonucleotides prevent this, allowing expression of active SMN. The 2018 "Breakthrough" award winners, Adrian Krainer at Cold Spring Harbor and Frank Bennett at Ionis Pharmaceuticals, demonstrated efficacy of this approach in cell and animal models. "Importantly, the phase III trials in both infants and older children with SMA both showed efficacy," says Sumner, "and the FDA quickly approved nusinersen/Spinraza for all SMA patients in December 2016." A second therapy program that has advanced quickly and is on the verge of FDA approval is onasemnogene abeparvovec (Avexis 101). "In this case, the goal is to deliver exogenous *SMN1* cDNA by using the adeno-associated virus 9." Importantly, AAV9 was shown to target motor neurons effectively when administered intravascularly, particularly in young mice and primates. "When delivered one time to SMA mice, it markedly improves disease outcomes," says Crawford. A single-site clinical trial showed clinical efficacy in type I SMA patients, and a follow-up multisite study has confirmed these initial findings. Hopkins' Pediatric Neuromuscular clinical trials unit, headed by Crawford with the assistance of neurologist Jessica Nance, M.D., M.S., has had a major role in enabling clinical trials of both nusinersen and Avexis 101. A third type of SMN induction treatment is also being evaluated in clinical trials, principally in Europe. Roche Pharmaceutical and Novartis each have identified and are testing orally bioavailable, small molecule-splicing modifiers that have shown impressive efficacy in preclinical studies.

Looking Ahead

In the two decades since the gene was identified, SMA has moved from a little-known and hopeless malady to one commanding substantial attention at all levels of government, industry, and science.

Hopkins investigators participated in policy work that led the U.S. Secretary of Health and Human Services to add SMA to the Recommended Uniform Screening Panel for Newborns. "This will enable more patients to be treated very early in the disease," says Sumner. The future of SMA therapeutics is likely to include combined treatments that target distinct but complementary targets. Sumner's group recently identified a novel long noncoding RNA that represses *SMN2* gene expression, and has shown that targeting this lncRNA might boost the efficacy of *SMN2* splice-switching therapeutic strategies. In addition, there has been interest in combining SMN induction with strategies that promote muscle growth, with which Sumner has shown some success in severe SMA mice. Multicenter clinical trials of one such muscle-enhancing therapy, nationally directed by Crawford, will soon commence. "Future therapeutic development will also require a return to investigations of the fundamental cellular and molecular pathways disrupted by SMN protein deficiency," notes Crawford. New insights made by studying human tissues from the autopsy program will improve the current therapies and help identify novel therapeutic targets. "Another priority for future work must be to advance treatment of other hereditary diseases of motor neurons and peripheral nerves," Sumner says. As was the case for SMA, a critical starting point for developing treatment is pinpointing the genetic causes. Sumner's group continues to identify genetic causes of these diseases; recently, her laboratory has focused on transient receptor potential vanilloid 4 (TRPV4), as it is the only example of mutant ion channel-causing forms of distal SMA and hereditary motor-sensory neuropathy. Studies are ongoing in the Sumner laboratory to further investigate the mechanisms underlying "TRPV4opathies," and determine whether available small-molecule antagonists may serve as novel therapeutics for these disorders.

Success has raised an unanticipated challenge: SMA therapeutics are exceptionally costly.

"Success" of a therapeutic program of this magnitude has been associated with much attention, but

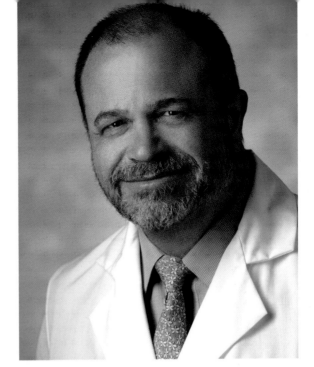

THOMAS CRAWFORD
The Hopkins SMA program has been highlighted nationally in the discussion of how society should pay for such lifesaving therapeutic advances, "especially as these now-proven technologies in SMA hold promise for a wide range of rare and not-so-rare diseases."

application of this success has raised an unanticipated challenge: SMA therapeutics are exceptionally costly. "Given the strength of beneficial effects, denial based upon cost is difficult to justify," comments Crawford, "but on the other hand, the cumulative costs to society are substantial. There is an emerging larger debate about how society should pay for advances of this nature, especially as these now-proven technologies in SMA hold promise for a wide range of rare and not-so-rare diseases." The Hopkins SMA program has been highlighted in local and national media to raise public attention to these issues. This attention has been matched by enthusiastic support from Hospital President Redonda Miller, and substantial commitment and financial backing from the Hopkins Health Care administration. The challenges of personalized medicine are sharply drawn by the SMA success. "SMA has become a key example of the quandary, permitting the issue to be addressed sympathetically in the public eye," Sumner adds.

The new therapies for SMA are exceptional but insufficient. Optimization of these therapies will require the interface of the human experience, modeling in animals, the emergence of laboratory biomarkers, and the ability to focus on the many interacting aspects of a single problem – something that is remarkably possible at Hopkins.

SELECTED REFERENCES

Sumner CJ, Crawford TO. Two breakthrough gene-targeted treatments for spinal muscular atrophy: challenges remain. *J Clin Invest* 2018; 128:3219-3227.

Crawford TO, Pardo CA. The neurobiology of childhood spinal muscular atrophy. *Neurobiol Dis* 1996;3:97-110.

Sumner CJ, Paushkin S, Ko CP. Spinal muscular atrophy: disease mechanisms and therapy: Elsevier, 2017.

Sumner CJ. Spinal muscular atrophy, John Griffin, and mentorship. *J Peripher Nerv Syst* 2012;17 Suppl 3:52-56.

Landoure G, Zdebik AA, Martinez TL, et al. Mutations in TRPV4 cause Charcot-Marie-Tooth disease type 2C. *Nat Genet* 2010;42:170-174.

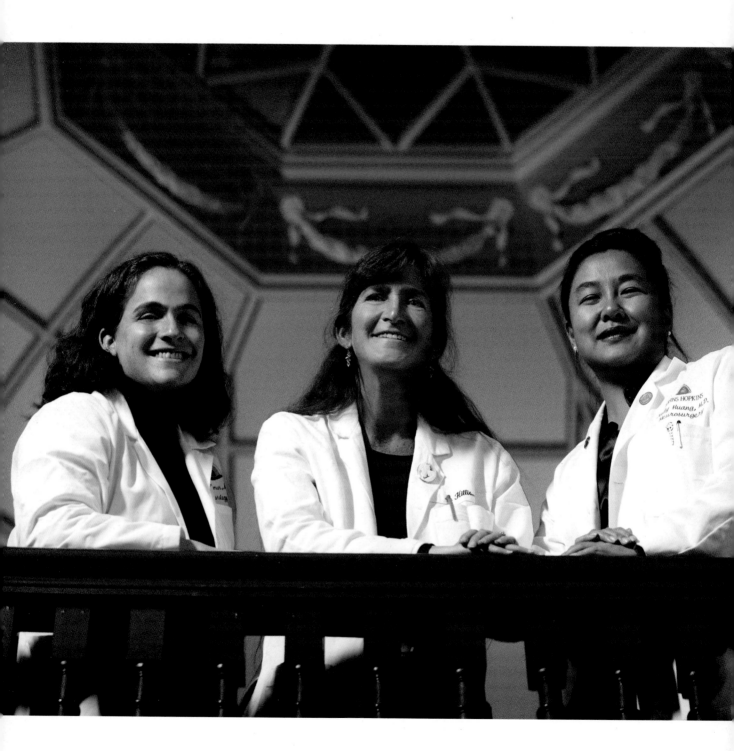

CHAPTER ELEVEN

CEREBROVASCULAR DISEASE: ADVANCING THE FIELD

Previous spread
Leaders of the Stroke
Team, from left: Rebecca
Gottesman, Director of
Research at Johns Hopkins
Bayview, Argye Hillis,
Director of the Cerebro-
vascular Division, and
Judy Huang, Vice Chair of
Neurosurgery. Innovative
research and treatment
at Hopkins is devoted to
reducing or even reversing
injury, restoring function,
and maximizing quality of
life for adults and children
after stroke.

Over the last half-century, the prevention, management, and treatment of strokes has changed dramatically. For many decades, cerebrovascular disease was managed in internal medicine departments – and strokes were observed, but not actively treated.

By contrast, we now have multidisciplinary Neurology teams with urgent, time-dependent consideration of interventions including endovascular therapies. Throughout this evolution, Johns Hopkins Neurology has provided cutting-edge diagnostic and interventional care, while playing a major role in discovery, and training new leaders in the field of cerebrovascular neurology.

In the 1960s, Abraham Lilienfeld, at the Hopkins School of Hygiene and Public Health (now the Bloomberg School), started to look at stroke in a different way. A member of the President's Commission on Heart Disease, Cancer and Stroke, Abe Lilienfeld emphasized the importance of prevention. When Guy McKhann came to Hopkins in 1969, this work laid the foundation for what is now a major program in stroke, combining both clinical care and research.

"The key principles," says Rebecca Gottesman, M.D., Ph.D., Director of Research at Johns Hopkins Bayview, with a joint appointment in Epidemiology at the Bloomberg School, "are that *stroke deficits may be due to **transient** alterations in cerebral perfusion; and **interventions** may reverse these deficits.*"

The work of Argye Hillis, M.D., who is Director of the Cerebrovascular Division, has emphasized the value of improving cerebral perfusion in rescuing these areas. Using brain imaging methods including MRI with perfusion weighting, Hillis, who also has joint appointments in Physical Medicine and Rehabilitation and in Cognitive Science at Johns Hopkins University, demonstrated that cognitive deficits after stroke could occur in areas of dysfunctional, but not infarcted, brain tissue. With Robert Wityk, M.D., Hillis studied the potential benefit of "induced hypertension" – augmenting blood pressure with intravenous fluids or pressor medications. Although induced hypertension is used only sparingly now, "permissive hypertension" – allowing blood pressure to run higher after acute stroke without direct interventions to augment it – is the standard of care for management of acute ischemic stroke.

Interventions in the stroke field are based on the concept that the outcome will improve with the increase of blood flow to the ischemic penumbra – the region of brain surrounding an infarct, which represents at-risk and dysfunctional but not infarcted tissue. Hillis' research revealed much of what is understood about the penumbra and its impact on tissue function.

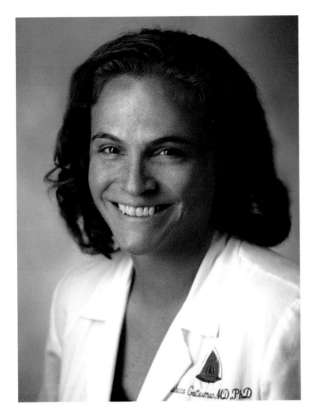

In 1996, the FDA approved the use of intravenous tPA (tissue plasminogen activator) to lyse the causative occluding clot. A "clot buster" drug, tPA is administered within a limited time period – four and a half hours – after the start of a clinical stroke, and establishing this window effected a major change in the pace and management of stroke patients. Stroke neurologists now have to be available at all hours for timely evaluation of stroke patients.

In addition, the most important new advance in acute management of stroke has been the demonstration of the benefit of mechanical thrombectomy in individuals with large artery occlusion and stroke symptoms. This intervention is based on the evidence that rapidly removing a clot to recanalize an occluded blood vessel will improve the outcome by restoring blood flow to the hypoperfused penumbra.

Rebecca Gottesman's work is minimizing brain damage from stroke, and also reducing vascular risks to lower the likelihood of dementia.

GENDER DIFFERENCES IN STROKE INJURY AND RECOVERY

Strokes are more common in younger men, but this reverses in middle age, with increased stroke risk, mortality and poor functional outcomes seen in elderly women.

Louise McCullough, M.D., Ph.D., who completed a Neurology residency at Hopkins and is now Chair of Neurology at the University of Texas-Houston, has made important contributions to the role of gender in the frequency and outcome of strokes. Strokes are more common in younger men, but this reverses in middle age, with increased stroke risk, mortality and poor functional outcomes seen in elderly women. McCullough's research has not only influenced stroke care, but has been an important factor guiding the NIH to require male and female animals in most pre-clinical experiments, and for explicit consideration of "sex as a biological variable" in NIH grant applications.

RISK FACTORS FOR COGNITIVE DECLINE AND DEMENTIA AFTER HEART SURGERY

The key studies conducted by Guy McKhann, in collaboration with cardiac surgeon William Baumgartner, Ola Selnes, Maura Grega, and Scott Zeger, provided important data on risk factors for cognitive decline in people with elevated vascular risk. Earlier studies had suggested that coronary artery bypass surgery, particularly cardiopulmonary bypass, led to higher rates of cognitive impairment and dementia. However, it was the controlled observational studies led by McKhann, in which patients with coronary artery disease treated with or without surgical intervention (bypass surgery vs. medical management) were evaluated over a six-year period that proved this was not the case.

McKhann's study demonstrated that cognitive decline in these patients was not specific to bypass surgery, but to the presence of vascular risk factors.

The implications of this study extended well beyond this particular surgical question and addressed the field of dementia more broadly. McKhann and colleagues showed that neurocognitive decline was most likely associated with vascular risk factors, including increased age and underlying cerebrovascular disease. Further, they suggested that moderating the cardiovascular risk factors might mitigate the decline in neurocognition in patients undergoing any type of cardiac surgical procedure.

Rebecca Gottesman, now Professor of Neurology, became involved in this study as a resident, and "found the concept that prevention of stroke might lead to prevention of dementia extremely appealing," she says. Her subsequent work has been primarily in epidemiologic studies, such as the Atherosclerosis Risk in Communities (ARIC) study, where it has been shown that vascular risk factors, especially in midlife, are important risk factors for cognitive decline over subsequent decades, and for mild cognitive impairment and dementia. Further, in an ancillary study to ARIC, she has demonstrated that higher midlife vascular risk – *more than later-life vascular risk* – indicated by increased amounts of hypertension, diabetes, hypercholesterolemia, obesity, and smoking, is associated with elevated late-life brain amyloid, the protein which is deposited in individuals in Alzheimer's disease (AD) and may play a role in the development of AD.

Other exciting findings: the recent SPRINT trial suggests that aggressive control of blood pressure not only reduces risk of cardiovascular disease but, in the as-yet-unpublished (but presented internationally) SPRINT-MIND trial, may reduce a combined outcome of mild cognitive impairment and dementia. Similarly, multimodal intervention trials in early dementia demonstrate that management strategies including controlling vascular risk factors, combined with other lifestyle and cognitive interventions, may reduce cognitive decline (studied in the FINGER trial, with the ongoing US POINTER trial addressing a modified intervention in the US).

"MINOR" STROKE

Marsh is studying subtle cognitive deficits in people who suffer small strokes.

Elisabeth Marsh, M.D., who has been at Hopkins as an undergraduate, medical student, neurology resident, fellow, and now faculty member, worked with Argye Hillis from her earliest days at Hopkins. Originally focusing on cognition, she collaborated with the pediatric epilepsy group in studies on cognition in patients who underwent hemispherectomy. She since has shifted her research to acute stroke care and recovery; particularly, Marsh is looking at subtle cognitive deficits in people who suffer small strokes. She is also studying interpersonal and behavioral issues that occur in these patients after strokes, hoping to understand the mechanisms of these subtle deficits and to guide rehabilitation. Marsh has worked with Rafael Llinas to establish a post-stroke clinic at Bayview, the BaSIC clinic, where patients' recovery trajectories are carefully followed and where these "minor" issues are studied in greater detail. Under the leadership of Llinas and Marsh, Bayview has developed an outstanding center for stroke care

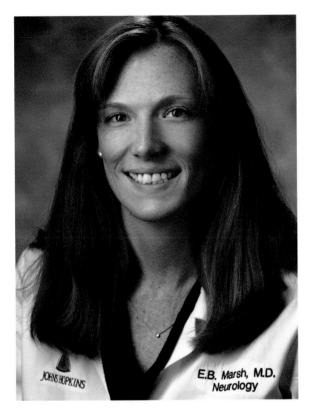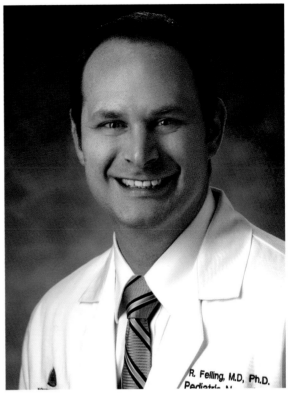

Elisabeth Marsh (left) established a post-stroke clinic at Bayview with Rafael Llinas. At this BaSIC clinic, patients' recovery trajectories are carefully followed, and "minor" interpersonal and behavioral issues are studied in detail. Ryan Felling (right), who directs the Pediatric Stroke Program, studies basic mechanisms of repair after ischemic injury.

and research. Both Johns Hopkins Hospital and Johns Hopkins Bayview are Comprehensive Stroke Centers, which means they provide a high level of care, with cutting-edge interventions, for the highest-acuity stroke patients.

PEDIATRIC STROKE

Pediatric stroke was a new field when Lori Jordan, M.D., Ph.D., a pediatric neurology resident, undertook a stroke fellowship at Hopkins.

She focused on intracerebral hemorrhage in babies and children, and the risk factors and outcomes associated with this devastating condition, and then studied the cerebrovascular consequences of sickle cell disease. Now, as Director of the Pediatric Stroke Program at Vanderbilt, she studies novel imaging techniques in sickle cell disease in children. The Pediatric Stroke Program at Hopkins has remained active, with its Director, Ryan Felling, M.D., Ph.D., studying recovery and the basic mechanisms of repair after ischemic injury, and Lisa Sun, M.D., investigating chemotherapy-associated cerebrovascular complications in children as well as evaluating motor recovery after pediatric stroke.

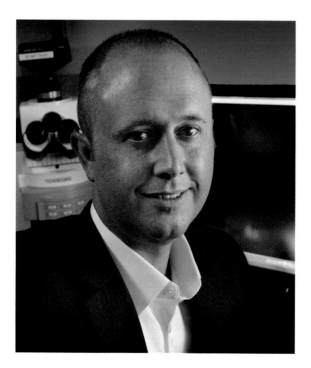

Steve Zeiler is working to lengthen the critical recovery period after stroke.

The Sheikh Khalifa Stroke Institute, launched early in 2018, embodies the importance of stroke care and research in medicine today.

With institute leadership by Justin McArthur, and center leadership by Argye Hillis and Pablo Celnik, M.D., Director of the Department of Physical Medicine and Rehabilitation, the center concentrates on delivery of stroke care and early recovery. Mona Bahouth, M.D., is focusing on the best systems of care for stroke management and early recovery, and the best ways to deliver simple interventions that can make big improvements in the outcome of stroke patients.

STROKE RECOVERY AND REHABILITATION

Beginning in the early 2000s, the Neurology Department began to pursue studies in recovery of language, cognition and motor function after stroke. Argye Hillis (see above) has investigated mechanisms and prediction of recovery from aphasia using careful behavioral characterization, complemented by functional, structural, and perfusion brain imaging. More recently, she has begun using non-invasive brain stimulation to augment language rehabilitation.

Inspired in part by Hillis' work, John Krakauer, M.A., M.D., came to Hopkins from Columbia University in late 2010 to set up a parallel program in motor recovery after stroke, founding and directing the Brain, Learning, Animation and Movement (BLAM) Lab in April 2011. Krakauer has created a remarkable program that asks new questions about how we learn motor skills, such as: "Why does it take so long to become an expert musician or athlete?" and "What is it that practice is making better?" Krakauer believes that motor learning has become separated from the rest of cognitive neuroscience, but "in our view, motor skill requires just as much 'cognition' as any other activity, such as chess, mathematics or language." Also, "lab-based motor learning tasks have predominantly focused on adaptation or sequence learning. We think that tasks need to be more multifaceted, like sports, and tracked over longer periods. We are currently developing video games to accomplish this."

Soon after his arrival, Krakauer, the John C. Malone Professor of Neurology, Neuroscience, and Physical Medicine and Rehabilitation, led the first multi-center, multi-modal study of the natural history of arm and hand recovery

The first game designed by KATA was centered on a physical simulation of a dolphin, based in part on research conducted at the National Aquarium in Baltimore. The game was used in a small pilot clinical trial of early stroke therapy with positive results.

after stroke. This study has led to new insights about inter-hemispheric interactions, mirror movements, and the dissociability of recovery from strength and dexterity. It also laid the groundwork for an acute interventional trial involving an animated dolphin (see below).

A critical aspect of the Hillis and Krakauer labs is that, in parallel to the more applied questions, they also conduct cognitive neuroscience research in healthy subjects; "predicated on the idea that rigorous clinical investigation in neurology depends on concomitant strong basic neuroscience," Krakauer explains. "Thus, BLAM lab also pursues studies in experimental and computational motor control and motor learning in healthy humans." In addition, Krakauer has mentored Steve Zeiler, M.D., Ph.D., and helped him create a mouse model of stroke that has already made important discoveries about the critical recovery period after stroke. Zeiler's Stroke Recovery Laboratory is working to lengthen the window of time for recovery of motor skills – which, Zeiler says, "is essential to rehabilitation and the restoration of a meaningful life."

In 2012, Krakauer co-founded the KATA project, in conjunction with Omar Ahmad, Ph.D., a computer scientist and Director of Innovative Engineering in the Department of Neurology, and software architect Promit Roy. The goal of the KATA project was to design a new form of "neuro-animation" that would allow patients to "experience motivating and immersive environments that are both motorically and cognitively challenging," Krakauer says. The originality and therapeutic potential of the animation was noted by Ed Catmull, President of Pixar and Disney Animation. The first game designed by KATA was centered on a physical simulation of a dolphin, based in part on research conducted at the National Aquarium in Baltimore. The game was used in a small pilot clinical trial of early stroke therapy with positive results that are being written up currently. The gaming software led to creation of a start-up company that was acquired in 2018, with the goal of combining the best of academia and industry.

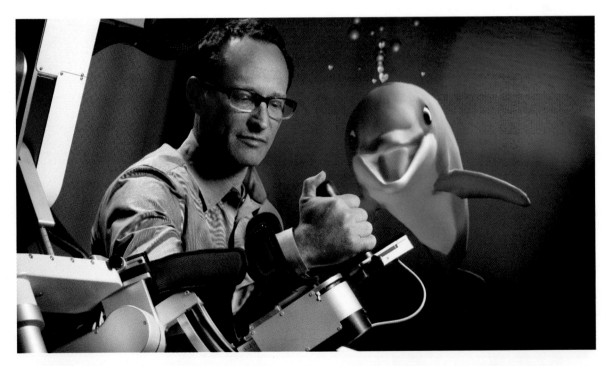

John Krakauer's Brain, Learning, Animation and Movement (BLAM) Lab includes not only physician-scientists, but experts in robotics, computer programming, animators, physicists and others working to develop innovative ways – such as an interactive video game involving an animated dolphin – to help patients recover movement after stroke.

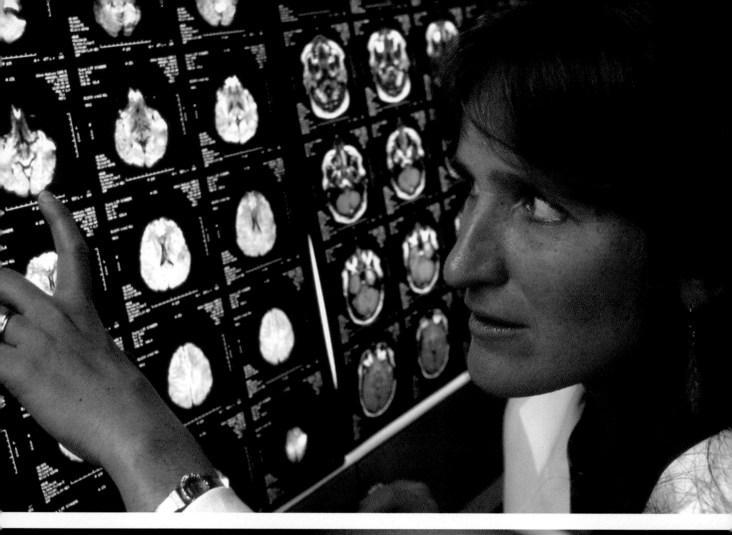
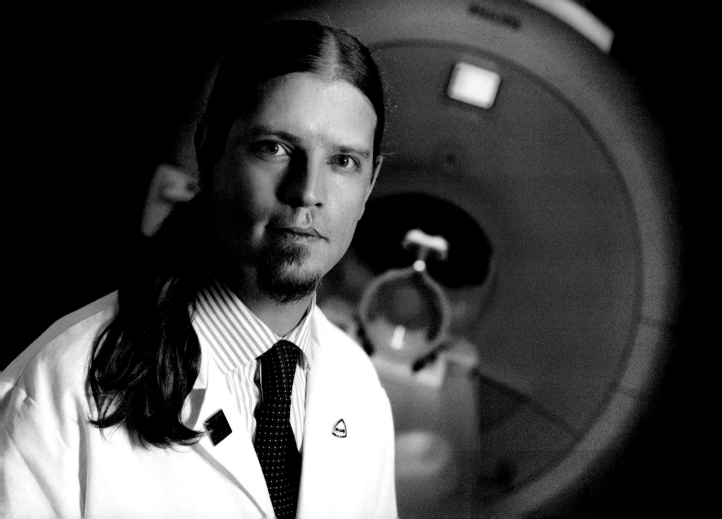

CHAPTER TWELVE

NEUROIMAGING: VIEWING THE FUTURE

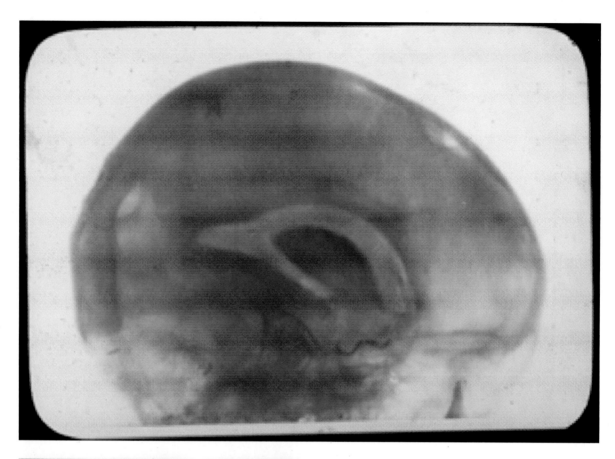

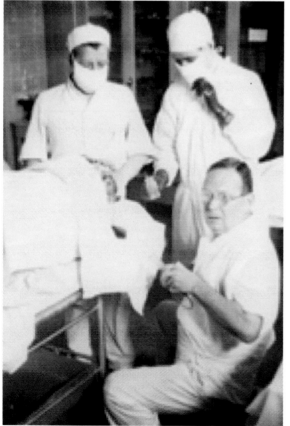

THE FIELD OF NEURORADIOLOGY WAS BEGUN BY HOPKINS NEUROSURGEON WALTER DANDY. At left, in this photo from 1946, Dandy (seated) is shown performing ventriculography at Johns Hopkins Hospital. Above, in this air ventriculogram taken from Dandy's lantern slide collection, the lateral ventricle is well seen. *(Photos were rediscovered by David Solomon and Ari Blitz in the Alan Mason Chesney Medical Archives, while they were investigating Dandy's role in the early evaluation of hydrocephalus with Daniele Rigamonti). Reproduced with permission.*

Previous Spread: Argye Hillis (top) and her colleagues used MRI studies to define the neural networks underyling normal language, attention, and even empathy. Richard Leigh (bottom), working with Peter Barker, identified a way to measure blood-brain barrier disruption in acute stroke patients, and thereby estimate the risk of hemorrhagic complications.

EARLY DAYS

Johns Hopkins Hospital was an early adopter of medical imaging. According to the minutes of the Medical Board from April 7, 1896, less than a year after Wilhelm Roentgen's discovery of the X-ray, it was William Osler who proposed the purchase of an X-ray machine.

Before the Department of Radiology began in 1946, imaging at Hopkins was performed by surgeons. Although it is not recorded when the first images of the head were taken, it was Harvey Cushing, future neurosurgeon, who made the first X-ray examination in 1897 as a Hopkins surgical resident: early evaluation of the intracranial contents was extremely limited, with mass effect and midline shift sometimes evident through asymmetric position of the pineal calcification. A few years later, another Hopkins neurosurgeon, Walter Dandy, performed the first studies to evaluate the intracranial contents in living patients – replacing cerebrospinal fluid (CSF) with air, thereby providing contrast between the brain and surrounding structures (also discussed briefly in Chapter One). Dandy first injected air directly into the ventricular system (ventriculography) in 1916, and then via the lumbar subarachnoid space (a technique later known as pneumoencephalography). Dandy's article, published in 1918 in the *Annals of Surgery*, has been described as having "signified the birth of neuroradiology." Both of Dandy's inventions preceded the invention of cerebral angiography by Egas Moniz in Lisbon in 1927. Together, pneumoencephalography and angiography became the standard neuroradiologic means of evaluation of the intracranial contents throughout much of the early to mid-twentieth century.

The early years of Johns Hopkins Neurology preceded the advent of modern cross-sectional medical imaging. Neurology residents routinely injected dye into the carotid arteries of patients undergoing cerebral angiograms and even, when the need arose, carried out pneumoencephalograms themselves – as neurology resident David Zee and medical student Neil Miller successfully did at Baltimore City Hospital. One area in which imaging excelled in those early days was in radionuclide cisternograms, done to establish the diagnosis of normal pressure hydrocephalus. This was due to the pioneering efforts of Johns Hopkins' Henry Wagner, M.D., whose work expanded upon that of Giovanni de Chiro at the National Institutes of Health. Wagner is widely considered to have been one of the founders of nuclear medicine.

In 1973, Guy McKhann attended a meeting of the American Neurological Association, at which a lecture announced the arrival of computed tomography (CT) of the brain. It was immediately clear to Guy that "this was the future," he says, and he was determined to bring it to Hopkins as soon as possible. But when he returned to Baltimore, Guy encountered lack of interest from Neuroradiology to obtain a CT scanner at Hopkins. Undaunted, he appealed to Robert M. Heyssel, Director of the Hospital, and Martin Donner, head of Radiology, explaining the potential of CT scanning, and persuaded them to purchase a machine for $380,000 from the British Company EMI, which was keen to sell its product in the States. The first CT scanner was installed in the basement of the Blalock building, while an "enlarged bathroom" on the sixth floor served as an access point for results. For the next two years, CT scans could only be obtained by first requesting a neurology consultation, and neurologists interpreted the scans. In about 1976, a national debate erupted concerning who had the right to read CT scans. Although Martin Donner was sympathetic to the practice of neurologists reading the scans, he felt obliged to conform with the national norms, and the control of CT scanning and reading shifted to neuroradiologists.

The first major studies using this scanner were of children with epilepsy by resident David Bachman, neuroradiologist Fred ("Ted") Hodges, and John Freeman. Structural abnormalities were detected in 30 percent of the 98 children scanned – an important insight, pointing to the future role of neuroimaging in epilepsy.

In 1975, feeling pressure about the potential costs of CT scanners, Lee Bahr and Ted Hodges in neuroradiology published a paper of the Hopkins experience, justifying the cost-benefit of the procedure. Thus, thanks to the foresight of Guy McKhann, from the outset neuroimaging has been a core interest of Johns Hopkins Neurology – not just in patient care, but also in many research studies.

Within a decade, CT was joined by MRI and PET scanning. Currently, Hopkins possesses more than a dozen MRI scanners, including a powerful 7T scanner for human subjects and even more powerful magnets for animal experiments. There is a tradition of collaboration between Neurology and Neuroradiology, which has witnessed such important technical milestones as the development of diffusion tensor imaging (DTI) fiber tracking, pioneered by Susumu Mori; amide proton transfer imaging, pioneered by Peter van Zijl, allowing for pH-weighted imaging; and advances in nuclear magnetic resonance (NMR) spectroscopy, pioneered by Peter Barker, allowing for neurotransmitter imaging. These and other imaging techniques have been applied to a range of disease states.

NEUROIMAGING STROKE

Systematically combining MRI and behavioral studies in stroke patients with cognitive deficits, Hillis and her colleagues were able to define the neural networks underlying normal language, attention, and even empathy.

Hopkins Neurology residents and faculty applied MRI to their questions concerning stroke soon after technological advances were made. Using serial perfusion-weighted MRI, Argye Hillis, Peter Barker and colleagues identified regions of hypoperfused cortex in acute stroke patients whose lexical deficits or hemispatial neglect reversed with successful reperfusion. Systematically combining MRI and behavioral studies in stroke patients with cognitive deficits, Hillis and her colleagues were able to define the neural networks underlying normal language, attention, and even empathy. Following up on work by Guy McKhann and colleagues that demonstrated cognitive deficits after coronary artery bypass operations, Hillis, Barker and colleagues demonstrated postoperative diffusion-weighted brain abnormalities in the MRIs of such patients, in whom no neurological defects were evident.

As a stroke fellow at Hopkins, Richard Leigh, working with mentor Peter Barker, identified a way to measure blood-brain barrier (BBB) permeability from standard perfusion-weighted MRI sequences. Applying such blood-brain permeability imaging to acute stroke, they found severe focal BBB disruption to be a risk factor for hemorrhagic complications in the treatment of acute stroke (see photo).

Blood-brain permeability imaging has also demonstrated how mild, diffuse BBB disruption in acute stroke can be reversible following successful reperfusion. It is currently being used to study the pathogenesis of white matter hyperintensities, which are associated with stroke, with disease affecting the cerebral small vessels, and vascular dementia.

Using high spatial resolution imaging (discussed below), Bruce Wasserman developed new methods for characterizing features of carotid atherosclerotic plaque that are indicative of stroke risk. Wasserman, with Robert Wityk, evaluated patients with little-to-no detectable plaque on carotid angiography – introducing a paradigm shift in managing low-grade carotid disease that has become accepted by contemporary standards. After further optimizing these techniques to image intracranial vessel walls, Wasserman teamed up with Steven Zeiler to identify potential biopsy targets in the setting of suspected CNS vasculitis. Together, they established a new protocol for patients suspected of having this disease that is now considered a preferred approach.

As the Sheikh Khalifa Stroke Institute at Hopkins is launched, these new MRI techniques will be employed in the acute stroke setting. They promise many new insights for understanding the pathogenesis of ischemic brain disease.

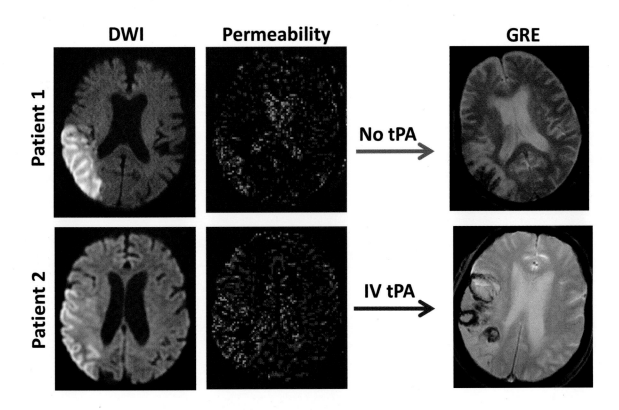

RICHARD LEIGH, WORKING WITH MENTOR PETER BARKER, FOUND SEVERE FOCAL BBB DISRUPTION TO BE A RISK FACTOR FOR HEMORRHAGIC COMPLICATIONS IN THE TREATMENT OF ACUTE STROKE.

Above, two patients presenting with similar strokes both demonstrate focally severe BBB disruption on permeability imaging (red voxels). In patient 1, intravenous tPA was not given, and follow-up imaging shows only minor asymptomatic hemorrhagic changes. In patient 2, administration of intravenous tPA was followed by severe symptomatic intracranial hemorrhage. Note that the permeability scans were not available at the time these two patients were treated; future research is focusing on determining if BBPI (blood brain permeability imaging) can guide treatment decisions in this way. *DWI: diffusion weighted images; GRE: gradient echo images.*

NOVEL METHODS OF BRAIN IMAGING

Conventional MRI is based on signals recorded from the protons of water molecules. Newer methods allow researchers to use MRI to detect protons attached to other molecules. Using this approach, Peter van Zijl and colleagues developed the technique called amide proton transfer weighted (APTw) MRI. This approach was first translated into clinical practice by Jaishri Blakeley, working with Jinyuan Zhou, who used it to measure amide concentration in brain tumors – thereby identifying optimal biopsy sites within heterogeneous malignant brain tumors, and distinguishing recurrent cancer from radiation-induced injury (see Chapter 8).

APTw MRI can also be used to measure the rate of hydrogen ion transfer, allowing for measurement of tissue pH. With Peter van Zijl and Jinyuan Zhou, Richard Leigh translated this approach into clinical use in patients suffering from ischemic stroke. Cerebral ischemia results in accumulation of lactic acid which, in turn, decreases tissue pH. Thus, using pH-weighted MRI (pHWI), the metabolic state of brain tissue at risk of infarction can be assessed. The photo on this page shows an example of pHWI in a patient with a right hemisphere stroke, and compares the relative extent of tissue affected by lactic acidosis (pH Lesion), cell death (Diffusion Lesion) and impaired vascular perfusion (PWI).

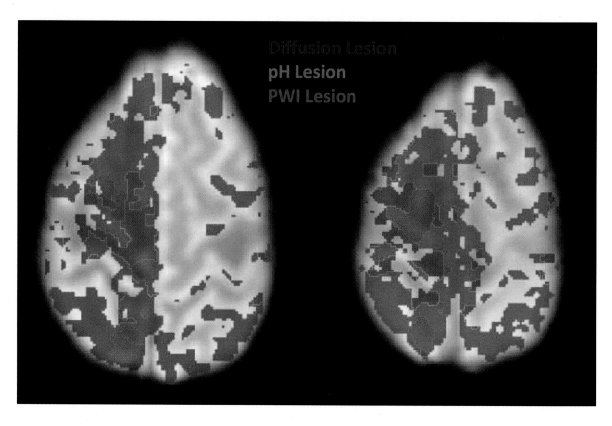

pH-WEIGHTED MRI (PHWI), CAN ASSESS THE METABOLIC STATE OF BRAIN TISSUE AT RISK OF INFARCTION.

Magnetic resonance images of a patient's right hemisphere stroke comparing the extent of cell death (Diffusion Lesion), impaired vascular perfusion (PWI lesion) and lactic acidosis in the penumbra (pH Lesion). *Courtesy of Peter van Zijl, Jinyuan Zhou, Hye-Young Heo, Alan Huang, and Richard Leigh.*

NEUROIMAGING DEMYELINATING DISEASES

A collaboration among Daniel Reich (then a resident in the short-lived combined neurology/radiology/neuroradiology program), Peter Calabresi, Susumu Mori, Peter van Zijl, Seth Smith, Kathleen Zackowski, and their colleagues applied diffusion tensor imaging (DTI) to map lesions in various functional systems of patients with multiple sclerosis (MS). They then built a natural history cohort to study the relationship between functional system MRI findings and clinical outcomes in MS. This work was done on research scanners at the F. M. Kirby Research Center for Functional Brain Imaging at the Kennedy-Krieger Institute. Example results are shown in the photo on this page. That project, still ongoing after 15 years, has spurred several dozen papers. The cohort has been invaluable in the training of many clinical and research fellows.

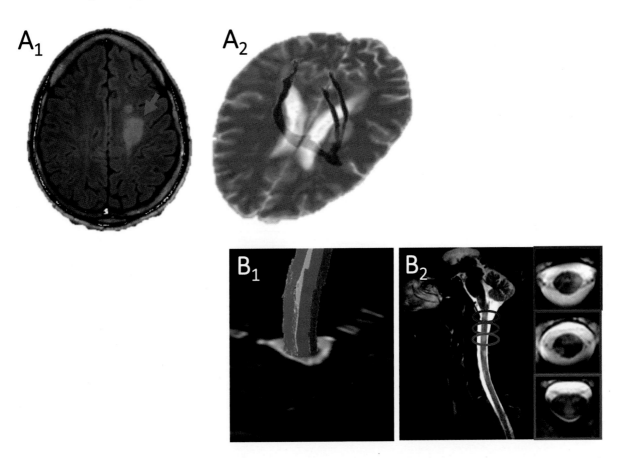

QUANTITATIVE MRI CAN BE USED TO ASSESS THE INTEGRITY OF FUNCTIONAL SYSTEMS IN MS.
Top left: A 33-year-old man presented with right hemiparesis, due to an acute inflammatory demyelinating lesion (yellow arrow) affecting the left corticospinal tract (T2-FLAIR MRI). Top right: Diffusion tensor imaging (DTI) allows reconstruction of the course of the corticospinal tracts (red), and shows that the left corticospinal tract is affected as it passes through the lesion. Bottom left: In the spinal cord, DTI can be used to reconstruct the locations of the major white-matter columns, including the lateral columns (yellow and red), dorsal columns (green), and anterior columns (cyan). Bottom right: Spinal cord fiber tracking can be especially informative when combined with high-resolution T2*-weighted gradient-echo MRI with magnetization transfer preparation, which allows outstanding delineation of focal spinal cord lesions in a 31-year-old with relapsing-remitting MS. The Hopkins/KennedyKrieger Institute-developed T2*-weighted gradient-echo imaging sequence, without or with magnetization-transfer preparation, leading to visualization of approximately three times as many spinal cord MS lesions (including new lesions) as conventional approaches.

High Spatial Resolution Imaging

With increasing MRI field strength and application of 3-D imaging techniques, a greater degree of anatomic precision has become possible: we can now see clinically relevant details that used to be beyond the reach of imaging. Ari Blitz, working with Nafi Aygun and colleagues, brought high-resolution 3-D MR imaging into routine clinical practice by devising a protocol and means of interpretation for evaluating the skull base and cranial nerves. Previously, evaluation of the cranial nerves was principally limited to the brainstem and cisterns. This work allows for visualization of the cranial nerves along nearly the entirety of their course – allowing for unprecedented detection of cranial nerve abnormalities (see photo on this page). This approach has allowed for greater precision in the diagnosis of patients with cranial nerve deficits, as well as improved surgical planning, in concert with Gary Gallia, with fewer post-operative deficits.

Blitz, working with David Solomon, Abhay Moghekar and Daniele Rigamonti, also developed a standardized clinical imaging approach, including high-resolution imaging, to evaluate patients with suspected normal pressure hydrocephalus, with focus on the detailed evaluation of the ventricular system and subarachnoid space. This has been adopted at multiple other institutions nationally and worldwide, and echoes Walter Dandy's original approach.

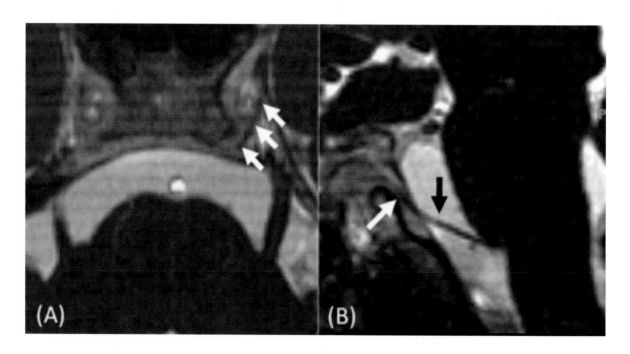

WITH INCREASING MRI FIELD STRENGTH AND APPLICATION OF 3-D IMAGING TECHNIQUES, A GREATER DEGREE OF ANATOMIC PRECISION HAS BECOME POSSIBLE. WE CAN NOW SEE CLINICALLY RELEVANT DETAILS THAT USED TO BE BEYOND THE REACH OF IMAGING.

Several-day history of abducens palsy on the right. Standard protocol MR imaging was unremarkable. Post-contrast isotropic constructive interference in steady state (CISS) images. (A) Axial image. The left interdural abducens nerve CN VI (arrows) is well visualized, extending through Dorello canal into the cavernous sinus. The right abducens nerve is not visualized in the cavernous region because of pathologic enhancement. (B) In sagittal oblique reformatted views, cisternal CN VI (black arrow) and the proximal interdural CN VI segment are seen, with an abrupt transition to the region of pathologic enhancement (white arrow). Tolosa-Hunt syndrome was suggested. (Reproduced with permission from Blitz AM et al., *Neuroimaging Clinics*. 2014; 24: 17-34.).

The full potential of MRI and CT has yet to be realized. It may be that these techniques are still in their infancy.

Since those early attempts to image the nervous system by Cushing and Dandy, our abilities to visualize its structure and function have grown enormously. However, the full potential of MRI and CT has yet to be realized. It may be that these techniques are still in their infancy: witness the recent development of ways to measure brain pH and permeability of the blood-brain barrier on MRI. As in other fields, progress in neuroimaging at Hopkins has been facilitated by collaborations among investigators with diverse talents and knowledge, and by the warm collegiality of the Hopkins community.

SELECTED REFERENCES

Blitz AM, Ahmed AK, Rigamonti D. Founder of modern hydrocephalus diagnosis and therapy: Walter Dandy at the Johns Hopkins Hospital. *J Neurosurg* 2018 Oct 19;1:1-6.

Blitz AM, Macedo LL, Chonka ZD, Ilica AT, Choudhri AF, Gallia GL, Aygun N. High-resolution CISS MR imaging with and without contrast for evaluation of the upper cranial nerves: segmental anatomy and selected pathologic conditions of the cisternal through extraforaminal segments. *Neuroimaging Clinics.* 2014 Feb 1;24(1):17-34.

Dandy WE. Ventriculography following the injection of air into the cerebral ventricles. *Ann Surgery.* 1918; 68: 5.

Di Chiro G. Observations on the circulation of the cerebrospinal fluid. *Acta Radiologica. Diagnosis.* 1966; 5(P2): 988-1002.

James AE, DeLand FH, Hodges FJ, Wagner HN. Normal-pressure hydrocephalus: role of cisternography in diagnosis. *JAMA* 1970; 213: 1615-22.

Leigh R, Jen SS, Hillis AE, Krakauer JW, Barker PB. Pretreatment blood-brain barrier damage and post-treatment intracranial hemorrhage in patients receiving intravenous tissue-type plasminogen activator. *Stroke.* 2014; 45:2030-5.

Leigh R, Knutsson L, Zhou J, van Zijl PC. Imaging the physiological evolution of the ischemic penumbra in acute ischemic stroke. *J Cerebral Blood Flow & Metabolism.* 2018; 38: 1500-1516.

Lindgren, Erik. "A History of Neuroradiology" in Newton T, Potts DG, editors. *Radiology of the Skull and Brain.* Mosby; 1971.

Rekate HL, Blitz AM. Hydrocephalus in children. In *Handbook of clinical neurology* 2016 Jan 1 (Vol. 136, pp. 1261-1273). Elsevier.

Reich DS, Smith SA, Zackowski KM, Gordon-Lipkin EM, Jones CK, Farrell JA, Mori S, van Zijl PC, Calabresi PA. Multiparametric magnetic resonance imaging analysis of the corticospinal tract in multiple sclerosis. *Neuroimage* 2007; 38: 271-9.

Wasserman BA, Wityk RJ, Trout III HH, Virmani R. Low-grade carotid stenosis: looking beyond the lumen with MRI. *Stroke.* 2005; 36: 2504-13.

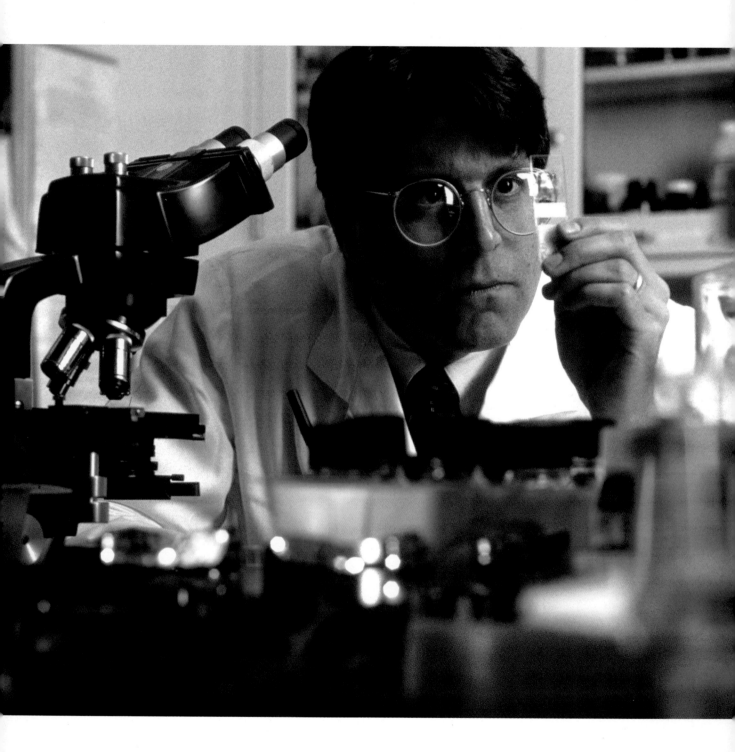

CHAPTER THIRTEEN

AMYOTROPHIC LATERAL SCLEROSIS (ALS)

Previous spread:
Jeffrey Rothstein designed
and is leading "Answer
ALS," a large, multi-center
study to collect biofluid,
tissue, and iPS cells, as
well as clinical information.
Its mission is to define
biological subgroups and
pathways in sporadic and
familial ALS.

Motor neuron disease has been a subject of keen interest and study in the Department of Neurology since the 1980s. Research in ALS has followed two somewhat parallel tracks involving both clinical and basic science.

CLINICAL RESEARCH: RECOGNIZING THE INFLAMMATORY COMPONENT

Early clinical studies in ALS evaluated the role of possible immunological abnormalities in this neurodegenerative disease. "Even back then," says Dan Drachman, "it was widely recognized that there was an inflammatory component to the pathology of ALS in both spinal cord and cortex." For example, animal models that resembled ALS could be produced by repeated inoculation with isolated motor neurons; further, our experience in autoimmune-based therapies in neuromuscular diseases allowed us to test the role of autoimmunity in ALS. However, "early clinical trials in ALS were often poorly designed," lacking matched-placebo groups, adequate methods of dosing, and evidence of efficacy of the immunosuppressive treatments. In the mid-1990s, Drachman and colleagues carried out a well-designed clinical trial of the immune-suppressing therapy, total lymphoid irradiation, that was far ahead of its time. "Although this was a period when many ALS trials were focused only on survival," comments Drachman, "our trial included appropriate immune markers to prove the efficacy of immunosuppression. We had multiple outcome measures, including muscle strength using dynamometry, decades ahead of its popularization." Most trials today, 25 years later, have caught up – routinely including such functional outcomes. The result showed that effective immune suppression did not change the course of the disease, essentially ruling out a primary role for autoimmune pathogenesis of ALS.

During the early to mid-1990s multicenter clinical trials of peripherally administered neurotrophic factors were carried out, with factors such as CNTF (Ciliary Neurotrophic Factor) and IGF-I (Insulin-like growth factor 1). Neuromuscular Division faculty served as local PIs in some of these trials, which were unfortunately negative.

After years of discouraging results, the first positive trial of ALS drug therapy came in the 1990s, with the international pharmaceutical trial of Riluzole, by Rhone Poulenc Rorer. Johns Hopkins was one of five sites in the U.S. to test this drug; in fact, the use of Riluzole in ALS was based in part on research by Neuromuscular faculty member Jeffrey Rothstein, Director of the Robert Packard Center for ALS Research (see below), who served as the local PI for this trial. In 1995, Riluzole became the first FDA-approved drug for ALS. "We waited another 25 years before a second drug, Radicava, was approved by the FDA for ALS treatment," says Rothstein.

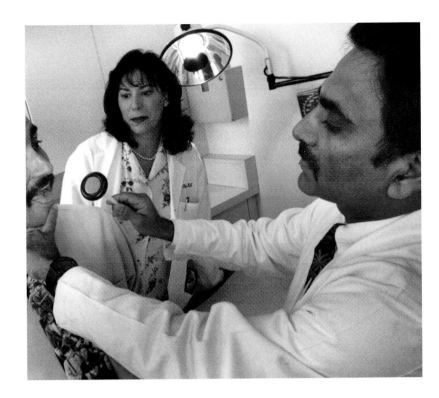

Vinay Chaudhry, right, and Lora Clawson have extensive experience with ALS clinical trials, reflecting the great growth of clinical and basic ALS research.

But momentum in this disease was beginning to build. Because of *in vitro* and animal models used to study ALS pathophysiology, numerous candidate drugs came to clinical trial between 1995 and 2005. "We saw a huge growth in the number of clinical trials based on apparent benefit in animal models," Rothstein adds, with the Neuromuscular Division playing an important leadership role in many of them. Rothstein was the local PI for trials of Topiramate, the Sanofi Aventis compound; Celebrex, with Dan Drachman as co-PI; the Lilly AMPA glutamate receptor antagonist; and Novartis TCH 346. Of all those trials, only the Lilly compound, LY300164, showed borderline positive phase 2 efficacy. Disappointingly, it later failed to show efficacy in an international phase 3 trial run by Teva. Celebrex (celecoxib) was another disappointment – particularly, notes Drachman, because it had seemed so promising in preclinical studies. "It worked spectacularly in the mouse SOD1 ALS model, delaying the symptoms of ALS more than any other drug that has been tried," he says. "I did a 300-patient trial in humans with ALS, but it did not do any good, possibly because we were obliged to limit the dose. We measured the possible metabolic effect of Celebrex by assaying prostaglandins in the spinal fluid. They should have been elevated in ALS, and should have gone down as a result of Celebrex treatment – but neither was the case, so we never knew whether more Celebrex would have worked in people with ALS as it did in the mice."

Since 2005, there has been an enormous growth in ALS clinical trials at Hopkins, with participation by multiple Neuromuscular faculty including Rothstein, Nicholas Maragakis, M.D., Director of the ALS Center for Cell Therapy and Regeneration Research and co-Medical Director of the ALS Clinic; Andrea Corse, M.D.; Vinay Chaudhry, M.B.B.S., M.D.; and Brett Morrison, M.D., Ph.D. Importantly the increase in Neuromuscular faculty participating in these clinical trials reflects the great growth of clinical and basic ALS research. The trials are managed by Lora Clawson, R.N., who has extensive experience with both ALS and clinical trials, and is Director of ALS Clinical Care at Hopkins. A partial list of agents used in those trials includes: Talampanel (Teva); SB109 (Sangamo); SOD1 antisense (Biogen and Ionis, still ongoing); C9orf72 antisense (Biogen, still ongoing); Anti-nogo antibody (GSK); and Tirasemtiv (Cytokinetics). We also are participating in a multicenter muscle exercise trial.

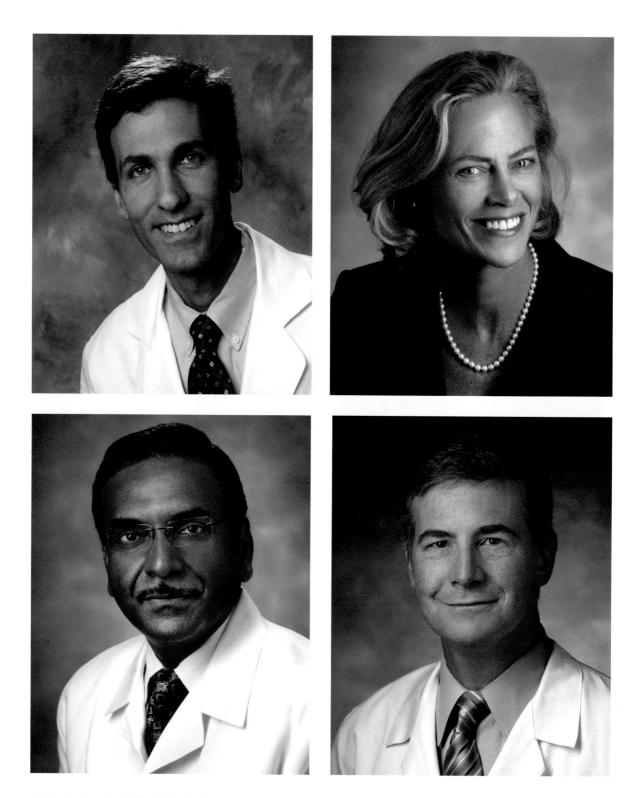

(clockwise from top left): Nicholas Maragakis, Andrea Corse, Brett Morrison and Vinay Chaudhry, clinician-scientists who are driving the Neuromuscular Division's progress in understanding ALS, with the hope for finding better treatment, prolonging life and improving quality of life.

Does ALS Differ from Person to Person?

The largest clinical research study in ALS history recently began at Johns Hopkins.

This multicenter study, called "Answer ALS," designed and led by Jeff Rothstein, is a longitudinal program designed to collect biofluid, tissue, and iPS cells, as well as clinical information. Its long-term mission is to define biological subgroups and pathways in sporadic and familial ALS. The program is enrolling 1,000 ALS patients (sporadic and familial) and 100 control patients at eight centers in the U.S. Patients are followed for at least one year and undergo repeated clinical examinations, including motor and cognitive evaluation (using ALSFRS and cognitive scales). Biological specimens of serum and CSF are collected and stored at all visits. The trial is also using smart-phone technology: each patient gets an iOS/Android app, by which data on motor activity, respiration, speech and cognition are collected every week, in partnership with IBM Watson for data analytics. Each patient and control will have whole-genome sequencing done, in collaboration with the New York Genome Center. Additionally, peripheral blood mononuclear cells (PBMCs), collected at the initial visits, are converted to iPS cell lines that are then differentiated into iPS spinal motor neurons; CNS tissue samples will be collected at autopsy. The investigators will carry out genetic and metabolic profiling on iPS-derived motor neurons; this includes RNA transcriptome, epigenomic/ATAC sequencing, proteome and metabolome analytics. "Our hope," says Rothstein, "is to be able to use precision medicine in ALS, to determine specific subgroups of patients who may respond to treatment differently, and to gain insight into new, more patient-specific ways to treat this disease."

Basic ALS Research

Early motor neuron disease research in the Department of Neurology began with work by Jack Griffin, Donald Price, and neuroscientist Don Cleveland (now at the University of California-San Diego). Early studies by Griffin investigated the response of motor neurons and their axons to injury. Then, in collaboration with Cleveland, Griffin developed and analyzed some of the first models related to intermediate filament proteins, which ultimately led to the development of surrogate transgenic motor neuron disease models in mice. "These early investigations provided insight into the responses of motor neurons to injury," says Rothstein, "and the potential link between neurofilament pathology seen in ALS and experimental animal models. Interestingly, now 30 years later, neurofilament proteins are serving as surrogate markers of *in vivo* neuronal injury in patients," and also help predict a patient's response to therapy.

Excitotoxicity and ALS

How does ALS begin? Insight into the pathogenesis of ALS in humans began at Hopkins in the late 1980s, as Jeff Rothstein and colleagues investigated the possible role of excitotoxicity in motor neuron degeneration. In 1989, Rothstein's lab first identified abnormal increases of the CSF excitatory amino acids, glutamate and aspartate, in ALS patients who had developed the disease sporadically, and this observation was validated in a cohort of hundreds of French ALS patients a decade later. Rothstein and colleagues found the underlying cause of aberrant glutamate to be a loss of functional astroglial glutamate transport; they first detailed the substantial role of astroglia in the pathogenesis of ALS in 1994. To understand the mechanism of glutamate transport defects and to screen for candidate drugs, Rothstein's lab developed an organotypic spinal cord culture system. Their high-throughput screen demonstrated that ceftriaxone and related beta lactam antibiotics could mitigate astroglial dysfunction. This finding resulted in a large clinical trial that was positive in its phase 2 component, but failed in phase 3. Several other drugs later went on to clinical trials through this system, including riluzole, topiramate, gabapentin, Celebrex, and LY300164 (AMPA antagonist).

ABERRANT RNA METABOLISM AND ALS

In the late 1990s, in attempting to define the underlying pathogenic cascade that leads to defective astroglial glutamate transport, the Rothstein lab identified pathways of aberrant RNA metabolism, including abnormal intron retention and exon-skipping in a subset of ALS patients. They first defined abnormal RNA metabolism in astroglia as a pathogenic event in sporadic ALS. In some ALS patients, the defect in a specific glutamate transporter, EAAT2, appeared to be the cause of astroglial dysfunction.

A decade later, a critical abnormality was found to result from a mutation in the C9orf72 gene (see below). The Hopkins team was part of a large consortium led by neurologist Bryan Traynor, M.D., Ph.D., a senior investigator and Chief of the Neuromuscular Diseases Research Section at the NIH (National Institute on Aging Laboratory of Neurogenetics), and an adjunct faculty member in the Hopkins Department of Neurology. In 2011, Traynor discovered that a mutation in C9orf72 (an increase of the two nucleotide repeats: G-G-G-G-C-C in a non-coding region of a gene in chromosome 9) was the cause of a common familial form of ALS (originally discovered in familial ALS in Finland); this mutation is also found in sporadic ALS. The ALS and basic science community aggressively sought to understand the pathophysiology of this gene defect – responsible not only for ALS, but also present in fronto-temporal dementia.

Fortunately, the Rothstein lab had already induced pluripotent cells from these patients, and two years later used these artificial spinal cord cells to discover a candidate antisense oligonucleotide therapy that can target the pathogenic mutation and mitigate the injury that this novel human cell system revealed. In 2015, the Rothstein lab, using the iPS cell platform, and the lab of Thomas Lloyd, M.D., Ph.D., using the C9 drosophila model, collaboratively were able to show that the core pathophysiology injury from the C9 mutation was the disruption of nuclear transport and the nuclear pore complex. Tom Lloyd's lab, using the C9orf72 fly model, discovered that a class of drugs that altered nuclear export could mitigate the nuclear transport defects and protect against overall neuronal injury. Those data, along with others, led to plans by Biogen to initiate a new ALS clinical trial with the nuclear transport-modulating drugs. The Rothstein lab, collaborating with other departments at Johns Hopkins, went on to discover that nuclear transport and the nuclear pore complex were implicated in other neurodegenerative diseases, including Huntington's and Alzheimer's.

MODEL SYSTEMS, GLIAL BIOLOGY AND STEM CELLS

In further exploration of the defect in ALS glia, Hopkins researchers defined astroglial pathways that may be contributing to or causing neurotoxicity in ALS. Starting first with astroglial glutamate transporters, the Rothstein lab systematically investigated the basic biology of all glutamate transporters in the CNS. In studies using both rodent and human models, they discovered that EAAT2 was an astroglial-specific transporter – and that loss of this essential function and protein was characteristic of ALS and could be a substantial contributor to neuron degeneration.

To develop better model systems beyond transgenic mouse models, Rothstein and Maragakis spearheaded a national effort to build large banks of the first ALS iPS cell lines from familial and sporadic ALS patients, and to make this unique human cell library available for scientists worldwide. As the role for astroglia in ALS became a central interest in the field, the Maragakis lab began work on astroglial stem cells and progenitors, and showed that ALS astrocytes themselves could induce focal neurodegeneration in the spinal cord – strongly suggesting that astrocytes could play an important role in ALS pathogenesis. This group later showed that another defect in astrocytes – not just loss of EAAT2, but the interconnectivity of astrocytes, through a GAP junction-based syncytium – could also be a contributing factor in the development of ALS.

HOPKINS COORDINATED/SPONSORED ALS RESEARCH WORLDWIDE: ROBERT PACKARD CENTER FOR ALS RESEARCH

The Robert Packard Center has raised more than $100 million, distributed to more than 100 scientists worldwide and engaging more than 1,000 postdoctoral fellows, graduate students and staff in its mission.

In 2000, Jeff Rothstein founded the Robert Packard Center for ALS research. This unique philanthropic endeavor funds ALS preclinical research, with the goal of finding effective drugs for ALS and new ways to mitigate the progression of this devastating disease. This collaborative Center funds research by basic and clinical investigators at Hopkins and elsewhere with the goal of elucidating pathogenic pathways involved in ALS, to develop preclinical models and to use them for therapeutics and biomarker discovery. Investigators are required to attend monthly meetings at Hopkins, and to collaborate. This remarkable Center has raised more than $100 million, distributed to more than 100 scientists worldwide and engaging more than 1,000 postdoctoral fellows, graduate students and staff in this mission. The Packard Center has funded the work of many neurologists in the Neuromuscular Division, including Dan Drachman, Jeff Rothstein, Tom Lloyd, Charlotte Sumner, Nick Maragakis, Brett Morrison, Lyle Ostrow, Lindsey Hayes, Ahmet Hoke and Jack Griffin. This organization of committed researchers has been responsible for identifying the majority of disease-causing pathways, and has developed many of the preclinical models – including transgenic mice, flies, fish and human iPS cell lines – used by researchers worldwide. Many drugs that have been tested in ALS clinical trials have resulted from Packard Center-funded research.

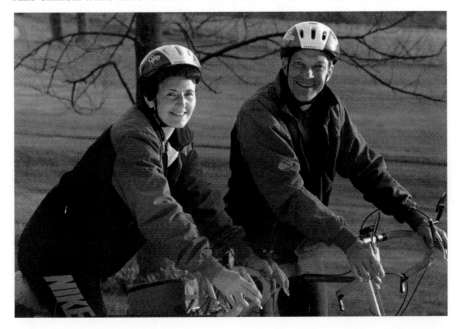

Nearly two decades before the Robert Packard Center began raising millions in desperately needed funding for ALS research, Dan and Jephta Drachman biked from Baltimore to the Pacific Ocean, raising awareness and also $40,000, one mile at a time.

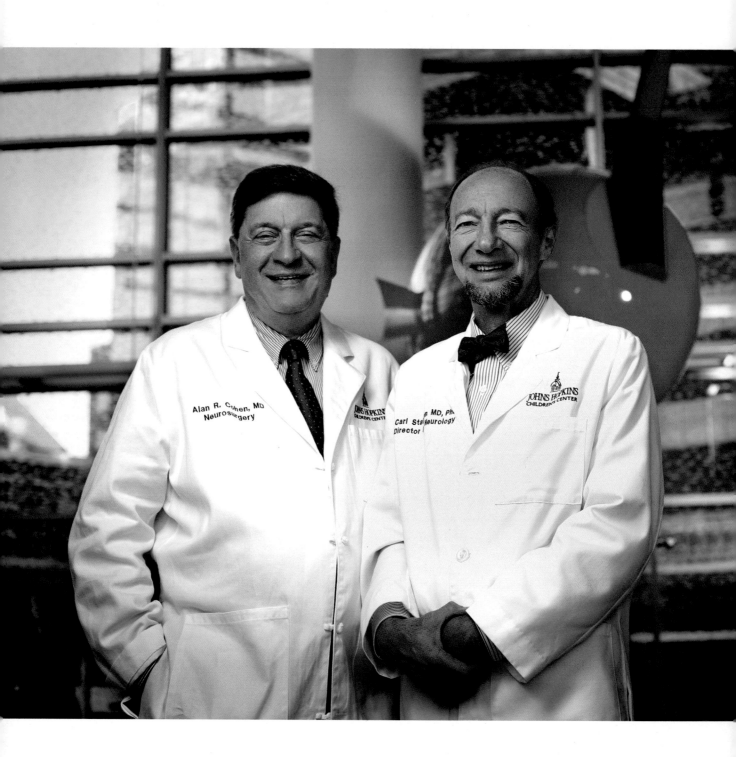

CHAPTER FOURTEEN

CHILD NEUROLOGY

Previous spread:
Alan Cohen, Director
of Pediatric Neurosurgery
and Carl Stafstrom,
Chief of the Division
of Child Neurology

The faculty of Johns Hopkins has always shown a strong interest in the neurological disorders of childhood – beginning with William Osler, who wrote a monograph, The Cerebral Palsy of Children.

Frank Ford (see Chapter 1), outstanding diagnostician and Chief of the Division of Neurology between 1932 and 1952, won international fame for his 1937 book, *Diseases of the Nervous System in Infancy, Childhood and Adolescence.* Ford built a team of neurologists with expertise in childhood disorders. These included David Clark, who established a birth defects center, and John Menkes, who went on to champion the newly emerging field of errors of inborn metabolism. After Ford retired, Clark and Menkes each moved on to lead other institutions, causing a hiatus in the momentum of academic child neurology at Hopkins, with Frank Schuster as acting chair. This hiatus ended for good in 1969, when Guy McKhann, a pediatric neurologist, was chosen to lead the new Department of Neurology.

MODERN CHILD NEUROLOGY COMES TO HOPKINS

Guy McKhann was exceptionally qualified for his new job. The son of two academic pediatricians, he was mentored at Yale Medical School by Pediatrics Chair Robert Cooke, from whom he learned research skills. After Cooke moved to become Pediatrician-in-Chief at Hopkins, he recruited McKhann as a resident. Guy then trained in child neurology at Harvard with one of the founders of the field, Philip Dodge. The next three years of Guy's training turned him into a clinician-scientist: they were spent at the NIH, where he developed expertise in neurochemistry with Don Tower, and learned concepts of neurobiology from Milton Shy. He left Bethesda to become Director of Pediatric Neurology at Stanford University. He served in this job for seven years; during this time, he also practiced adult neurology, and was part of Stanford's strong program in neurobiology, which included Joshua Lederberg and Eric Shooter. At Stanford, Guy attracted a group of bright residents who wanted to become academic neurologists. Thus, Guy was a clinician-scientist who could care for both children and adults, and who had proven administrative capabilities. When he returned to Hopkins as the new Chair of Neurology, he brought several of his residents with him, including Alan Percy, Bill Logan, and Gary Goldstein (and eventually, medical students Larry Davis, Jack and Diane Griffin). He also brought two colleagues, Robert Herndon and pediatric neurologist John Freeman, a graduate of the Johns Hopkins School of Medicine, who was to become the first Director of the Division of Child Neurology.

THE DIVISION OF CHILD NEUROLOGY:
THE JOHN FREEMAN YEARS

John Freeman made major contributions that revolutionized the approach to childhood seizures.

During medical school, John Freeman's interest had been greatly influenced by David Clark, who became a mentor and was pivotal in his choice of child neurology as a specialty. When he finished his pediatric residency at Hopkins, Freeman went on to train with Sidney Carter, head of child neurology at Columbia-Presbyterian Hospital in New York. After two years of military service at Walter Reed Hospital, Freeman was recruited to Stanford University by McKhann, whom he had known during his time at Hopkins. When Freeman moved back to Baltimore, in 1969, he was well aware of the challenges needed in setting up a new Division of Child Neurology at Hopkins. As described in Chapter 2, many of the concerns about clinical facilities and space were ably negotiated by Guy McKhann, but little of the Frank Ford legacy remained. There were only three child neurology faculty: Samuel Livingston (champion of the ketogenic diet – see side story), Lydia Pauli, who ran the epilepsy clinic, and Frank Schuster, who had served as an acting director.

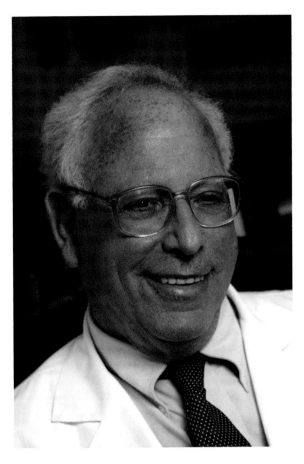

John Freeman founded the Pediatric Epilepsy Center, which now bears his name.

But any potential stumbling blocks were more than offset by McKhann's optimism and hard work, and were hammered out at his "kitchen table conferences" (see Chapter 2). The residency training program got off to a good start, immediately reflecting the strong influence of child neurology on the new Department. Of the first group of residents, four went on to become professors of pediatric neurology: Alan Percy, Mark Molliver, Ruthmary Deuel, and Gary Goldstein. They were soon followed by Gihan Tennekoon and Harvey Singer. All of them joined the faculty and went on to achieve distinguished careers in child neurology. Early on, Guy and others decided to combine pediatric neurology and pediatric neurosurgery patients into one service. Although the neurology residents spent a good deal of time doing routine ward work on neurosurgical patients, the result was that the patients received superb care, and the residents learned about neurosurgical issues.

The Division of Child Neurology also benefited greatly from its close, long-term partnership with the Kennedy Institute (now the Kennedy-Krieger Institute). Hugo Moser, a pioneering neurochemist, was recruited to head

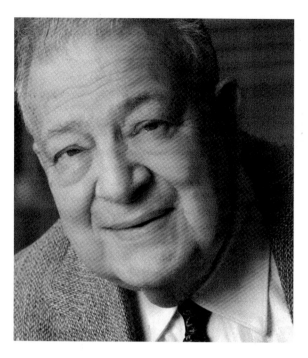

Hugo Moser, a pioneering neurochemist, was recruited to head the Kennedy (now Kennedy-Krieger) Institute, and made major contributions in understanding hereditary brain disorders.

the Kennedy Institute; his main research interest was in hereditary brain disorders, especially adrenoleukodystrophy. In 1988, an alumnus of the Hopkins Child Neurology program, Gary Goldstein, returned to become Director of the Kennedy-Krieger Institute, a post he held until 2018. Goldstein has made important contributions to understanding abnormalities of the blood-brain barrier. Goldstein, in turn, recruited Hopkins alumnus Michael V. Johnston to serve as Chief Medical Officer and Executive Vice President of the Institute. Johnston is a clinician-scientist with research interests in neuropharmacology, neuroprotection, and the developing brain. Later, Tom Crawford, who had developed an interest in muscular dystrophies under the influence of Daniel Drachman, would go on to make impressive contributions to the management of the spinal muscular atrophies (see Chapter 10).

One of John Freeman's initiatives was to develop a multidisciplinary birth defects clinic. Its staff included neurologists, neurosurgeons, orthopedists, urologists, and therapists, and the success of this program is reflected by the first published book on this approach. A seminal observation made by John Freeman – that children with meningomyelocele initially appeared to move normally *in utero*, but less so as pregnancy progressed – led him to postulate that exposure to amniotic fluid throughout the pregnancy damaged the spinal cord. Based on this insight, and on animal experiments to test the hypothesis, *in-utero* surgery has been shown to be helpful in selected cases. John's abiding interest in managing birth defects informed his later contributions to the field of bioethics.

John Freeman also made major contributions that revolutionized the approach to childhood seizures. He founded the Pediatric Epilepsy Center at Hopkins, and re-examined conventional treatment approaches: for example, he questioned the poor prognosis attributed to febrile seizures, leading to a major change in management, in which phenobarbital was no longer indicated. He also helped redefine the role of hemispherectomy in controlling unihemispheric epilepsy, and he promoted the important role of a ketogenic diet, administered by an informed nutritionist, in the treatment of seizures unresponsive to drug therapies. The ketogenic diet initiative (see side story) has led to a sustained program of productive clinical research. In addition, the Pediatric Epilepsy Center educated families of patients with epilepsy as well as professional colleagues. Even after his term as Director ended, John Freeman maintained a leading role in the Pediatric Epilepsy Center, which now bears his name.

THE HARVEY SINGER YEARS

Work led by Harvey Singer has transformed the way Tourette's syndrome is approached.

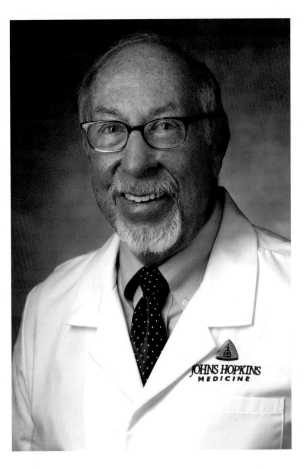

Guy McKhann's abiding influence on the Division of Child Neurology is evident in the choice of John Freeman's successor: Harvey Singer, an alumnus of the Hopkins Child Neurology program, who also embodies the example of the clinician-scientist. Starting during his residency, he took full advantage of the Hopkins research community, writing early papers on seizures in adolescents with John Freeman, on ocular motor apraxia with David Zee, and on embryogenesis of the spinal cord with Don Price. But soon his interest focused on movement disorders in childhood and adolescence – which had been a somewhat neglected topic – and especially on Tourette's syndrome. Working with a number of collaborators, including Ian Butler, Michael Johnston, and Joseph Coyle, he brought modern neuroscience to bear on Tourette's syndrome and the range of tics, vocalizations and abnormal movements that had been frequently described in children but seldom approached in terms of pathogenesis. Work led by Harvey Singer has transformed the way Tourette's syndrome is approached. In collaboration with alumni Andrew Zimmerman and Don Gilbert, and others, and using neuroimaging (both structural and functional), histopathological analyses, and immunological studies, Singer developed a consensus that *noninfectious autoimmune mechanisms* play a significant role in a number of movement disorders. The concept of autoimmune mechanisms has been extended to include a number of neuropsychiatric disorders, including autism. This collaborative research effort has resulted in the writing of a standard text, *Movement Disorders in Childhood*, coauthored by Singer and Don Gilbert.

Harvey Singer brought modern neuroscience to bear on Tourette's syndrome and the range of tics, vocalizations and abnormal movements that had been described in children but seldom approached in terms of pathogenesis.

Under Harvey Singer's directorship, the Child Neurology Residency Program expanded to three fellows per year. Singer also recruited faculty with broad clinical and research expertise. Importantly, he became the Training Director for the Neurological Sciences Academic Development Award (NSADA) beginning in 1993, which has promoted the careers of many young academic child neurologists. The contributions of these clinician-scientists are discussed in several chapters, including those on spinal muscular atrophy, stroke, and neuro-oncology.

The Diet that Changes Lives

ERIC KOSSOFF ON THE JOHNS HOPKINS KETOGENIC DIET CENTER

For decades, the ketogenic diet and Johns Hopkins have been synonymous. But we didn't invent the diet here: Russell Wilder, at the Mayo Clinic, did, back in 1921. However, our Center has helped perfect it, and certainly we have published the most about it (approximately 210 articles referenced from the JHH group on PubMed to date).

THE EARLY YEARS: HOWLAND, LIVINGSTON AND PAULI

Back in the early 1900s, Hopkins pediatrician John Howland started the first lab to evaluate why fasting worked for epilepsy. This subject hit close to home: Howland's brother, Charles, a wealthy New York lawyer, had a son with epilepsy who was cured by fasting. Charles wanted to know exactly why fasting worked, and donated $5,000 to help John learn more. Despite years of research, no explanation was found.

The clinical use of the ketogenic diet at Hopkins goes back to 1946, when Samuel Livingston became Chief of the Hospital's Epilepsy Clinic. Over the course of his long career, he and Lydia Pauli treated more than 33,000 patients with epilepsy and wrote several textbooks. Children were seen not only at the Hospital, but also at a private clinic at 1039 St. Paul Street (now a rowhouse) near Baltimore's Washington Monument. Pediatrician Jim Rubenstein recalls that in the 1970s, he would admit children to the "Livingston" unit of the Children's Center, where often these children would be having frequent seizures or dehydration from prolonged fasting – and Jim as a pediatric resident would have to intervene. Livingston only published a few letters to the editor from his vast experience, but in 1977, he reported in *Developmental Medicine and Child Neurology* that over 41 years of his career, he had treated 975 of 1,600 children with myoclonic epilepsy with the traditional ketogenic diet. He reported seizure-freedom in 54 percent and "marked improvement" in an additional 26 percent. This remains the largest single-center series ever reported. As new anticonvulsants became widely used in the 1970s and 1980s, and research waned, the ketogenic diet became less widely discussed in epilepsy books and at national meetings. Things were about to change dramatically.

JOHN FREEMAN AND MILLIE KELLY

In 1972, when Sam Livingston retired, John Freeman took over the ketogenic diet center, along with Millicent "Millie" Kelly, R.D., a dietitian who had worked with Livingston for many decades. According to John's autobiography, she had retired – but came back to work with him with the request that they "continued to do the diet 6-8 times per year"... and "only for the most difficult epilepsy patients."

In November 1993, John and Millie admitted a 20-month-old boy named Charlie Abrahams, after he had failed multiple medications, corpus callosotomy and treatment by an herbalist in Houston. Within days on the ketogenic diet, his multiple daily seizures stopped completely. Charlie's father, Jim Abrahams, a Hollywood movie producer (*Airplane, Naked Gun, Police Squad*), was upset that the diet was discouraged by their local neurologist – and that he had to "discover" it in the library. He created the Charlie Foundation to help get the word out about the ketogenic diet. A "Dateline NBC" special (1994), a movie starring Meryl Streep about the diet called ... *First Do No Harm* (1997), and then funding the first edition of The Epilepsy Diet Treatment (now in its 6th edition) were Jim's accomplishments during what was clearly the renaissance of the diet. The book's initial 1,500 copies sold out after the Dateline NBC special aired! Charlie, is now 25 years old and teaching elementary school kids in California.

EXPLOSION OF RESEARCH

Research quickly followed, and at a rapid pace. John Freeman created an IRB-approved database to maintain information on our JHH patients starting in late 1994. This remains in existence, with more than 1,000 children continuously enrolled so far. A multicenter study, the first of its kind, of 51 children was published in *Archives of Neurology* in 1998, with Patti Vining as the first author and John Freeman as the second author. At six months, 55 percent of the children had a greater than 50-percent seizure reduction – results that have been replicated many times since. That same year, the "150" study was published in *Pediatrics* by John and the team, reporting prospective results from Johns Hopkins from 1996-1998. To date, it has been cited 550 times in the literature.

Many other studies followed, including work at Hopkins by Steven Kinsman, Peter Kwiterovich, Cheryl Hemingway, Susan Furth, Margaret Pulsifer, Tracy Swink, and Don Gilbert. A randomized, double-blind, crossover study using saccharin in the active treatment arm and glucose in the control arm, funded by the NIH and and published in *Epilepsia* in 2009, remains the only blinded study of the ketogenic diet. Millie Kelly retired again, and was succeeded by Jane McGrogan R.D., working with Jane Casey, L.C.S.W., Heather Cass R.N., and research coordinator Paula Pyzik in the late 1990s.

The "face" of the ketogenic diet center was undoubtedly Diana Pillas, who helped plan admission groups of typically three to four families at a time, and most importantly, provided comfort and support to families and children from referral to diet initiation to follow-up. She unfortunately passed away in 2010, from breast cancer.

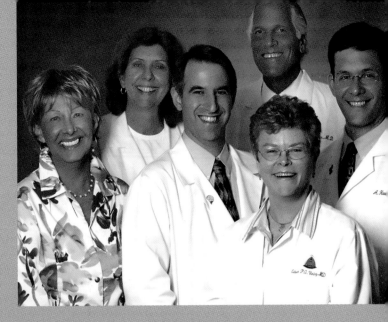

Members of the Ketogenic Diet Team, circa 2007, from left: Diana Pillas, Paula Pyzik, Eric Kossoff, James Rubenstein, Patti Vining, Adam Hartman

EXPANSION, COLLABORATIONS, AND NEW DIRECTIONS

In 2002, I joined the faculty after my Child Neurology Residency and then Pediatric Epilepsy fellowship with John Freeman and Patti Vining. I became interested in the diet after helping John with admissions and seeing occasional remarkable patient responses within days. When John Freeman stepped down as Division Director of Pediatric Epilepsy, Patti asked me to take over the ketogenic diet program formally in 2007. Jim Rubenstein joined as a second epilepsy neurologist to help with admissions and follow-up (he retired June 2017) and was succeeded by nurse practitioners Kathleen Naughton and Sarah Doerrer.

Zahava Turner was hired in 2005, and has remained the primary ketogenic dietitian ever since. She is now Assistant Professor of Neurology and Pediatrics, the only dietitian promoted as such at Johns Hopkins, and an author of 29 publications.

We have partnered since 2014 with Johns Hopkins All Children's Hospital in St. Petersburg, Florida, and they actively contribute to our IRB, research and clinical protocols.

TWO REMARKABLE PATIENTS

Two patients, whose stories have led to important progress in the use of the ketogenic diet, are Casey and Carson. In 2003, Casey was about to start the ketogenic diet for her epilepsy, but her mother wasn't clear on what the foods were. John Freeman suggested "reading about low carb foods in the Atkins book." Her mother took that as permission to start the Atkins diet, which she read about and implemented over a weekend. Casey's seizures stopped within two days. Casey's ketone test was very high on Monday morning. Casey remained on the diet for about three years and is now 21 years old. This "modified Atkins diet" ("MAD") has changed the paradigm for treating adolescents and adults with more "mild" epilepsies (such as absence and juvenile myoclonic epilepsy), using diets for conditions other than epilepsy (with appeal as a more feasible, less restrictive diet) and with now over 600 patients published, it appears to be essentially equivalent to the ketogenic diet.

In 2007, Carson, a six-month-old infant, was brought to the JHH emergency department with new-onset infantile spasms. This extremely severe and potentially devastating form of epilepsy responds well to the ketogenic diet, but it is typically used for only the more refractory cases (compared to steroids or vigabatrin). Drs. Freeman and Vining had tried the diet as a first-line therapy a few times before, but the positive results in Carson were dramatic. Her parents – motivated, like Jim Abrahams, to "get the word out" – created the Carson Harris Foundation.

BASIC SCIENCE

Eighty years after the first use of the ketogenic diet, Adam Hartman decided to study the effects of the diet in mice, also examining the benefits of intermittent fasting (which we have tried in children too!), and discovering D-leucine as a novel anti-seizure drug through his research into the diet. The new Chair of Child Neurology, Carl Stafstrom, is continuing studies into the mechanisms of action of the diet by evaluating the compound 2-DG (2-deoxy-glucose) as a glycolysis inhibitor.

THE DIET IN ADULTS

For many years, we considered using the ketogenic diet in adults with epilepsy. And why not? Their epilepsy can be very drug-resistant, many pediatric epilepsy syndromes continue into adulthood, and children grow up and need adult epilepsy care at age 18. However, neurologists specializing in epilepsy in adults were skeptical about the ketogenic diet – until Mackenzie Cervenka started her adult epilepsy fellowship in 2008, and then joined our faculty in 2010. Her interest in seeing adults for dietary therapy started immediately, as did the world's first Adult Epilepsy Diet Center. To date, Cervenka and her team – adult dietitian Bobbie Henry-Barron and her associate, Diane Vizthum, medical office coordinator Joanne Barnett, and nurse Rebecca Fisher – have treated more than 300 adults with ketogenic diets.

LOOKING AHEAD

Our dietary centers continue to grow and evolve. We have now published our sixth edition of the *Ketogenic Diets* book. The book has expanded its scope and authorship.

Over the past three years, Mackenzie Cervenka and I have been working with the International League Against Epilepsy (ILAE) and other groups to help bring the diet to groups worldwide.

—Eric Kossoff

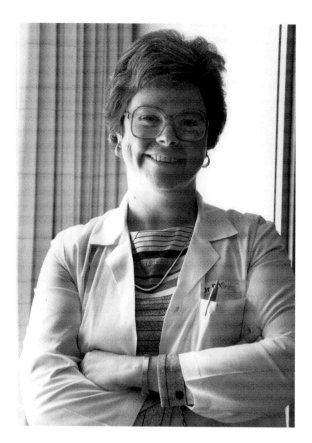

Patti Vining took over as Director of the Division of Child Neurology for two years, strengthening the partnership with Kennedy-Krieger and developing a new relationship with Hopkins' All Children's Hospital in Florida.

THE DIVISION OF CHILD NEUROLOGY 2011-PRESENT

When Harvey Singer stepped down in 2011, Patti Vining Directed the Division of Child Neurology for two years, strengthening the partnership with the Kennedy-Krieger Institute and developing a new relationship with Hopkins' All Children's Hospital in St. Petersburg, Florida. Vining also promoted the careers of residents and young faculty, sustaining NIH training grant funding with the collaboration of Michael Johnston. Johnston's pioneering research has applied pharmacology and molecular biology to study genetic disorders and excitotoxic injury; his work has led to the concept that critical and sensitive periods of brain development in health and disease can create "windows of opportunity" for neuromodulatory interventions that are not commonly seen in adult brain.

After Vining stepped down in 2013, Carl E. Stafstrom was appointed Chair of the Division of Child Neurology. Stafstrom's research expertise is in epilepsy, including investigating the mechanism by which ketogenic diets suppress seizures (see side story). Seizure-inhibiting diets now include the modified Atkins diet and the low-glycemic index treatment. One possible mechanism of action of these diets is in partially inhibiting glycolysis, which reduces seizure susceptibility in animal models. One glycolytic inhibitor, 2-deoxy-d-glucose (2DG), increases the threshold for seizures in animals, and may eventually prove useful in the clinical management of some forms of epilepsy.

In many ways, general acceptance of the place of the ketogenic diet in the management of epilepsy is a tribute to the persistent, scholarly, research endeavors that the Division of Child Neurology faculty have pursued over the past half-century, due to a team effort by clinician scientists, dieticians, nurses and therapists – very much as Guy McKhann had originally conceived.

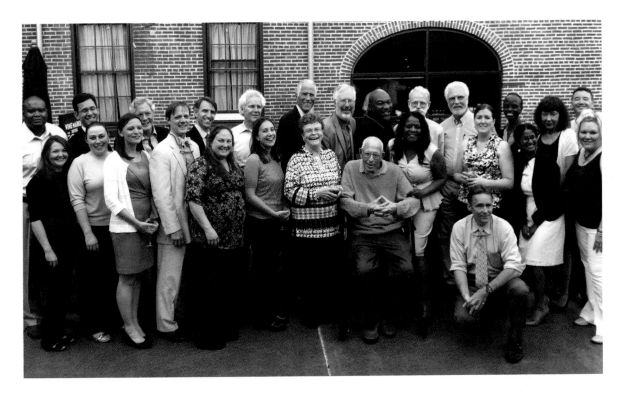

Retirement party for Patti Vining in 2013, held at the Wine Market in Federal Hill.

SELECTED REFERENCES

Freeman JM. 2007 *Looking Back: A Career in Child Neurology*. Booksurge Publishing, Charleston SC.

Ismail FY, Fatemi A, Johnston MV. 2017. Cerebral plasticity: Windows of opportunity in the developing brain. *European J Paediatric Neurol.* 21: 23-48

Shao LR, Rho JM, Stafstrom CE. 2018. Glycolytic inhibition: A novel approach toward controlling neuronal excitability and seizures. *Epilepsia Open.* 2018 Aug 19;3(Suppl Suppl 2):191-197, PMID 30564778.

Singer HS. 2017. Autoantibody-Associated movement disorders in children: Proven and proposed. *Semin Pediatr Neurol.* 24:168-179.

Vining EPG. 2016. Chapter 24: *Neurology*. In: Dover G. & Winkelstein J. (eds). If Only Walls Could Talk. The Johns Hopkins Children's Center, 1964-2012. Johns Hopkins Department of Pediatrics, Baltimore, MD.

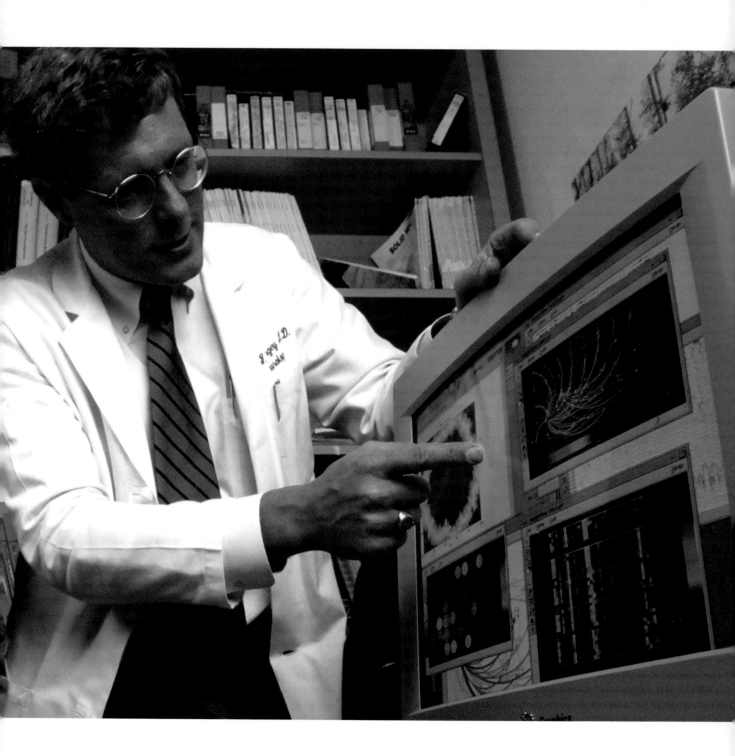

CHAPTER FIFTEEN

EPILEPSY

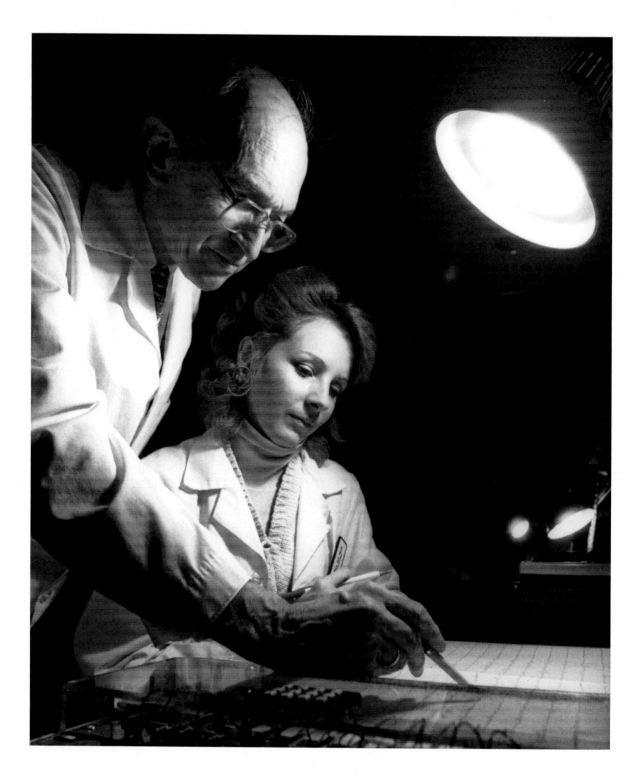

Above: Ernst Niedermeyer, pictured with Mary Ann Smith, was the preeminent electroencephalographer of his time.

Previous spread: Greg Bergey and his research group have studied neural network models and seizure dynamics from intracranial recordings.

In 1969, treatment for epilepsy therapy was limited. There was no CT, no MRI, and just a few effective antiepileptic drugs (AEDs) were available. EEG was an important diagnostic tool, used for epilepsy and other neurologic disorders. Only a few neurology departments were doing continuous monitoring and epilepsy surgery.

This soon began to change for the better. Beginning in the 1970s, imaging with brain CT, and later MRI, plus advances in continuous digital EEG monitoring led to much-improved assessment of patients with focal epilepsy, and increased implementation of epilepsy surgery. Since 1993, more than 15 new AEDs have been approved for epilepsy therapy, along with new modalities for neurostimulation. Faculty in the Hopkins Department of Neurology have played important roles in this dramatic evolution of therapy.

EPILEPSY FACULTY EXPANDS FROM JUST ONE

When Guy McKhann started the Department of Neurology, there was only one faculty member specializing in adult epilepsy: fortunately, this faculty member was Ernst Niedermeyer (see side story), who would become an internationally renowned expert on EEG. In fact, Niedermeyer became the preeminent electroencephalographer of his time. He served as Director of the EEG Laboratory at Hopkins, and also cared for epileptic patients. Largely self-taught, he wrote 240 papers on EEG, and was author or editor of six books including the masterpiece, *Electroencephalography: Basic Principles, Clinical Applications and Related Fields* (co-edited with Fernando Lopes Da Silva). First published in 1982, this became the leading EEG text, with the fifth edition under his editorship published in 2005, when he was 85 years old. The book is now in its sixth edition.

In his early years at Hopkins, Niedermeyer worked with neurosurgeon Earl Walker to establish the epilepsy surgery program, with pioneering studies using depth electrodes and electrocorticography. He served as President of the American EEG Society and rose to full professor before retiring in 1997, and he stayed very active intellectually until he died at the age of 92.

John Freeman, who arrived soon after Guy McKhann in 1969, cared for children with epilepsy (see Chapter 14), and Robert Fisher came in 1982. Fisher had done graduate work at Stanford on cellular physiology, earning his M.D.-Ph.D. before coming to Hopkins for neurology residency. Bob Fisher's research activities included studies on thalamic stimulation for seizure control. He eventually left Hopkins for the Barrow Neurologic Institute, where he became Chair of Neurology. In 2000, he joined the Neurology Department at Stanford, where he has an endowed professorship and is Director of the Epilepsy Center. Fisher served as President of the American Epilepsy Society and has made a number of major contributions, most notably in the area of seizure classification and in the pivotal trials of anterior thalamic stimulation for the treatment of epilepsy.

Bob Fisher has made major contributions in the area of seizure classification and in the pivotal trials of anterior thalamic stimulation for the treatment of epilepsy.

Fisher was joined in 1986 by Ronald Lesser, who came to Hopkins from the Cleveland Clinic, and in 1987 by Bob Webber, a physicist who collaborated in the development of continuous video-EEG monitoring. Monitoring later evolved to the fully digital monitoring used today. Ron Lesser has published extensively,

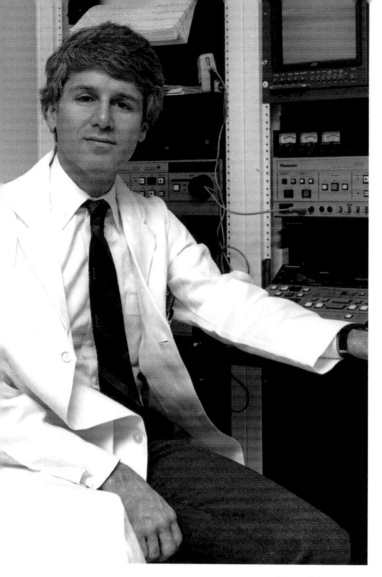

Ron Lesser's studies of termination of evoked discharges with excitatory stimulation have contributed to the basis for responsive neurostimulation.

particularly in the area of cortical stimulation and functional mapping. His studies of termination of evoked discharges with excitatory stimulation laid the groundwork for responsive neurostimulation. Peter Kaplan also came to Hopkins in 1987 and has been based at Bayview, where he is Director of the Epilepsy Service. He has published most notably in the areas of non-convulsive status epilepticus and seizure disorders in women.

Greg Bergey and the Epilepsy Research Laboratory determined stereotyped time-frequency onset patterns for a seizure focus in a given patient.

Greg Bergey, who also completed his Neurology Residency at Hopkins, was recruited in 1999 from the University of Maryland to return as professor and Director of the Epilepsy Center. He brought with him members of the Epilepsy Research Laboratory, including Piotr Franaszczuk and, later, Christophe Jouny. Here at Hopkins, their supported research has involved studies of neural network models and seizure dynamics from intracranial recordings. This group has applied various analytic techniques to study the dynamics of seizure onset, determining that there are stereotyped time-frequency onset patterns for a given seizure focus in a given patient. This has important implications for closed-loop stimulation therapy that relies on early seizure detection. Neurostimulation in the treatment of epilepsy has evolved beyond vagus nerve stimulation to include closed-loop responsive neurostimulation (RNS, Neuropace). For a decade, Bergey was involved in some of the earliest trials of RNS and played an important role in the later pivotal trials leading to FDA approval in 2013.

ADVANCES IN ANTI-EPILEPTIC THERAPY

The 1990s heralded an almost exponential growth in the number of new, FDA-approved antiepileptic drugs, and under the direction of Gregory Krauss, Hopkins has led in the development of many of them. Krauss (now a full professor, he joined the department in 1991, following residency and fellowship at Hopkins) conducted pivotal trials of a number of these second- and third-generation AEDs, including oxcarbazepine, vigabatrin, perampanel, and carisbamate. He has published landmark papers on the use of generic AEDs with greater adoption of their use.

Dietary therapy for the treatment of epilepsy at Hopkins dates back to the time of Samuel Livingston, and is discussed in greater detail in Chapter 14. Extensive use of the ketogenic diet, predominantly in children, by John Freeman and Patti Vining, made Hopkins a leader in this area. More recently, Eric Kossoff has been prominent in advocating ketogenic diet therapy. Working with Mackenzie Cervenka, he has pioneered using the modified Atkins Diet (MAD) in adults with drug-resistant epilepsy, and established the first adult epilepsy diet clinic. These therapeutic developments have made Hopkins the leading center for dietary therapy for epilepsy. Ketogenic diets are now used in other neurological disorders and in super-refractory status epilepticus. The dietary therapy team's services and research expanded in 2018, when Tanya McDonald joined the division after residency and fellowship at Hopkins.

EPILEPSY SURGERY

After Earl Walker, Sumio Uematsu became the head of adult epilepsy surgery, followed by Fred Lenz and Stan Anderson. When George Jallo left Baltimore to direct the Johns Hopkins All Children's Institute for Brain Protection Sciences in Florida, Shenandoah Robinson was recruited from Boston to head the Pediatric Surgery program. As mentioned in the Pediatric Neurology section (see Chapter 14), Hopkins was one of the early leaders in hemispherectomy.

Now, many patients who previously would have had intracranial grid or strip arrays have robotic stereo EEG recordings instead.

Many of our surgical referrals require intracranial monitoring, either with depth electrodes or subdural grid and strip arrays. Nathan Crone, who joined the Department in 1994 after fellowship, has coordinated functional mapping of our patients who require intracranial recordings. Now, many patients who previously would have had intracranial grid or strip arrays have robotic stereo EEG recordings instead. Joon Kang was recruited to join the faculty in 2016, after her epilepsy fellowship at Jefferson, to assist in these efforts with sEEG. She also has helped introduce laser ablative surgery for patients with mesial temporal epilepsy, as well as other focal lesion epilepsy. This minimally invasive surgery (typically one day in the hospital) is now used frequently in patients who otherwise would have undergone craniotomies for anterior temporal lobectomies.

RESEARCH

Nathan Crone's group, working with Stan Anderson of neurosurgery, has been studying high-frequency activity and the mind-brain interface.

The Johns Hopkins Epilepsy Center has a strong record of external research funding. Most notable is Nathan Crone's laboratory, which has been a leader in assessing gamma frequency activity in functional mapping of patients undergoing presurgical evaluations. These new methods greatly augment the data obtained with traditional stimulation techniques. Dana Boatman has had well-supported studies of auditory processing, which she has done with Nathan Crone and others. More recently the Crone group, working with Stan Anderson of neurosurgery, has been studying high-frequency activity and the mind-brain interface. Studies with Anna Korzeniewska, a physicist in the division, have focused on patterns of flow of seizure activity. In work with Greg Krauss, Crone is developing an Apple watch app for seizure detection in patients.

Training

Training of Epilepsy fellows is a key part of the mission of the Division, and the fellows play an important role in the care of patients in the Epilepsy Center. Since 2000, more than 80 percent of the epilepsy fellows trained at Hopkins have gone on to full-time academic positions. Some of our former fellows are already directing epilepsy centers at other institutions.

Clinical Services

Traditional EEG has continued at Hopkins, now in a fully digital format. Intraoperative monitoring, coordinated through the Epilepsy Division, was led initially by Robert Minahan, later by Jehuda Sepkuty, and then by Eva Ritzl, who has been instrumental in developing and directing the continuous EEG service at Hopkins. Continuous EEG is one of the most rapidly developing diagnostic areas, and Ritzl has been a national leader in this area. The activities of the Pediatric Epilepsy group are discussed in Chapter 14.

Summary

Since its very small start in 1969, the Epilepsy Division at Hopkins has grown to include 10 full-time clinical adult faculty, four full-time clinical pediatric faculty, three dedicated research faculty, and additional adjunct faculty. While EEG remains a core component of services, our division now includes an expanding Epilepsy Monitoring Unit, continuous EEG monitoring, and state-of-the-art diagnostic and surgical therapies such as stereo EEG, laser ablative surgery, and closed loop RNS. The Hopkins group remains at the forefront of translational research, and of delivering superb clinical care.

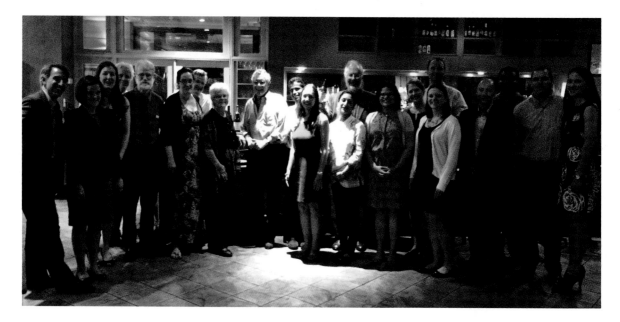

The Epilepsy Team in 2015, at a celebration honoring the graduating Epilepsy Fellows, held in the Inner Harbor.

Ernst Niedermeyer: From POW to Master of EEG

Ernst Niedermeyer, a pioneer in electroencephalography and world-renowned author of the top textbook in the field, became a doctor despite difficult odds – and an EEG expert out of necessity.

Born in Schoenberg (once in Germany, now part of Poland), Niedermeyer moved to Vienna with his family when he was 15. Soon afterward, his father, a physician brave enough to speak out against the Nazis, was sent to jail for three months. Niedermeyer finished high school and was promptly drafted into the German army – which allowed him to go to medical school briefly, until they learned that his mother's father was Jewish.

Because of this, Niedermeyer was considered "racially tainted and politically unreliable," according to his obituary in *The Baltimore Sun*, written by Frederick Rasmussen. So the Nazis sent him to the Russian Front, where he served in a Panzer division during the brutal winter of 1943-1944. He was wounded twice and then sent to France, where he was captured by Allied forces after D-Day.

As a captive, he cared for many wounded soldiers on board a ship bound for America and POW camp – where, his son, Franz Niedermeyer later recalled, he picked corn and made his fellow prisoners suspicious because "he attended Mass and read *The New York Times*." When the war was over, he returned to Austria and finished medical school at Leopold-Franz University in Innsbruck, earning his M.D. in 1947. He trained in neurology and psychiatry at the Hôpital de la Salpêtrière in Paris, then joined the faculty at Leopold-Franz University.

THERE, THANKS TO THE MARSHALL PLAN, SOMETHING HAPPENED TO CHANGE NIEDERMEYER'S LIFE FOREVER: THE HOSPITAL GOT AN EEG MACHINE. THE TECHNICIAN WHO WAS SUPPOSED TO OPERATE IT RESIGNED. NIEDERMEYER LEARNED HOW TO USE IT BECAUSE HE HAD TO.

During this time, he became increasingly interested in epilepsy. "He essentially embraced the first generation of EEG technology of the 1930s through the 1950s, and was instrumental in transforming it into an extremely useful diagnostic and research tool," Franz Niedermeyer recalled.

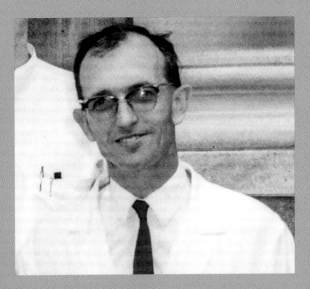

Ernst Niedermeyer, 1964

Niedermeyer came to America again, this time as a faculty member at the University of Iowa, and then he came to Hopkins in 1965 as electroencephalographer-in-chief – a position he would hold for 35 years.

Although Niedermeyer officially retired from Hopkins in 1997, he remained extremely active in the field until shortly before his death, continuing to read clinical EEGs, to publish research papers, and to write and contribute to textbooks – including five editions of his outstanding book, *Electroencephalography*; the book is now called *Niedermeyer's Electroencephalography*. In addition to being extremely knowledgeable about medicine, the American Civil War, operas written by Mozart, and the Baltimore Orioles, Niedermeyer was a gifted classical pianist, a mountain climber, and passionate hiker.

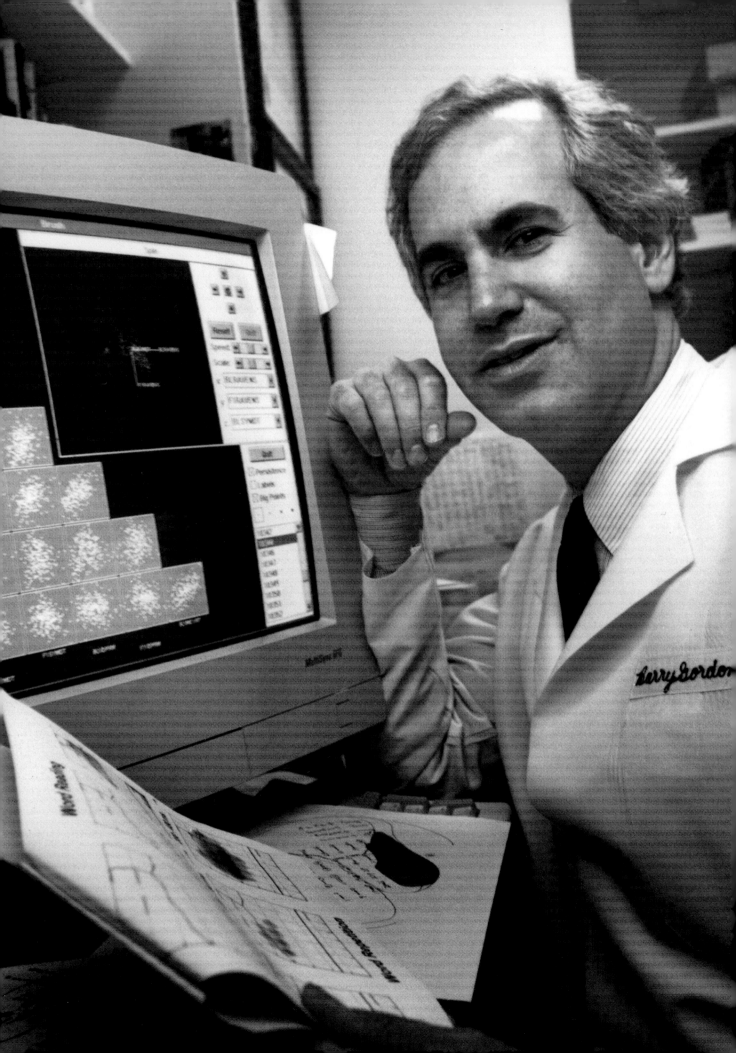

CHAPTER SIXTEEN

COGNITIVE NEUROLOGY

previous spread

BARRY GORDON
Barry Gordon, pioneer in cognitive neurology, opened the Memory Clinic with the goal of focusing on disorders of language and of memory, "particularly, the problems of differentiating normal memory from early pathologic changes, as well as understanding the basis for profound amnesia."

EARLY DAYS

The field of behavioral neurology was re-energized in the early 1970s by the discovery of critical associations between behavior and neuroanatomic features, such as disconnections of different regions of the brain.

In 1973, Oscar Marin, M.D., left Jefferson Medical College to establish a Behavioral Neurology program in the Johns Hopkins Department of Neurology. Marin, says behavioral neurologist and cognitive neuroscientist Barry Gordon, M.D., Ph.D., "had long been interested in using clinical neurological observations to understand behavior, particularly cognition."

Although Marin had extensive training in classical neuroanatomy and neuropathology, he was skeptical about how well neuroanatomy alone could explain many neurobehavioral conditions, Gordon continues. Marin's strategy was to give "at least equal weight to the purely psychological aspects of cerebral function and dysfunction – not just their neuroanatomic aspects."

Marin established a neuropsychology lab at Baltimore City Hospital with two psychologists, Eleanor M. Saffran, Ph.D. and Myrna F. Schwartz, Ph.D, in association with Alfonso Caramazza, Ph.D., and Rita Berndt, Ph.D. They studied a variety of aphasic conditions and related disorders to understand what cognitive operations were normally responsible for language and related functions, and what underlying impairments were involved in overt disorders.

Gordon, who was a medical student at Jefferson Medical College, had done a neurology rotation with Marin in 1972. "I was impressed with Dr. Marin's plans, and with the neurology program Guy McKhann had established at Hopkins." Gordon came to Hopkins as a Neurology resident in 1974. When he finished his residency in 1977, he began working with Marin's group at Baltimore City Hospital, and earned his Ph.D. in experimental psycholinguistics at Johns Hopkins University. Gordon soon became the acting director of the Neurology program at Baltimore City Hospital, when Saffran, Schwartz and Marin left Hopkins.

"THE MEMORY CLINIC"

When the Adolph Meyer Building opened in 1982, four rooms were set aside for behavioral neurology. Gordon wanted to offer a clinical service to diagnose and manage problems in behavioral neurology, and also to use patient material for research to understand and possibly treat these conditions. From the outset, he planned to focus on disorders of language (aphasia) and of memory, "particularly, the problems of differentiating normal memory from early pathologic changes, as well as understanding the basis for profound amnesia."

Gordon's new program – officially named Cognitive Neurology/Neuropsychology, and known colloquially as "The Memory Clinic" – offered both consultative and neurologic primary care services. "We hired Barbara J. Mroz as a neuropsychology testing technician," Gordon says, "and she proved essential to our early clinical and research successes." Ola Selnes, Ph.D., whose background was in linguistics, neurolinguistics, and neuropsychology, joined the division in 1983, and the clinic grew to include Deborah Hasenauer, Sharon Powell, R.N., Sarah Reusing, and others. The program became part of Hopkins' first Alzheimer's Disease Research Center (ADRC) grant, and also carried out clinical trials of anticholinesterases and other drugs to treat early, mild Alzheimer's disease.

Ron Lesser introduced to Hopkins the technique of implanting subdural electrode arrays, for recording epileptic activity and also for mapping language and other functions.

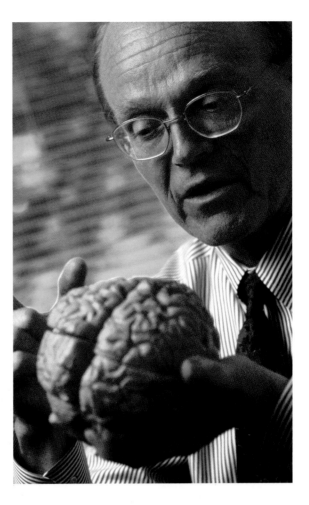

OLA SELNES
Selnes brought to Cognitive Neurology expertise in linguistics, neurolinguistics, and neuropsychology.

Neurologist Ronald Lesser, M.D., whose specialty is epilepsy, introduced to Hopkins the technique of implanting subdural electrode arrays – for recording epileptic activity and also for mapping language and other functions – to help with planning for patients whose conditions might benefit from surgery. Gordon's group, which by then included John Hart, M.D., joined with Lesser and the other epileptologists to offer clinical services for the patients with epilepsy, along with research on the patients' representations of language and other functions, using the cortical stimulation and cortical recording techniques.

Hart also began employing the newly developed technique of functional MRI (fMRI) in the assessment of cerebral functions and their neuroanatomic associations. Dana Boatman, Ph.D., joined the division in 1990, with a specialty in audition and speech perception. Nathan Crone, M.D., came to Hopkins as a fellow, and continued the development of electrocortigraphic recording through the implanted electrode arrays.

THERAPEUTIC COGNITIVE NEUROSCIENCE

Thanks to the generosity of two families, the Cognitive Neurology program began research initiatives in 1996 aimed at enhancing speech perception, communication, and ultimately oral language production in individuals with autism. In 2000, Gordon received an endowed Chair in Therapeutic Cognitive Neuroscience; a substantial gift established a Therapeutic Cognitive Neuroscience Fund for the program. As these names suggest, the ultimate goal of these efforts would always be the *treatment* of disorders of language, memory, and other cognitive functions. Their underlying *mechanisms* — both psychological and neural —would be studied, and this knowledge would then be used to guide rational treatment approaches.

The ultimate goal of these efforts would always be the treatment of disorders of language, memory, and other cognitive functions.

This goal has remained steadfast, even as the structure of the program has evolved over the years. Dana Boatman became director of the auditory neurophysiology clinic and laboratory; and Ola Selnes, who had been doing groundbreaking studies in the neuropsychological effects (or lack of effects) of conditions such as cardiopulmonary bypass and HIV infection (in conjunction with Guy McKhann, Justin McArthur, and others), transferred his clinical efforts to the Division of Medical Psychology of the Department of Psychiatry. Nathan Crone became director of the Cognitive Neurophysiology Laboratory in 2001, and has continued developing methods to analyze and interpret EEG recordings.

OUTREACH IN NEW YORK

In 2000, as part of the Cognitive Neurology program, Gordon started a full-time educational program in New York City for one nonverbal person with low-functioning autism. This program now serves not only the one individual – who has learned to speak – but also other people with developmental disabilities. The New York site is also the focus of research efforts aimed at improving communication, cognitive control, and other issues of autism and related conditions, complementing the research carried out in Baltimore.

In 2000, Gordon started a full-time educational program in New York City for one nonverbal individual with low-functioning autism. This program now serves not only that person – who has learned to speak – but also others with developmental disabilities.

In recent years, the program has expanded several areas of research and established new ones, including studies of visual and language abilities and disabilities of individuals with Autism Level 3. Gordon's group has developed methods for assessing familiarity and comprehension that do not require traditional overt responses, including pupillometry, eye movements, and various scalp EEG and evoked potential measures. Boatman continues to collaborate on auditory electrophysiology studies of real-world listening in people with autism and other developmental disorders.

Besides testing a variety of behavioral methods for enhancing cerebral functions, since 2008 the program has been researching transcranial direct current stimulation as a potentially effective and

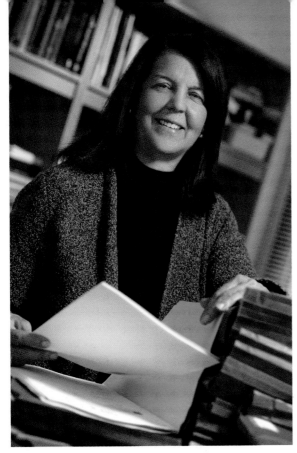

MARILYN ALBERT
Marilyn Albert's research focuses on integrating careful clinical and cognitive evaluations with imaging and other biomarker studies, and is aimed at prediction of disease – particularly, on understanding the very earliest phases of Alzheimer's.

safe method of modulating cerebral functions. This work was initially conducted through a partnership with David J. Schretlen, Ph.D., and colleagues.

In 2014, Nazbanou "Bonnie" Nozari, M.D., Ph.D., began investigating the psychological mechanisms involved in word production and in executive control, in neurotypical speakers as well as in people with aphasia. In 2016, the Division began an extensive collaboration with cognitive neuroscientist Jordan Grafman, Ph.D., of Northwestern University, focusing on understanding executive disorders and potential explicit and implicit ways of teaching and guiding behaviors. The program recently expanded its educational and research efforts at the New York site, increasing the number of classes (with a research focus) and participants.

For a more detailed version of this history, as well as most current efforts, people, and publications of the Division, go to http://web.jhu.edu/cognitiveneurology.

DIVISION OF COGNITIVE NEUROLOGY

In 2003, Jack Griffin, then Chair of the Department of Neurology, recruited Marilyn Albert, Ph.D., to establish a Division of Cognitive Neurology. In addition to Gordon, several senior investigators who were already at Hopkins had extensive experience in this area, including Argye Hillis, Ola Selnes, Dana Boatman, and Ned Sacktor.

Hillis's primary interest was initially in the language disorders following stroke – most often, left hemisphere stroke. Originally trained as a speech pathologist before she went to medical school, Hillis conducted a series of important studies examining the impact of raising blood pressure in the acute stroke setting, gauging its potential benefits by following subtle improvements in the patient's language. Her studies suggested that elevating blood pressure reduced damage to the hypoperfused tissue surrounding the stroke – thereby reducing the severity of the language impairment. Eventually, her interests in post-stroke syndromes broadened to include studies of spatial neglect and studies of affective disturbances following stroke. She also became interested in the gradually evolving language disorders sometimes seen early in the course of neurodegenerative disorders including frontotemporal dementia and Alzheimer's disease.

Ola Selnes worked with Guy McKhann, William Baumgartner, and their team, studying the cognitive outcomes of coronary artery bypass surgery. Their seminal study revealed that the surgery itself did not adversely influence the cognitive status of patients over the long term. Instead, the patients'

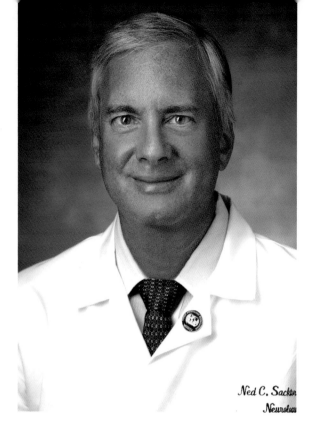

Ned C. Sacktor
Neurology

NED SACKTOR
Sacktor leads pioneering studies in the U.S. and Africa to understand the impact of HIV on cognition.

underlying vascular pathology turned out to be the key determinant of ultimate cognitive function (see Chapter 11). They also focused on cognitive deficits related to vascular disease, but from a different perspective, looking at cognitive impairments following cardiac bypass grafting (also discussed in Chapter 11).

Dana Boatman focused on cognitive deficits at the other end of the age spectrum: she studied children with severe epilepsy and the cognitive deficits following surgery. Through detailed assessments, she showed the remarkable brain plasticity of these children, whose cognitive skills had reorganized over time after surgery, including hemispherectomy.

Ned Sacktor's primary interest has been in the cognitive impairments associated with HIV. As part of the team of investigators associated with the HIV Center, he has carefully delineated the impact of HIV on cognition. At first, these studies were mainly conducted in patients from the Greater Baltimore area. They since have expanded to involve HIV patients in Africa, where Sacktor also oversees a series of unique longitudinal studies.

NEUROIMAGING AND COGNITIVE NEUROSCIENCE

The field of cognitive neuroscience has grown exponentially in recent years, in large part due to the remarkable insights provided by modern neuroimaging. John Desmond, M.S., Ph.D., who was recruited to Hopkins in 2006, applies contemporary functional neuroimaging techniques. His primary research interest is in the role of cerebro-cerebellar networks on cognition, which he has studied with carefully designed activation paradigms, using functional magnetic resonance imaging (fMRI). He has demonstrated convincingly that the cerebellum is important for much more than the regulation of movement and balance: it also plays a major role in working memory. Building on this imaging platform, his colleague Cherie Marvel, Ph.D., has been examining patients in the Ataxia Center. She has shown that – in addition to having progressive problems with balance – they also have cognitive deficits, which were largely under-recognized until now.

Marilyn Albert's research represents another trend in the field: the integration of careful clinical and cognitive evaluations with imaging and other biomarker studies, aimed at prediction of disease. In this case, the focus is on understanding the very earliest phases of Alzheimer's. Before coming to Hopkins, Albert led a large longitudinal study at Massachusetts General

Hospital of people with mild cognitive impairment, who underwent clinical and cognitive assessments, as well as MRI and SPECT scans and quantified EEG. Several years after coming to Hopkins, Albert re-established a cohort of cognitive-normal individuals (75 percent with a family history of dementia) who had been followed at the NIH (starting in 1995). The biomarker collection that was begun at the NIH was ahead of its time: it included cognitive testing, MRI scans and the collection of blood and also cerebrospinal fluid. "Many of the participants have now been followed for over 20 years," Albert notes, "and a substantial number have progressed from normal cognition to mild cognitive impairment, as well as dementia." This has permitted a unique series of studies, using biomarkers collected when participants were cognitively normal, to predict development of clinical symptoms five and 10 years later. This study is an excellent example of an approach that is increasingly used in the study of other neurodegenerative disorders (such as Frontotemporal Dementia and Parkinson's Disease), which develop over many years, if not decades. "The overall goal is be able to identify accurately which cognitively normal individuals are likely to progress over time," Albert continues.

"With the increasing focus on research in these disorders, we hope that improved treatments will be found – and when that time comes, early and accurate intervention will be critical."

In 2010, Albert became the Director of the Johns Hopkins Alzheimer's Disease Research Center, following more than two decades of leadership by Don Price in Neuropathology (see Chapter 18). "The overarching goal of the center is to provide infrastructure for research in Alzheimer's disease and related disorders throughout the institution, as well as mentorship for junior investigators," Albert says. "This goal is greatly facilitated by the fact that leadership roles within the center span four different departments," including: Constantine Lyketsos, M.D. (Psychiatry), Abhay Moghekar, M.B.B.S., (Neurology), Philip Wong, Ph.D., (Neuropathology), Juan Troncoso, M.D., (Neuropathology) and Karen Bandeen-Roche, Ph.D. (Biostatistics). "Through our team, collaboration across the institution has accelerated, and more investigators have become focused on the diagnosis and treatment of Alzheimer's and related disorders."

This integration of activities is also reflected in the establishment of the Memory and Alzheimer's Treatment Center at the Johns Hopkins Bayview Campus (see Chapter 19). Led by Lyketsos, the Center is jointly staffed by faculty from the Departments of Psychiatry, Neurology and Geriatrics. It sees more than 3,000 patients with memory disorders each year, and serves as a prototype for the development of integrated clinical care for patients with chronic neurological disorders.

LOOKING AHEAD

Understanding cognition, and reducing the impact of diseases that cause cognitive deficits, requires the integration of many approaches, says Albert. "Interdisciplinary collaboration, as we have had in many of our studies over the last 15 years, is essential." New studies will integrate careful clinical and cognitive assessments with state-of-the art neuroimaging, biomarker development using blood and CSF, neuropathology, neurogenetics, molecular and cellular model systems, and biostatistics. "The collaborative environment at Johns Hopkins makes this integration possible, and will ultimately lead to important insights into the causes of these disorders, and new ways to treat them."

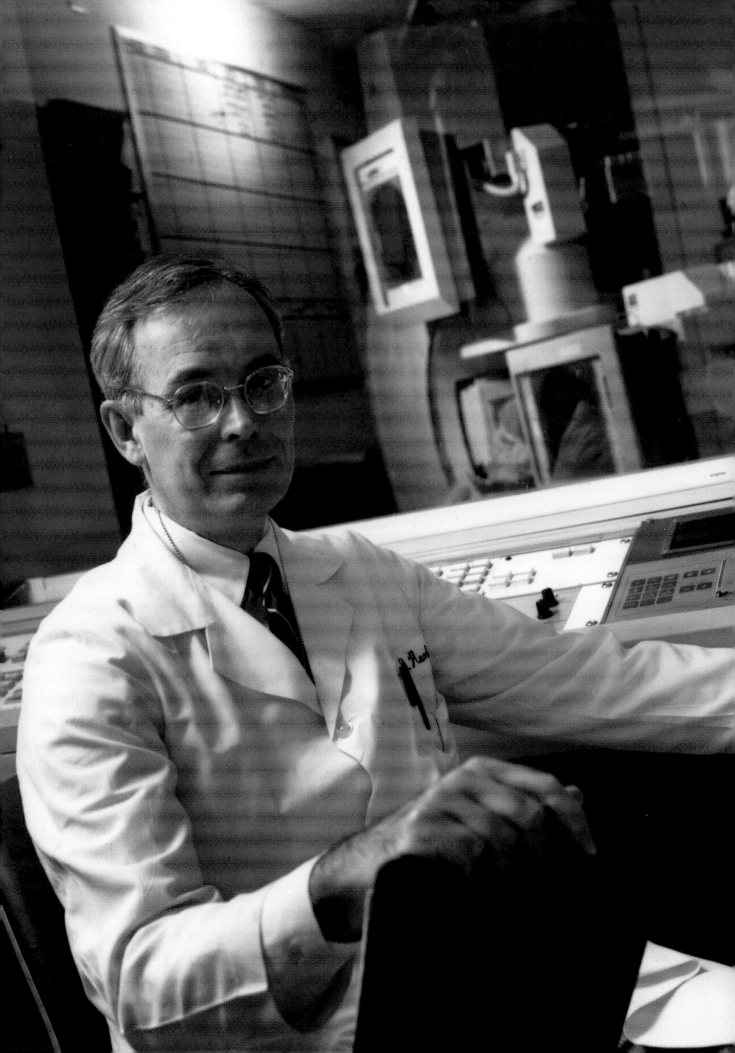

CHAPTER SEVENTEEN

NEUROCRITICAL CARE UNIT (NCCU)

Before 1982, there was no Neurocritical Care Unit at Johns Hopkins.

Acute neurological disorders such as brain hemorrhage, status epilepticus, subarachnoid hemorrhage, brain infections and respiratory failure associated with neurologic disease were cared for in the Medical intensive care services of Johns Hopkins and Baltimore City Hospitals, with advice provided by a consultant neurologist in both the MICU and SICU. Neurosurgery attending physicians performed two to three craniotomies a week, and these patients were cared for in the SICU by neurosurgery residents. Approximately 20 ruptured aneurysms were treated a year.

In 1982 Don Long, Guy McKhann, Chip Moses, and the Director of Nursing, Shirley Sohmer, began discussions with Johns Hopkins Hospital to start a Neuro ICU – one of the first such units in the country – and they had a candidate in mind to become its founding director: Daniel Hanley. A graduate of Cornell University Medical College, Hanley had completed his medical internship and residency at New York Hospital and a Kettering Research Fellowship at the Sloan-Kettering Institute, and was Board-certified in internal medicine. In New York, he had been trained in intensive care by some of the leaders in critical care medicine: Joseph Parrillo, Henry Murray and Henry Masur. Dan Hanley had come to Hopkins for his residency in Neurology and research fellowships in the Departments of Neurology and Anesthesia. Hanley was interested in applying emergency treatment principles to brain injuries, and at Hopkins, he was encouraged to start a career in academic medicine by Dan Drachman and by John Freeman, who introduced him to Mark Rogers, the first chair of the new Anesthesia and Critical Care Medicine (ACCM) Department.

The Hospital approved the idea of the NCCU, with some caution: After Long, McKhann, Moses and Rogers overcame the objections of the Department of Medicine, the Hospital funded a "temporary," four-bed, 20-by-24-foot ICU on Halsted 6, with renewal conditional on fiscal and clinical performance.

The newly recruited NCCU nurse, Judith "Ski" Lower, carried out months of careful planning (see side story). When Hanley started, he and anesthesiologist Cecil Borel took turns, alternating two-week segments of 24/7 call. The first NCCU patient was a man in acute coma, with elevated intracranial pressure due to a large intracerebral hemorrhage; he soon died. The first patient transferred from out of state was a 23-year-old woman with a brain abscess, who recovered completely, but slowly.

"Beginning in 1985, we obtained three successive, five-year NIH program project grants," says Hanley, the Legum Professor in Neurological Medicine, professor in Anesthesiology and Critical Care Medicine, Neurosurgery and Nursing, and Director of the Division of Brain Injury Outcomes. "We also received a large award for NCCU translational research and training under the guidance of Mark Rogers, Guy McKhann, Richard Johnson and Richard Traystman." Advances in multiple areas of Acute Care Neurology included the use of calcium antagonist therapy for vasospasm secondary to subarachnoid hemorrhage, brain protection for cardiac arrest, and plasmapheresis for Guillain Barré syndrome.

"Initially, NCCU fellows came from outside Johns Hopkins," including the Mayo Clinic, Stony Brook, Indiana University, University of Michigan and University of Maryland, Hanley notes. But this soon changed: "With our NIH grants and foundation support," including funding from the Eleanor Naylor Dana Trust, Hanley developed the Neurocritical Care Fellowship Training Program, "a combined

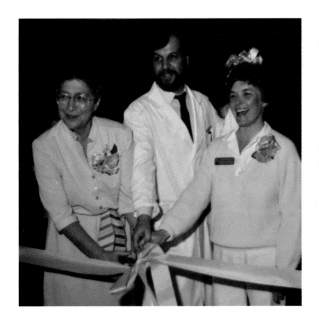 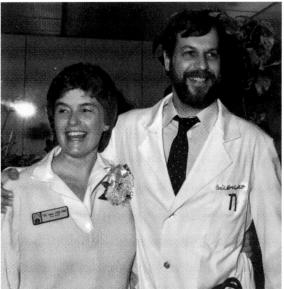

clinical and research program requiring two years of experience, including ICU, OR and molecular physiology research. We initiated and developed programs in blood-brain barrier, brain electrical monitoring, intracranial pressure monitoring, ventilator care for neuromuscular disease, ICU-based Guillain Barré management, intra-arterial thrombolysis for basilar stroke, support for brain tumor surgery and a Critical Care curriculum for Neurosurgery and Neurology residents."

As Interest in acute neurocritical care grew, more Hopkins Neurology residents chose critical care training. The NCCU became even busier: "NCCU support was being required for care of patients with inflammation or infection, and for clinical trials in stroke, cardiac arrest, epilepsy, and neuromuscular disease." The NCCU was also in frequent use "for post-operative care for neurosurgical patients, and for patients with ventilatory and consciousness impairments."

In 1990, its "temporary" status long gone, the NCCU was given permanent financial support from the Hospital, and in 1992, it expanded to an eight-bed unit on Meyer 7. "Referrals of critically ill, acute neurologic patients from the mid-Atlantic region increased with recognition of our centralized neurocritical care services and knowledge of new therapies available," says Hanley. In 1994, the NCCU expanded again, adding six intermediate-care beds. The expanded services allowed Clinical Neurosciences to recruit special interventionalists, including Haring J.W. Nauta (vascular neurosurgery), Gerard Debrun (catheter-based neurovascular interventions), Henry Brem (neurosurgical oncology), Ron Lesser and Fred Lenz (epilepsy monitoring/epilepsy surgery).

DEDICATION CEREMONY
March 8, 1985: Cutting the ribbon at the launch of the new Neurocritical Care Unit. Shirley Sohmer, Director of Neuro Nursing, anesthesiologist Cecil Borel, and Judith "Ski" Lower, NCCU Nurse Manager. In those early days, Borel and Dan Hanley alternated two-week segments of 24/7 call.

Previous spread:
Dan Hanley, founding director of the NCCU.

Interest in acute neurocritical care grew, and more Hopkins Neurology residents chose critical care training. The NCCU became even busier.

Meanwhile, Don Long developed combined Neurosurgery programs with Otolaryngology-Head & Neck surgery and Orthopedic Surgery, each providing patients for a growing intra-operative neuro-monitoring service and postoperative care. "We supported four to six fellows a year in the two-year NCCU training program," Hanley says. These fellows received broad exposure to all elements of ICU and brain disorders, which led to recruitment of Hopkins NCCU trainees by other major research institutions. With academic career paths combining neuroscience and clinical care increasingly well-defined at the research university level, NCCU clinical electives and fellowships became popular among Johns Hopkins medical students and residents. "We developed a Joint Neurology, Neuro-Anesthesia-Neurocritical Care fellowship and began training dual-specialty physicians," including John Ulatowski, Marek Mirski, and Laurel Moore.

The NCCU faculty grew to six members, and Hanley initiated a clinical research group "to perform investigator-initiated research and to join NIH- and pharma-sponsored clinical trials." This group was led by Alex Razumovsky and Karen Lane, clinical researchers with expertise in transcranial Doppler, and neuro-genetics research, respectively. Two junior faculty, Neal Naff and Michael Williams, initiated an FDA-sponsored orphan drug program to investigate minimally invasive, catheter-based thrombolytic therapy for intracerebral hemorrhage. The research group members have become national leaders in intracerebral hemorrhage, subarachnoid hemorrhage and hydrocephalus research. The NCCU faculty, widely recognized for research, clinical and teaching expertise, also established Neurocritical Care sections of the American Academy of Neurology, the American Neurological Association, and the Society for Critical Care Medicine.

"As Chairman of Neurology, John Griffin gave the NCCU Director the opportunity to pursue translational research full-time," Hanley says. "With Neurology Department support, the research division of the NCCU became a full-time clinical trials organization." Research support for this new group came from Jeffrey and Harriet Legum and the France Merrick foundation.

Marek Mirski, M.D., Ph.D., returned from the University of Hawaii, where he directed a statewide NCCU, and became the new Director of the Johns Hopkins NCCU. During his tenure, the NCCU expanded to the Weinberg Building and to Johns Hopkins Bayview Medical Center, and the NCCU Nurse Practitioner Program was developed. The NCCU faculty and fellowship expanded dramatically. Mirski became the first Thomas and Dorothy Tung Professor of Neuro Anesthesia Research. In 2017, after another extensive national search, Jose I. Suarez, who had trained as a fellow at the Hopkins NCCU from 1996 to 1998, was recruited from Baylor College of Medicine to become the Director of the Neurocritical Care Division. Suarez, President of the Neurocritical Care Society, is also the founding chair of the Neurocritical Care Research Network, made up of 230 sites worldwide.

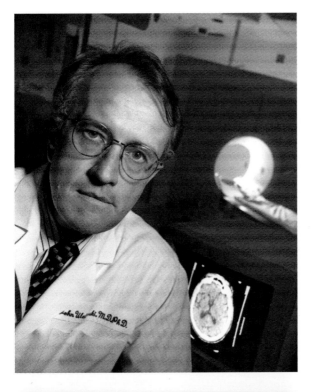

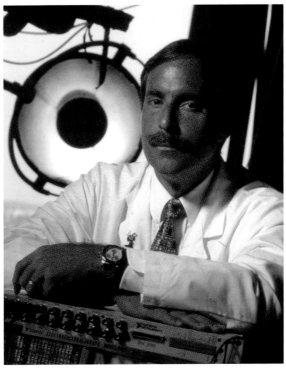

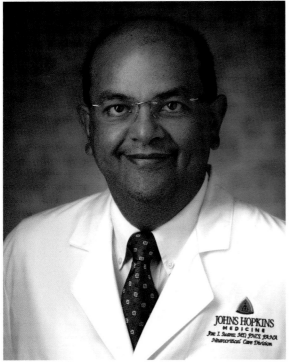

(clockwise from top left):

John Ulatowski is one of the world's leading investigators into the regulatory mechanisms of cerebral blood flow and oxygen delivery to the brain.

Marek Mirski is the inaugural recipient of the Thomas and Dorothy Tung Professorship in the Department of Anesthesiology and Critical Care Medicine. Under his tenure as NCCU Director, the NCCU expanded to the Weinberg Building and to Johns Hopkins Bayview, and the NCCU Nurse Practitioner Program was developed.

Jose Suarez, a fellow in the Hopkins NCCU from 1996 to 1998, under the tutelage of Dan Hanley and John Ulatowski, came back in 2017 to serve as Director of the Neurocritical Care Division.

When the NCCU Began

Judith "Ski" Lower asked for, and received, flexibility, permission to think outside the box and freedom to pilot new ideas.

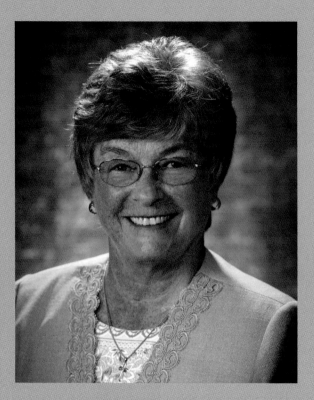

It was 1982. I received a call from the Director of Neurology Nursing, asking me to interview for the position of Nurse Manager – whose responsibility it would be to hire, educate, establish protocols and help design The Johns Hopkins Hospital's first intensive care unit for the neuro population.

I interviewed with Dr. Guy McKhann, head of Neurology, Dr. Donlin Long, head of Neurosurgery and Shirley Sohmer, director of Neuro nursing. It was Dr. Long who sold me on accepting the job, as he described his vision of developing a Center of Excellence for this population that would become a model for others. I assured both him and Ms. Sohmer they would have the beginning of that within two years – but that I needed flexibility, permission to think outside the box and freedom to pilot new ideas. Thankfully, they both said yes. But I don't think either one was prepared for what we would do, how we would do it, and how differently we would do it.

Challenges: Our beginning wasn't smooth. There were multiple challenges, and I was brand new to this hospital with its decentralized organizational structure operating in its traditional "Hopkins Way." Some of these challenges included:

A severe national nursing shortage. In addition, we knew that working with neuro patients was not the desired career path for many nurses, who had received little education and training in this specialty, and little exposure to this patient population in their schools of nursing. Many predicted that we would fail. Thankfully, I had little difficulty hiring the 11 nurses I needed – although only two had previous neuro experience, and one had ICU experience.

No physical space had been allocated for this new unit. We totally underestimated how territorial folks would become when faced with the loss of any space on their unit to another service and were not prepared for what happened. One ICU was asked to let us use four beds in the back of their unit while our unit was being built... NO!! The compromise was to offer us two semi-private rooms with the wall between them knocked down on the Intermediate Care Unit. The only bathroom and locker room was across the hall from our unit, but we were denied access.

OUR RESPONSE? WIN THEM OVER WITH KINDNESS... AND WE DID!

Later that year, when one of our nurses committed suicide, their staff offered to cover our entire unit so that we could all attend the funeral together. It was a beautiful, healing gesture, and all was well after that.

Trust. On our first day of actually expecting a patient directly from the Operating Room, we waited and waited and waited, but he never came. Why? The house staff and attending did not "trust" us to care for their patient because they did not know us. The new nurses were devastated! Our response? Educate, educate, educate, and show them what we were prepared to offer their patients and them. Our staff had had four weeks of classes in neuro, and one each of respiratory and cardiac. A competency exam was given each year that they had to pass with 80 percent to remain in the unit. But how do we translate our knowledge to the house staff? The pattern at that time was for the house staff to come to the unit a half-hour before their formal rounds, and copy all the data from the nurse's flow sheet that they would need to present the patient to the attending.

WE WAITED AND WAITED AND WAITED, BUT THE PATIENT NEVER CAME. WHY? THE HOUSE STAFF AND ATTENDING DID NOT "TRUST" US TO CARE FOR THEIR PATIENT BECAUSE THEY DID NOT KNOW US. OUR RESPONSE? EDUCATE, EDUCATE, EDUCATE.

I proposed a pilot where the nurse who had been with that patient all night and knew him best would present the DATA and any trends to the medical team, and let the house staff present their opinions, conclusions, questions to the attending. The nurses for the most part cared for the same patient from admission to transfer, in order to maintain continuity and prevent the patient and family from having to adjust to several new nurses each day. It also facilitated their knowledge of the patient so they could also present the history and trends. Together, the RNs and MDs developed the template for that report. The nurses quickly learned HOW to present a patient to the physician succinctly and with confidence. I will forever be grateful for them allowing us to do this and for their patience while some of the nurses worked through a learning curve. Also helping was that there were some exceptional Chief Residents. In addition, after 18 months of working with neuro patients, one could sit for the *national* CNRN (certified neurological RN) exam, which most did. We provided a review course for them over some potluck dinners. In time, we had Hopkins neuro ward nurses, pharmacists and physical therapists join us, as well as nurses from other Baltimore hospitals.

What to name the new unit? NICU (neonatal ICU) was taken. I asked for NCCU (Neurocritical Care Unit), knowing that critical care was a strong draw for nurses, and wanting to demonstrate that most of the challenge with this patient population was extensive knowledge of anatomy and the patient's neurological exam, being able to pick up on the subtle changes, and knowing what it meant and what to do. And that could be as exciting and rewarding as having lots of surgical dressings, drains, and equipment, because it depended specifically on the nurse's knowledge and ability to apply it.

No full-time present Medical Director. Dr. Dan Hanley had been named, but the Unit needed someone until he was ready to take on the role in three months. Dr. Chip Moses, Vice Chair of Neurology, assumed that role temporarily. He checked in on us and we met occasionally. In retrospect, I consider that a blessing in disguise, for as an experienced ICU nurse and manager, I knew what needed to be done to create that promised Center of Excellence, and he gave me that freedom.

Quality Improvement: One of our favorite sayings was (author unknown) "Yesterday's Excellence is Today's Standard, and is Tomorrow's Not Good Enough." We constantly searched for ways to make everything we did just a little better. It became one of the building blocks to the unit's success.

In time. the demands for both ICU and progressive care beds for neuro patients allowed us to expand from the initial four beds, to eight, then 12 beds and eventually to develop a new Brain Rescue Unit (for strokes). Again, that name was chosen to demonstrate the exciting advances made in the management of stroke patients. The BRU moved to one of our neuro wards and the NCCU/NPCU was housed in the same area – a total of 22 beds where it remained until the newly constructed Clinical Care Tower opened and all ICUs moved to that new building.

I retired in 2005, and I miss it every day.

–Judith "Ski" Lower, M.S.N., C.C.R.N., C.N.R.N.

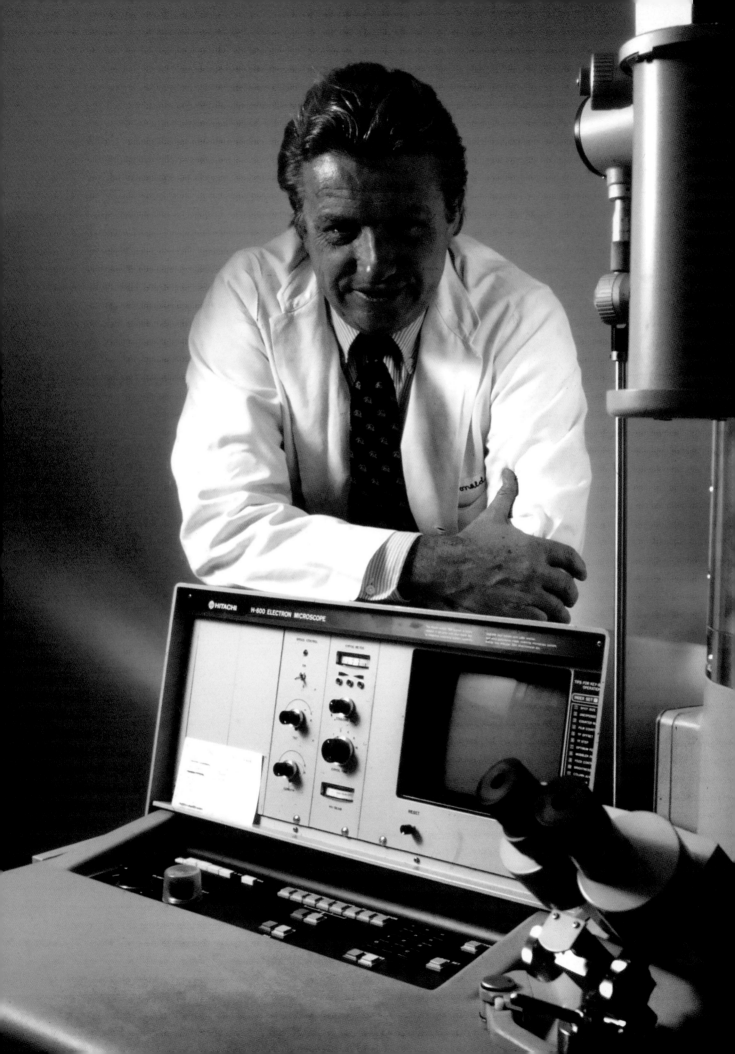

CHAPTER EIGHTEEN

NEUROPATHOLOGY: THE MOLECULAR NEUROSCIENCE OF DISEASE MECHANISMS

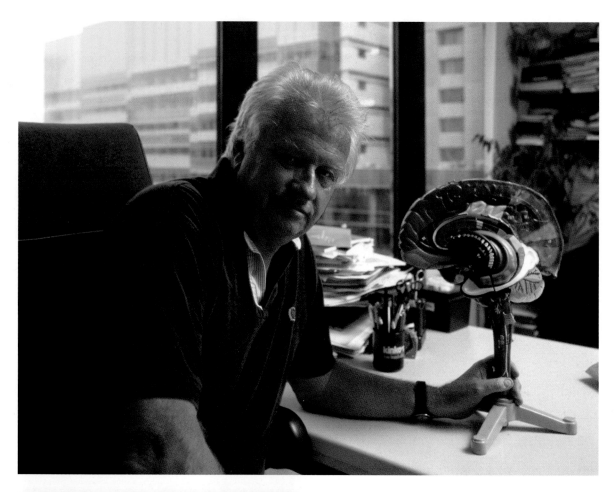

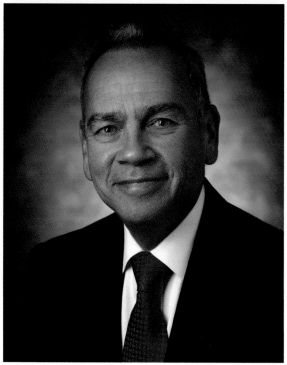

Top: Don Price attributes his early successes to the encouragement of Guy McKhann and a close-knit group of bright, young investigators, who shared their ideas – often, as they carpooled from Columbia.

Bottom: Juan Troncoso, who had trained in both neurology and neuropathology, started and developed the Alzheimer's Disease Research Center.

NEUROPATHOLOGY: THE MOLECULAR NEUROSCIENCE OF DISEASE MECHANISMS

It all started with Guy McKhann's recruitment of Donald L. Price in 1971.

Previous spread:
DON PRICE
Clinical brilliance, combined with infectious enthusiasm and energy.

Every university department of neurology relies on neuropathologists, who serve as valued colleagues in the management of patients, and who are indispensable for teaching medical students, residents, fellows and faculty. However, when the Department of Neurology started in 1969, there was no formal section of Neuropathology at Johns Hopkins Hospital. This might seem somewhat surprising, given the high academic profile of the Department of Pathology, started by William H. Welch, one of the Hospital's "Big Four" founding medical faculty.

During the early days of the Department of Neurology, residents collaborated with Bruce Konigsmark on classifying cerebellar degenerations; after he moved, curious neurologists turned to Richard Lindenberg, a forensic pathologist for the Medical Examiner's Office, whose academic interests included neuro-ophthalmology. But soon, Hopkins Neuropathology would become a powerhouse of molecular neuroscience that would shape the careers of generations of Neurology clinician-scientists. The beginning of this impressive rise can be dated to Guy McKhann's recruitment of Donald L. Price in 1971.

A MODERN NEUROPATHOLOGIST

At the time of his recruitment, Don Price was an Assistant Professor of Neurology and Neuropathology at Harvard Medical School. Trained in neurology by Raymond Adams, and in neuropathology by E. P. Richardson, he had also learned techniques of cell biology from Keith Porter, and anatomy from Walle Nauta at Massachusetts Institute of Technology. During his military service at the National Naval Hospital, Price became interested in peripheral nerve injuries in soldiers returning from Vietnam. Back at Harvard, he collaborated with Porter in studies of experimental neuronal injury and regeneration in frogs, using radiolabelled amino acids and electron microscopy. This approach – developing animal models for a range of human diseases – would prove important for his future research at Johns Hopkins. But Price also brought to Hopkins an attribute as important as any of his scientific training and expertise: his ability to write. At Wesleyan University, he had studied English literature and the classics; at one point, he had even been set on moving to Columbia University to work with the prominent European scholar, Jacques Barzun. His natural gift for writing was honed by crafting grant applications with his well-funded scientific mentors at Harvard. Price also gained experience developing teaching programs at the National Institutes of Health, while he was at the Naval Hospital.

The Prices soon fell in love with Columbia – then a new, growing, planned community that offered good public schools. Columbia was to prove an important factor in other early recruitments, including those of Jack and Diane Griffin, David Zee, Robert Herndon, Gihan Tennekoon, and Mahlon DeLong.

Despite the excellence of his academic environment in Boston, a combined recruiting effort at a national meeting by McKhann, Dick Johnson, and Dan Drachman persuaded him to move to Hopkins – although his wife, Helen, viewed it as a "two-year trial period" to see how things worked out. The Prices often had travelled through Baltimore on their trips to Boston and Cape Cod from the Naval Medical Center in Bethesda, and they did not regard it as an attractive city in which to live. However, they soon fell in love with Columbia, Maryland, a new and growing planned community that offered good public schools. Columbia later proved an important factor in other early recruitments, including those of Jack and Diane Griffin, David Zee, Robert Herndon, Gihan Tennekoon, and Mahlon DeLong.

On his first visit to Hopkins, as David Zee relates, Don Price was invited to supervise a brain-cutting session with Neurology faculty and residents. The patient had presented with acute coma, from which he had awakened. However, he had been left with deficits in both right and left visual hemifields, and soon died. Price predicted an embolus to the top of the basilar artery as the cause of the initial coma. Then, he hypothesized, the thrombus later fragmented, causing the patient to wake up, and embolic infarction of occipital cortex had caused the visual defects. To the delight of the audience, Price turned out to be right on all counts. At that very first session, Price displayed his clinical acumen, infectious enthusiasm and energy that would prove a magnet for many individuals interested in research into neuro-degenerative disorders.

Other early recruits with research expertise came to work with young staff in Price's lab. Robert Herndon brought skills with the electron microscope that were put to work in Richard Johnson's lab – demonstrating, for example, that inclusion bodies were aggregates of viral material. Hugo Moser, who had been directing a metabolic unit in Boston focusing on metachromatic leukodystrophy, came a year after Price. Some of Price's early collaborations included work with Guy McKhann and Gihan Tennekoon, studying optic nerve development with a focus on primordial glial cells and their lineage. Price also worked with many basic scientists already at Hopkins: one was David Bodian, chair of Anatomy and a pioneer in the study of polio virus, who was a great over-the-microscope teacher of young individuals interested in the neurosciences. Another was Vernon Mountcastle, whose influence was crucial in founding the Department of Neurology.

THE NEUROPATHOLOGY-NEUROLOGY COLLABORATIONS

Encouraged by McKhann, Price quickly filled the void in "real neuropathology" at Hopkins. He soon made critical contributions to both neuropathology and neurology by winning two federal grants: a T32 training grant, to fund fellows' research, and a program project grant to study the regeneration of motor neurons following axonal transection. These two grants (the training grant was renewed several times) allowed Price to hire and to train a generation of young neurologists and neuroscientists.

One of the first trainees was Jack Griffin, who became fascinated by the potential for experimental axonal transection in understanding clinical neuropathies. Griffin, Price recalls, "was wonderful, out of Stanford," where he had worked with Lucien Rubinstein. "He saw the beauty of the peripheral nervous system, and what you could do: you could damage the nerves, you could watch them regenerate, repair." Price adds that "Jack came with curiosity and skills: he knew how to use a microscope." Based on observations of the temporal course of tetanus following injection of a peripheral limb, Griffin and Price hypothesized that there must be retrograde axonal transport of the toxin. One of their first collaborations confirmed this, and they later demonstrated that the distribution of tetanus toxin at presynaptic terminals was similar to that of the inhibitory transmitter glycine – and thus, ideally positioned to choke off excitation. In collaboration with Dan Drachman, they described fast axonal transport in motor neurons, and soon recognized that studying axonal transport was of central importance for understanding mechanisms of regeneration of nerves following injury.

Jack Griffin "saw the beauty of the peripheral nervous system, and what you could do: you could damage the nerves, you could watch them regenerate, repair... Jack came with curiosity and skills: he knew how to use a microscope."

Serendipitously, the latest techniques in axonal transport came knocking on Price's door in the form of molecular scientist and cell biologist Paul Hoffman, M.D., Ph.D. With Ray Lasek at Case Western Reserve University, Hoffman had used radioactively labeled axonal polypeptides, identified on gels, to study slow axonal transport of microtubule and neurofilament proteins. Hoffman was welcomed into the Price lab and soon contributed to a number of studies with Griffin and Price. This led to clarification of how the neurotoxin ß,ß'-iminodipropionitrile (IDPN) caused proximal axons to become distended with neurofibrillary pathology: by selectively impairing slow axonal transport. It also supported the hypothesis that neurofilaments are major intrinsic determinants of axonal caliber in large myelinated nerve fibers. In collaboration with Lasek, the Hopkins group demonstrated how, during development, the velocity of slow axonal transport reflects the level of maturation of the neuron. Hoffman also applied this technique to study mechanisms of optic disc swelling with Harry Quigley, anticipating his transition to a career in ophthalmology.

THE BRAIN OF A PATIENT WITH ALZHEIMER'S DISEASE

In the late 1970s, Neurology resident Peter Whitehouse joined Price's lab and, with Arthur Clarke, studied the brain of a patient with Alzheimer's disease, comparing the findings with those of age-matched control subjects. The difference was striking: the brain of the patient with Alzheimer's had lost almost all neurons in the nucleus basalis of Meynert. Drawing on modern anatomical studies, suggestions by Joseph Coyle, who had studied cholinergic systems, and Mahlon DeLong's studies of the activity of single neurons, an influential hypothesis was forged. This proposed that the *basal nucleus provides an important, cholinergic drive to neocortex, distinct from thalamic inputs.* It was the first insight that involvement of a subcortical structure, with a specified neurotransmitter (acetylcholine), could play an important role in the pathogenesis of Alzheimer's disease. The concept also carried over to other neurodegenerative disorders, such as the dementia that can occur in Parkinson's disease. These discoveries were followed by a series of studies concerning the pathogenic mechanisms of neurodegenerative disorders, including processes causing dementia and amyotrophic lateral sclerosis, to which members of the Department of Neurology contributed. This progress ultimately led to the development of animal models for these disorders, allowing study of methods that might slow the disease progress, such as administering nerve growth factor (NGF) in the Alzheimer's model, and using glial cell-derived neurotrophic factor (GDNF) to rescue axotomized motor neurons. In parallel with the development of these murine models, a study of rhesus monkeys as old as 28 years, by a team including veterinarian Linda Cork, scientist Larry Walker, and neurologist William Mobley, demonstrated impaired cognition, with neuropharmacological and pathological findings similar to those of human Alzheimer's disease.

The difference was striking: the brain of the patient with Alzheimer's had lost almost all neurons in the nucleus basalis of Meynert.

THE BALTIMORE LONGITUDINAL STUDY ON AGING

In the early 1980s, leaders of the National Institute on Aging's Baltimore Longitudinal Study of Aging, which began in 1958, approached Price with an intriguing idea: they proposed a collaboration to study the brains of cohort participants who had died. At the time, Price was caught up in the many scientific projects of the lab, but Juan Troncoso, M.D., who was also trained in neurology and neuropathology, was able to step in and start what was to become the Alzheimer's Disease Research Center. Later, cognitive neuroscientist Marilyn Albert, Ph.D., joined the team, which has made major contributions to that field.

GENETIC MODELS OF NEURODEGENERATIVE DISEASE

In the early 1990s, the focus of the Price lab moved to harnessing the potential of genetic models of neurodegenerative diseases. Linda Cork had already worked with Price and Griffin in developing a model for hereditary spinal muscular atrophy in Brittany Spaniels (see Chapter 10). However, the development of a genetic model for ALS based on mutant superoxide dismutase 1 (SOD1) in mice opened the way for generating genetic rodent models for a number of neurodegenerative diseases.

Jeff Rothstein, a Hopkins Neurologist with expertise in neurochemistry, was one of a team to capitalize on the potential of these models. Moving forward from this mutant SOD1 model, in collaboration with Don Cleveland, Sam Sisodia, Mike Lee, David Borchelt and Philip Wong, he generated transgenic models for forms of ALS, Alzheimer's disease, Parkinson's disease, dentatorubral-pallidoluysian atrophy (DRPLA), and Huntington's disease.

The beta-amyloid protein, derived from a larger amyloid precursor protein (APP), is the main component of senile plaques in Alzheimer's disease. Price comments: "We were among the first to generate mice carrying the human APP gene. We also clarified the roles of presenilin 1 and 2 (PS1 and PS2), mutations of which had been identified in familial Alzheimer's disease." PS1 and PS2 are enzymes that normally cleave APP to produce beta-amyloid. "We then made transgenic mice co-expressing two familial Alzheimer's disease variants, one in APP and one in PS1," Price continues. "We found that they developed numerous amyloid deposits much earlier than of age-matched mice expressing the APP variant alone." These results provided evidence for the view that one pathogenic mechanism by which mutant PS1 causes Alzheimer's disease is to accelerate the rate of beta-amyloid deposition in brain. "We then knocked out the PS genes, and demonstrated that these mutants failed to produce beta-amyloid protein, because they lacked the enzymes to make the cuts in APP. So what this did was to focus people's attention on inhibiting or modulating those enzymes, which is still an active area of research, and allowed the Alzheimer's field to blossom."

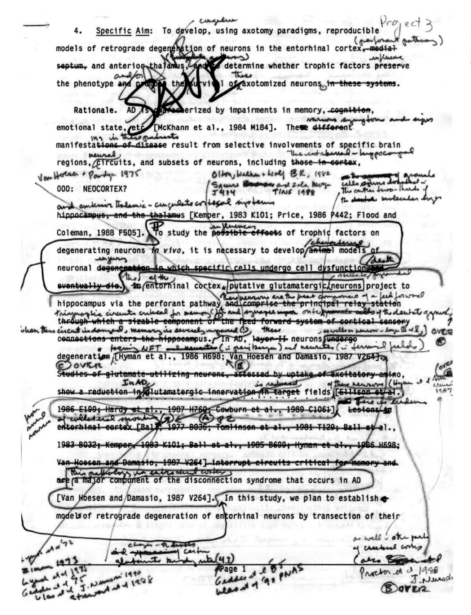

HOW TO WRITE A SUCCESSFUL GRANT APPLICATION
This draft of a grant proposal from Don Price's lab shows the essential process of critically editing, re-editing, and re-re-editing the research rationale to get it right.

DeLong used the MPTP model to discover that lesions of the subthalamic nucleus reverse the clinical signs of parkinsonism – thereby opening up the field for modern interventional treatment of Parkinson's disease.

An Experimental Model for Parkinson's Disease

In the fall of 1978, Price had heard, through a colleague, Eduardo Eidelberg, of a young man who had self-injected a drug that he had synthesized, which had induced parkinsonism. He had been found dead in the grounds of the National Institutes of Health. Autopsy findings, reported by Glenn C. Davis and colleagues, and reviewed by Price, showed typical appearances of Parkinson's disease, including dramatic loss of neurons in the substantia nigra with Lewy body inclusions. The responsible toxin was later identified by J. William Langston as 1-methyl-4-phenyl-1,2,3,6-tetrahydropyridine (MPTP). A primate model for Parkinson's disease was developed by R. Stanley Burns and his colleagues at the NIH. Eidelberg, working in San Antonio, Texas, had duplicated these results and offered Price the opportunity to study the neuropathological changes in the macaques' brains. In collaboration with Cheryl Kitt, Price applied immunocytochemical methods and demonstrated that axonal pathology was conspicuous in the nigrostriatal pathway. The development of an animal model for Parkinson's disease was a time of great excitement and fostered frequent discussions with Mahlon DeLong, who was a neighbor of Price's, both at Hopkins and at home. DeLong had trained as a Hopkins neurology resident, and Price had known him since his days at Harvard. DeLong ultimately used the MPTP model in a different strain, African green monkeys, to discover that lesions of the subthalamic nucleus reverse the clinical signs of parkinsonism – thereby opening up the field for modern interventional treatment of Parkinson's disease.

The Legacy of Collaborations between Neuropathology and Neurology

Contributions by Price and his colleagues have had a huge impact on the development of the Department of Neurology, both by training young neurologists and collaborating with faculty. Some of his trainees have gone on to become departmental chairs and win prominence as basic scientists and clinicians. Most remain active researchers in the neurosciences. Price has received numerous honors and awards for his research. He attributes early successes to the encouragement of Guy McKhann, Dick Johnson, and a close-knit group of bright, young investigators, who shared their ideas – often, as they carpooled from Columbia. He credits the progression of research interests of his lab to being sufficiently enlightened to recognize the potential of new techniques, and identifying young investigators who could apply them to the thorny group of neurodegenerative disorders, whose study he has championed. Don Price's legacy is his trainees, but also the tradition of open inquiry, curiosity, and fun that he imbued in his colleagues, that seems likely carry on way beyond the first 50 years of Neurology and Neuropathology at Johns Hopkins.

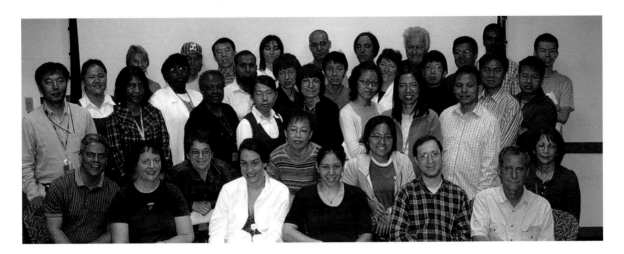

Members of the Division of Neuropathology group in 2008

Don Price's legacy is his trainees, but also the tradition of open inquiry, curiosity, and fun that he imbued in his colleagues.

SELECTED REFERENCES:

Price DL and Griffin J: Neural transport of tetanus toxin. *Science* 192: 159, 1976.

Griffin JW, Hoffman PN, Clark AW, Carroll PT and Price DL: Slow axonal transport of neurofilament proteins: impairment by ß,ß'-iminodipropionitrile administration. *Science* 202: 633-635, 1978.

Whitehouse PJ, Price DL, Clark AW, Coyle JT and DeLong MR: Alzheimer's disease: evidence for selective loss of cholinergic neurons in the nucleus basalis. *Ann. Neurol.* 10: 122-126, 1981.

Lamb BT, Sisodia SS, Lawler AM, Slunt HH, Kitt CA, Kearns WG, Pearson PL, Price DL and Gearhart JD: Introduction and expression of the 400 kilobase precursor amyloid protein gene in transgenic mice. *Nature Genetics* 5: 22-30, 1993.

Borchelt DR, Lee MK, Slunt HH, Guarnieri M, Xu Z-S, Wong PC, Brown RH Jr, Price DL, Sisodia SS and Cleveland DW: Superoxide dismutase 1 with mutations linked to familial amyotrophic lateral sclerosis possesses significant activity. *Proc. Natl. Acad. Sci. USA* 91: 8292-8296, 1994.

Wong PC, Pardo CA, Borchelt DR, Lee MK, Copeland NG, Jenkins NA, Sisodia SS, Cleveland DW and Price DL: An adverse property of a familial ALS-linked SOD1 mutation causes motor neuron disease characterized by vacuolar degeneration of mitochondria. *Neuron* 14: 1-20, 1995.

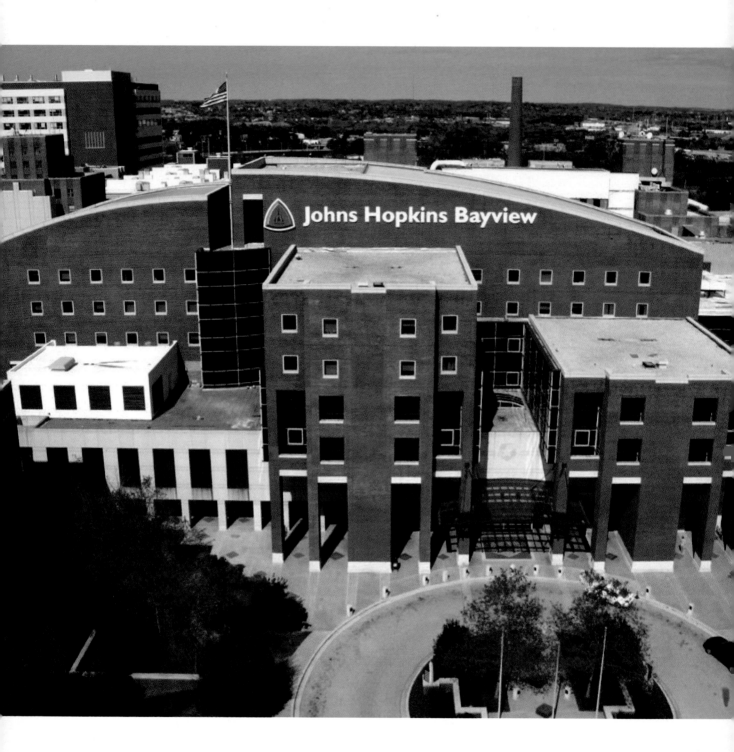

CHAPTER NINETEEN

EXPANSION TO BAYVIEW

BALTIMORE CITY HOSPITALS

Johns Hopkins neurologists were no strangers to the place now known as Johns Hopkins Bayview Medical Center.

They had been there for decades, starting back when it was the Baltimore City Hospitals (plural because it had both a general hospital and a chronic hospital that included a nursing home). Many Hopkins medical students did rotations there, and some of its physicians also held faculty appointments at Hopkins.

Though it served a great need, City Hospitals was a massive financial drain on Baltimore, losing millions each year; in 1984, mayor William Donald Schaefer sold it to Johns Hopkins. Hopkins expanded its mission to the 130-acre East Campus – which, for a decade was called The Francis Scott Key Hospital.

Under its various names, this hospital on Eastern Avenue – once at the outskirts of Baltimore – has long played an important role in Maryland and beyond: it housed the country's first intensive care unit, and was the birthplace of cardiopulmonary resuscitation techniques. It began as the Baltimore City and County Almshouse in 1773, well over a century before Johns Hopkins Hospital opened in 1889. In 1911, Thomas R. Boggs, M.D., who was trained at Hopkins, became Baltimore City Hospitals' Physician-in-Chief, and Arthur M. Shipley, M.D., became Surgeon-in-Chief.

With the arrival of Guy McKhann and the establishment of the Department of Neurology, Neurology faculty members carried out intermittent teaching and consultation at Baltimore City Hospitals, or the "East Baltimore campus." In 1973, Oscar Marin was appointed Chairman of Neurology there. Marin, originally from Chile, had been trained at Harvard's Boston City Hospital by Derek Denny-Brown and by Paul Yakovlev, and had a special interest in cognitive neurology (see Chapter 16). He recruited Eleanor Saffran, Ph.D., and Myrna Schwartz, Ph.D., experimental psychologists who studied language mechanisms, and they developed collaborations with the Hopkins Psychology Department. Soon, Fernando Miranda, M.D., Barry Gordon, M.D., Ph.D., Richard Allen, Ph.D., Frank Baker, M.D., and Margit Bleecker, M.D., joined the East Baltimore campus's Neurology group. In 1973, Marin hired Sylvia Parham as the first EEG technician, and she is still an exceptional member of the Bayview staff, having taught EEG to generations of Hopkins Neurology residents.

When Oscar Marin left Baltimore in 1979 to develop a Cognitive Neuropsychology laboratory at Oregon Health Sciences University, Barry Gordon served as interim Chair of Neurology, and then Mahlon DeLong, M.D., served as Chair of Neurology from 1980 to 1985, when he was recruited to Emory University; DeLong won the Lasker Award in 2014 for his work on deep brain stimulation of the subthalamic nucleus in Parkinson's Disease (see Chapter 7).

In 1982, Gordon started a cognitive neurology clinic known as "The Memory Clinic" (see Chapter 16) on the East Baltimore campus. The goal was to have a unified clinical and research effort, "where each would inform the other," he explains. This clinic ultimately contributed to Hopkins' first Aging & Disability Resource Center grant, and was the precursor of the current Alzheimer's Disease and Memory Disorders Center at Bayview.

FRANCIS SCOTT KEY MEDICAL CENTER

In 1984, when Hopkins bought it, the Baltimore City Hospitals' name was changed to Francis Scott Key Medical Center. At that time, Margit Bleecker was in charge of the Neurology Service. Her primary interest was in Neurotoxicology and Occupational Neurology, with special interests in the toxic neurological effects of arsenic, organophosphates, and lead. Claudia Kawas, M.D., joined the group as director of Cognitive Neurology, and worked predominantly with the important Baltimore Longitudinal Study of Aging.

Kawas continued the tradition of outstanding Cognitive Neurology, becoming a nationally recognized expert in Alzheimer's disease, correlating cognitive loss and neuropathological changes. Her most important contributions have been the identification of risk factors for Alzheimer's disease, and the understanding of biomarkers, risk factors and "super agers," who live far longer than the average population and who maintain intact mental acuity. George Ricaurte, M.D., Ph.D., came from Stanford, and works on neurotoxicology of non-human primates.

JOHNS HOPKINS BAYVIEW MEDICAL CENTER

Margit Bleecker stepped down in 1990 and started the Center for Occupational & Environmental Neurology, which is still active today. She was succeeded by Peter Kaplan, M.B.B.S. In 1994, Hopkins completed a $60 million, six-story, 221-bed hospital tower on the campus, and Francis Scott Key was given the new name of Johns Hopkins Bayview Medical Center; the department moved into the new building. Under Kaplan's leadership, Neurology at Bayview became a multispecialty group, able to care for a wide range of neurological disorders. Kaplan expanded EEG, EMG, and the stroke service. The new inpatient unit opened, as did the Bayview Neurocritical Care Unit, with neurosurgeon Alessandro Olivi, M.D., as its director.

Kaplan instituted Neurology Grand Rounds and research conferences at Bayview on a regular basis. Special interests at Bayview now include stroke, movement disorders, EMG, epilepsy, Alzheimer's disease and aging, AIDs dementia, sleep disorders, and restless leg syndrome. Ned Sacktor, M.D., has made major contributions to the study of AIDs dementia. Christopher Earley, M.B.B.Ch., Ph.D., and Richard Allen, Ph.D., have developed expertise in Sleep Neurology and restless leg syndrome. Rafael Llinas, M.D., was recruited from Harvard and developed the first Joint Commission-certified stroke center within the Health system.

In 2005, Richard O'Brien, M.D., Ph.D., became Chair of Neurology at Bayview. He established multidisciplinary clinics, including the Headache Center, led by Jason Rosenberg, M.D., the CSF Disorders Center under Abhay Moghekar, M.B.B.S., and the Johns Hopkins Myositis Center.

Kawas is interested in learning from "super agers," who live far longer than the average population and who maintain intact mental acuity.

Kaplan expanded EEG, EMG, and the stroke service. The new inpatient unit opened, as did the Bayview Neuro-critical Care Unit.

O'Brien established multidisciplinary clinics, including the Headache Center, the CSF Disorders Center, the Myositis Center, and the Johns Hopkins Bayview Memory Center.

Previous spread:
It began as the Baltimore City and County Almshouse in 1773, became Baltimore City Hospitals, then changed names again to Francis Scott Key Medical Center in 1984, when Johns Hopkins bought it. Now it is Johns Hopkins Bayview Medical Center and the home of some flagship programs in Neurology.

Together with Constantine (Kostas) Lyketsos, M.D., M.H.S., O'Brien started the multidisciplinary Johns Hopkins Bayview Memory Center, where patients with a variety of dementing disorders are followed by neurologists, psychiatrists and gerontologists. He brought Michael Polydefkis, M.D., to direct the EMG laboratory and continue small fiber neuropathy research. The multidisciplinary Myositis Center includes Antony Rosen, M.D., and Lisa Christopher-Stine, M.D., M.P.H., of Rheumatology, Sonye Danoff, M.D., Ph.D., of Pulmonology, and Andrew Mammen, M.D., Ph.D., of Neurology. The Myositis Center was responsible for discovering the role of antibodies to HMG CoA reductase in the pathogenesis of statin myopathy. Rich O'Brien left Hopkins in 2014 to be the first chairman of Neurology at Duke University.

Rafael Llinas was named Interim Chair in 2014, and since 2016 has served as Chair of the Neurology Department at Bayview. He also is Director of the Johns Hopkins Neurology Residency Program. His chairmanship has seen tremendous advances in management of stroke (see Chapter 11): in 2015, published studies demonstrated the advantages of thrombectomy plus TPA. Elisabeth Marsh, M.D., medical director of Bayview Medical Center's Stroke Program, instituted rapid and efficient thrombectomy for stroke treatment, and Johns Hopkins Bayview has been certified by the Joint Commission as a Comprehensive Stroke Center. Nauman Tariq, M.B.B.S., significantly expanded a three-person operation into the Johns Hopkins Headache Center, a multidisciplinary clinical service that also includes psychologists and pain interventionalists. Tom Lloyd, M.D., Ph.D., is the Neurology Director of the Myositis Center, and faculty including Rebecca Gottesman, M.D., Ph.D., Aruna Rao, M.B.B.S., Steven Zeiler, M.D., Ph.D., and Emily Johnson, M.D., continue to contribute to the knowledge of neurological function and disorders.

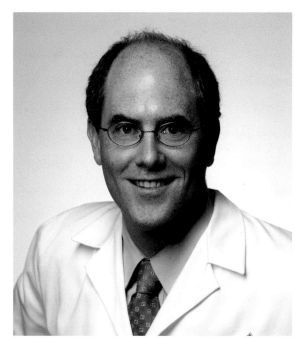 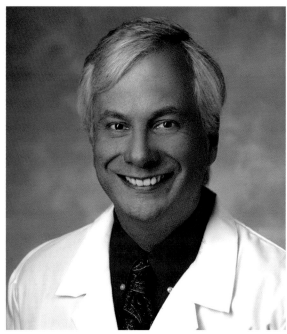

Andrew Mammen, left, co-founding member of the Johns Hopkins Myositis Center, and Rafael Llinas, Chair of the Neurology Department at Bayview.

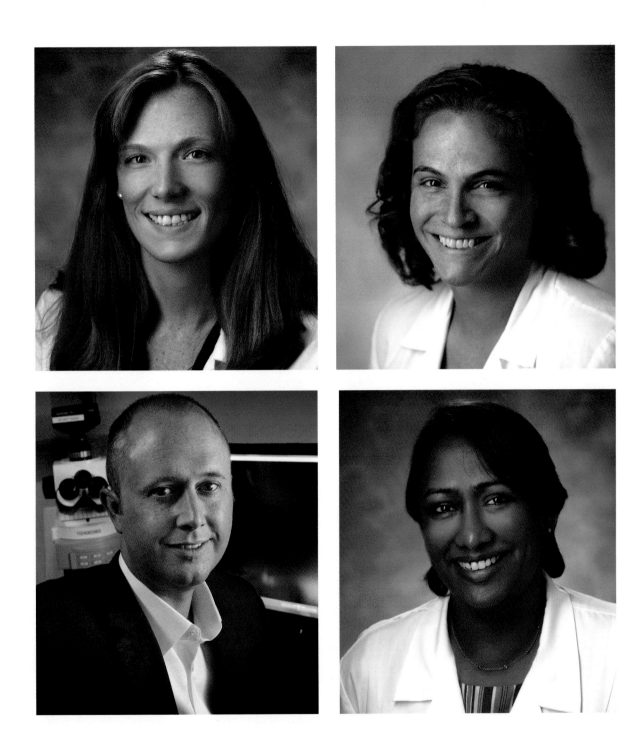

Among our outstanding faculty at Johns Hopkins Bayview are (clockwise from top left):
Elisabeth Marsh, Rebecca Gottesman, Aruna Rao, Steve Zeiler

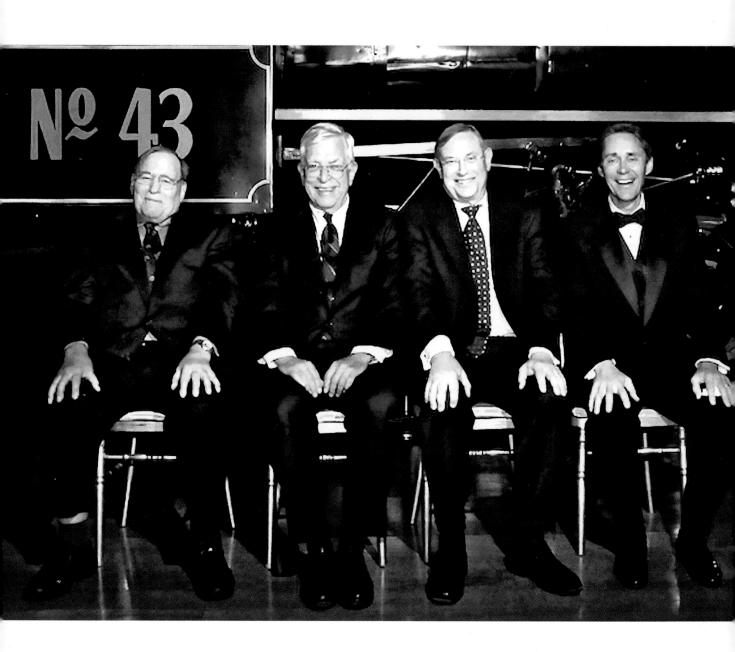

CHAPTER TWENTY

THE ALUMNI OF JOHNS HOPKINS NEUROLOGY

Top: The class of 2017 at the top of the Dome.

Bottom: Three of the Four Chairs: Griffin, McArthur, and Johnson.

Opposite spread: The Four Chairs. From left: Guy McKhann, Dick Johnson, Jack Griffin, and Justin McArthur. Photo taken by Eva Feldman at the B & O Railroad Museum, during the 2009 meeting of the American Neurological Association.

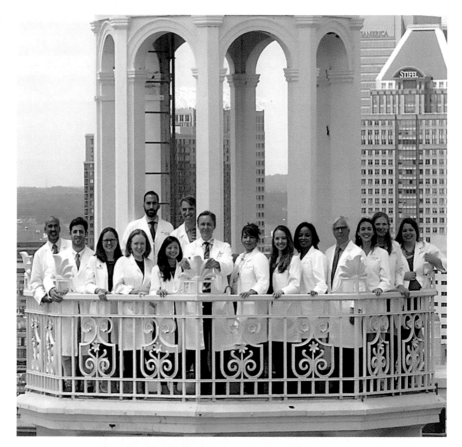

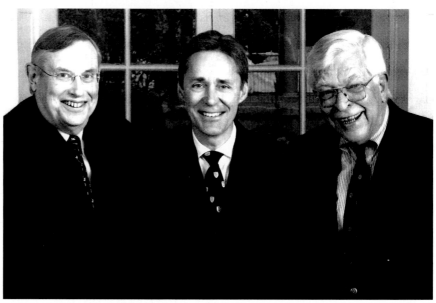

THE ALUMNI OF JOHNS HOPKINS NEUROLOGY

Although born late, our Department is a child of the bourgeoning neurosciences, and has ridden the wave of discovery during the last half- century.

What is the intellectual legacy of the Department of Neurology? The reputation and influence of a department rest on its faculty and trainees who make discoveries that gain widespread attention, teach at national meetings, win research funding, and serve on government bodies that evaluate research proposals. Faculty who make themselves freely available to teach, and set a personal example of dedication to patient care, imbue the tradition of the clinician-scientist. Departments at many academic medical centers throughout the world could claim these characteristics. So: what qualities set Johns Hopkins Neurology apart? Here are some important ones. If you think of others, we encourage you to go online (www.hopkinsmedicine.org/neuro/50th) and tell us about them!

The breadth of our scholarly output, which spans the broad fields of neurology and the neurosciences, and which we've described in this book.

The warm collegiality between faculty and trainees that extends throughout the University, its *esprit de corps*. This quality is born of an open community with diverse views, where we can set aside ego and enter into open discussions, using our creativity. Ideally, dogmas, conventional wisdom, and pet theories are set aside as we make novel suggestions, and then listen as colleagues run with those ideas to see where they might lead, and review them critically. Such is the recollection of many Hopkins trainees since the beginning of the department, perhaps best exemplified by memories of exchanges of ideas in the doctors' dining room.

The remarkable growth of the Department, capitalizing on the conceptual and technological advances that progress brings. In this regard, any history of an academic department has to be cast against what is happening generally in the scientific community – for example, how much use has been made of advances such as brain imaging and the internet. Although new discoveries are crucial – and Johns Hopkins Neurology has opened many new fields – equally important is the insight to realize that a new technique is well suited to address an important issue. Although born late, our Department is a child of the bourgeoning neurosciences, and has ridden the wave of discovery during the last half-century.

The way the Department reaches out to be inclusive – a family – for of all its employees and support staff. Such mutual respect, openness and trust maximizes team effort and enhances our mission. Although such camaraderie and outreach can evolve from a grass-roots level, Johns Hopkins Neurology has been fortunate in having leaders who inspire team spirit. A related attribute is the contributions that the Department makes to the community in Baltimore and Maryland.

The scholarly achievements of our progeny – our residents and fellows. Over the past 50 years, the Neurology faculty have trained a large number of clinicians and research scientists. Many residents and fellows have become leaders in their field. Some have stayed on at Hopkins, but most have gone on to develop their own research careers at other institutions, contributing to clinical neuroscience at national and international levels. Equally important are our alumni who have practiced neurology in the community, maintaining warm relations with their former colleagues at Hopkins.

What follows is derived from the personal accounts of more than 100 alumni of Johns Hopkins Neurology who responded to our request for a summary of their main career and research achievements. We also asked for their reflections on how training at Hopkins has prepared them and influenced their intellectual growth. These individual accounts constitute the final chapter of this book, ordered chronologically to provide a series of snapshots of how the Department has evolved and flourished over a half-century.

"A Magical Place of Learning and Discovery"

From the outset, Guy McKhann and the Founding Faculty were on the lookout for bright young individuals who were curious about neurology and neuroscience, and their personal recruiting efforts proved very successful.

Residents or fellows joined the Department after coming to Hopkins as undergraduates, visiting students, Hopkins medical students, and M.D.-Ph.D. students. Others were attracted by the fame of Johns Hopkins, and the growing reputation of the department. McKhann, and soon Dick Johnson, Dan Drachman, John Freeman, Jack Griffin and others made exceptional efforts to recruit the best and brightest. For example: "As I was snowed in, Guy McKhann drove me back to his house, and he and his wife gave me a drink in front of his fireplace, fed me dinner, and late that night drove me to the airport. He was Chair and I was one of dozens of nameless applicants."

On entering the intellectual world of Johns Hopkins Neurology, many alumni were impressed by "a magical place of learning and discovery." Although they quickly realized the limits of their knowledge base, they were encouraged to ask questions, to challenge the status quo, and to look for themselves to answer the mysteries that they encountered. For many, a pivotal moment occurred during their residency that determined their future careers. This moment might have happened during the presentation of a patient to a faculty member, a journal club discussion, or through patient experiences shared with their peers. Here, mentors – in the Department, and also throughout the Hopkins community – created opportunities to follow through on nascent interests and develop career interests. They also accommodated and supported residents and fellows who decided to change their primary interest, and helped them transition to a position where they could make a new start. Such is the behavior of an academic department that functions as a family, assuming responsibility for its progeny, and helping them forward.

Our residents and fellows support and teach each other. "The greatest teachers, I felt, were my fellow residents, who had strong clinical and basic science backgrounds and tremendous academic aspirations." These bonds between residents and fellows continued after they graduated: "Watching the ever-increasing success of my co-residents and professors — many now close friends — is deeply inspiring."

Thus, even early on, "while learning the secrets and perils of clinical neurology, even without the help of CT, MRI, DNA sequencing etc., I obtained the clinical skills to continue my main field of interest: hereditary and genetic disorders."

"Guy allowed me to commit more than 90 percent of my time to research in Biochemistry in third year."

"Dick Johnson was my attending on my first month, and inoculated me with his infectious curiosity in tackling challenging cases."

"My mentor, Dan Drachman, watched me develop confidence for independent research, and in sprouting relevant clinical questions. This mindful guidance with a light touch was the key to develop and sustain my enthusiasm for the rest of my career to explore, learn, fail, and succeed."

"John Freeman encouraged me to be courageous and to challenge the status quo."

"I recall diagnosing a patient who presented with frontotemporal dementia to Dr. Griffin, which solidified my path towards becoming a cognitive neurology researcher."

"My first experience of Hopkins was in 1991 as a student, when I was lucky enough to meet Justin McArthur. We wrote a paper together on CMV encephalitis. Justin encouraged me to come back to Hopkins as a neurology resident in 1993."

Many other lessons were learned from mentors. They taught that ameliorating disease of patients is always the ultimate focus of research, and that there is always something one can do to improve a patient's lot. They stressed the importance of patient care and of teamwork between all the care providers. They pointed out that there need not be a conflict between clinical and scientific excellence, self-advancement and compassion. They taught the skills and ethics of research and the rich, bi-directional connection that can exist between clinical care and translational research. In this way, they taught the true meaning of the term 'clinician-scientist' and encouraged residents to publish their studies.

Residents and fellows also learned about collegial interactions: "During this time, I learned the importance of collaboration, both at JHU and outside." Importantly, Hopkins alumni were taught that, when they in turn became mentors, "unselfishly giving a boost to those early in their careers is one of the most rewarding services we can do."

In this way, the faculty laid the groundwork for many alumni to become competent neurologists

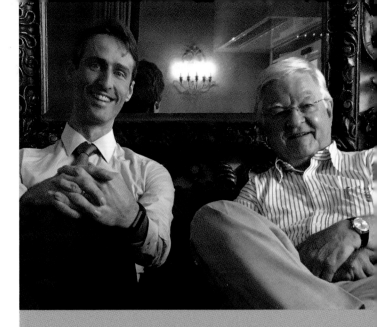

LOGAN SCHNEIDER (LEFT) **AND KLAUS TOYKA:** working on a new, more relevant type of neurologic exam training manual that reflects some "Street Fighter Neurology" style.

Mentorship and Collaboration

"It was quite a fortuitous encounter," says Logan Schneider. "I was attending the 80th Birthday Celebration and Symposium for Dr. Guy McKhann post-call during my JAR year. The reception table I sat at had Drs. Payam Mohassel and Felton (SARs at the time), as well as Prf. Dr. Klaus Toyka. We all got to talking about the neurological exam and how well trained we were."

Toyka mentioned that he was working on a syllabus to share the neurologic exam with trainees and non-neurologists. "I was particularly keen on this," Schneider continues, "as I had a desire to record all of the expertise that Hopkins Neurology was cultivating in me, and there is no better time than when in the trenches." Toyka said he saw the need for a new, more relevant type of neurologic exam training manual. "So we adapted the first drafts that had the traditional Neurologic Cerebration into a new format that reflected the 'Street Fighter Neurology' style of Dr. Raf Llinas." This project, and Toyka's mentorship, "sustained me through the many stressful days of clinical work as well as the rollercoaster of residency-based research efforts, because the project had multiple dedicated individuals to help keep it moving forward, and it leveraged the skills that I was learning and mastering throughout my residency training."

It seems likely that many research contributions made by alumni will, as the history of science tells us, eventually be recognized as pivotal events in the progress of medicine.

and independent clinician-scientists. Often these mentors remained as productive collaborators, interacting as colleagues and friends for many years. Some alumni have sent students from their own institutions to Johns Hopkins Neurology to train. Other alumni have returned as full-time or adjunct faculty. Collaborations between mentors and their students have led to a number of standard texts co-authored by our alumni, including an international collaboration on a neurology physical examination syllabus (see side story).

WHAT HAVE OUR ALUMNI GONE ON TO ACHIEVE?

Many have established, or are beginning, productive clinical and scientific careers. Some have stayed on as directors at Hopkins, while many have established new departments in other cities or countries. Our alumni have gone on to become lab chiefs and program directors, chairs of neurology and neuroscience departments, NIH program directors, editors of journals, leaders in the pharmaceutical industry, and university presidents.

We have produced public policy leaders who are influencing hospital systems, developing health access and community medicine programs, founding professional societies, promoting public intergenerational inner-city schools, directing drug safety at the Food and Drug Administration, serving as Vice President of the National Academy of Sciences, and becoming national, and international health research ambassadors.

Johns Hopkins Neurology alumni have made many discoveries, ranging from identifying mechanisms of neuronal death and protection to mechanisms of opiate addiction; understanding the role of autoimmunity in neuromuscular disease; creating models for viral disorders of the brain; defining new disease entities; and developing novel treatments for disabling disorders, such as gene therapy for neurodegenerative disorders of infants, new drugs to treat epilepsy; evidence-based therapy for stroke; and deep brain stimulation for movement disorders. In addition, it seems likely that many research contributions made by alumni will, as the history of science tells us, eventually be recognized as pivotal events in the progress of medicine. Our alumni have received many awards, including election to the Johns Hopkins Society of Scholars, the National Academy of Medicine, numerous distinguished international honors, and the Lasker-DeBakey Clinical Medical Research Award, to Mahlon R. DeLong.

WHAT DO OUR ALUMNI REMEMBER MOST ABOUT THEIR EXPERIENCE?

For many, "it is the only place I never left," because of lasting, productive friendships. It is a place where "I learned how to do research, its ethics and the value of collaboration, while making friendships that have accompanied me ever since." The Department of Neurology is remembered as a center whose reputation is justified by brilliant colleagues and a wealth of opportunities. It is a place that not only encourages inquiry, but is supportive of a change of plans. "The roots of my collaborative, multi-disciplinary approach to research originated at Hopkins." It is a place that demonstrates how a rich, bi-directional connection can exist between clinical care and translational research. A place that teaches "professionalism, empathy, humility, inquisitiveness, and, above all, persistence."

"Life is like a jigsaw puzzle – each piece is needed to form a complete picture. Hopkins has provided many of the pieces of my life that comprise that picture."

"This most exciting and inspiring period of my academic life."

"I have always felt that Hopkins Neurology was my second home."

"Few days pass without recalling my Hopkins experiences as influences on my life."

These extracts and quotes are just a representative sample of the personal accounts of Johns Hopkins Neurology alumni, which you'll find in Chapter 21. Taken together, these accounts summarize an important additional point about the development of research in the 21st century: It depends greatly on interactions – among the worldwide community of scientists; exchanges of ideas between trainees and visiting scientists from diverse backgrounds, conversations at conferences and via the internet. Based on all of these, Johns Hopkins Neurology is an important node in the worldwide scientific community; it trains, collaborates, and promotes research, and benefits from the productive collegiality that it fosters.

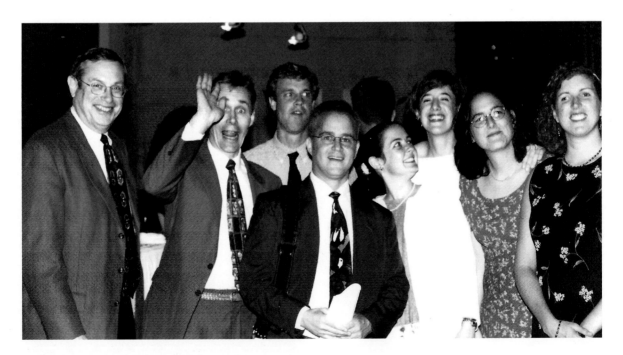

We work hard, but we also have fun together.

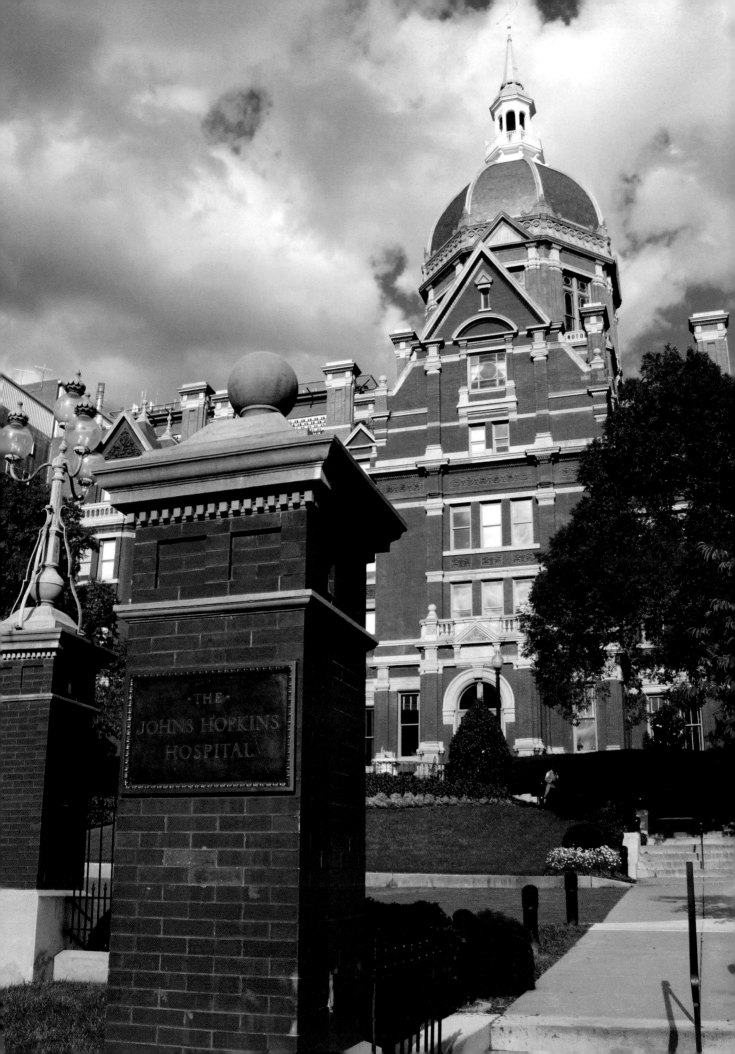

CHAPTER TWENTY-ONE

105 REFLECTIONS ON THE DEPARTMENT OF NEUROLOGY, FROM OUR ALUMNI

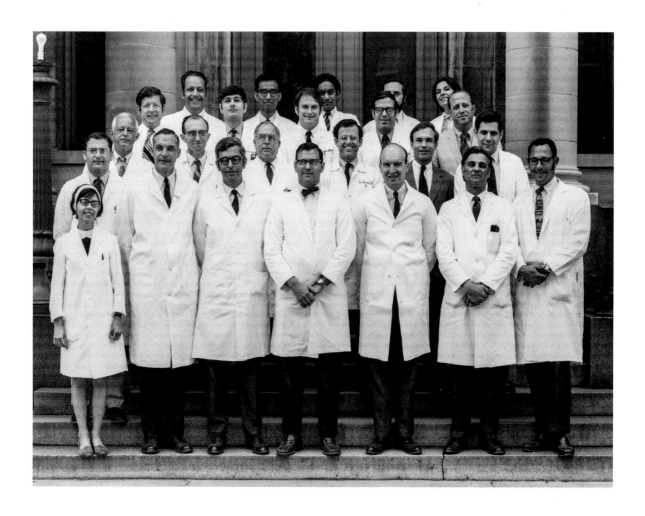

1969-1970

Front Row:
J. Benjamins
D. Drachman
R. Johnson
G. McKhann
R. Herndon
T. Preziosi
J. Freeman

Second Row:
L. Weiner
R. Teasdall
E. Niedermeyer
J. Magladery
D. Gilden
H. Moses
G. Goldstein

Third Row:
W. Logan
E. Meyer
K. Stecher
O. Limcaco
A. Percy
G. Tennekoon
H. Lipton
M. Molliver
R. Deuel
F. Schuster

Here are the personal accounts of 105 people who trained in the Department of Neurology as residents or fellows. Want to read more? Go online to www.hopkinsmedicine.org/neuro/50th, where you'll find selected publications, honors and awards, and more photos.

1969

Gary W. Goldstein, M.D.

President, Kennedy Krieger Foundation; Former President and CEO of the Kennedy Krieger Institute

My journey to Baltimore in 1969 to join the new Department of Neurology at Johns Hopkins was bittersweet. A year earlier, Guy McKhann and John Freeman had recruited me to Stanford for a fellowship in Child Neurology. The phone call from the two of them came in the spring of 1968, on the day of the last snow storm of the long winter in Minneapolis. I pictured Palm Drive leading to a hospital that looked like a resort. However, my first rotation was at the Palo Alto VA in Building D—the accurate inspiration for the book and movie, *One Flew over the Cuckoo's Nest*. The best experience there was the experimental use of L-DOPA for our own version of *Awakenings*. Guy took that summer to sail to Tahiti, and upon returning said to me, "Mate, you need to pack up. We are all moving to Baltimore." A city that was having riots and fires. My first assignment was to the newly created inpatient service on Nelson 2. Neurology was no longer a division of Medicine controlled by Osler Marines, and their most senior residents seemed unhappy about the change. Guy told me to not let them know that I (and he) were pediatricians. Every morning, we had Chief's Rounds in Guy's office and my attendings were Dick Johnson, Bob Herndon and Dan Drachman. The experience was so intense that I still remember most of the patients from that year and the battles with Osler residents, who were determined to fill our beds with difficult-to-place patients to close off admissions and keep complex neurology patients on the medical service. We successfully resisted. After a year, I was drafted and spent two years as the child neurologist for the 5th Army in Denver, completed my training at UCSF and began my faculty career in San Francisco. The next stop was Ann Arbor for 10 years and then, ever-my-mentor Guy, as chair of the search committee, brought me back to Baltimore in 1988 to the Kennedy Krieger Institute and Johns Hopkins. As of 2019, my goal is to establish a Foundation to support the clinical, educational and academic goals of the Institute.

Alan K. Percy, M.D.

Professor, Pediatrics, Neurology, Neurobiology, Genetics, and Psychology; Associate Director, Civitan International Research Center, University of Alabama at Birmingham

I was one of the original resident group at Johns Hopkins in 1969. We were thin in the first year, but expanded dramatically the second year with a notable cadre, including Jack Griffin, Dave Zee, and Gihan Tennekoon. During these two years, I was fortunate to continue research on neurodegenerative disorders begun at Stanford, continued at NIH with Roscoe Brady, and expanded by close collaboration with Mike Kaback in Pediatrics. During the third year, Guy allowed me to commit more than 90 percent of my time to research in Biochemistry under Bill Lennarz. There, I began a long, fruitful program with another post-doc, Skip Waechter, investigating the biosynthetic pathways of phospholipids in the CNS, among other systems. Thereafter, my faculty career began first in Los Angeles (UCLA) in 1972 and Baylor College of Medicine in 1979. An encounter with a young girl began the next thirty-five years of study of a rare neurodevelopmental disorder, Rett syndrome. After moving to head Child Neurology at UAB, this expanded increasingly, occupying me to the present. Those early years at Hopkins enriched my subsequent experiences with enduring friendships and continued inquiry into the neurodegenerative and neurodevelopmental disorders.

Gihan Tennekoon, M.B.B.S.

Professor, Neurology and Pediatrics, University of Pennsylvania

My Neurology residency was from 1969 through 1972. During this time, I had fantastic fellow residents with whom I have a maintained long friendships. Much of my learning of both adult and pediatric Neurology was from my fellow residents. These included Mark Moliver, Al Percy, Dave Zee and Jack Griffin, to name a few. There were others, including Ed Myer, who had a repertoire of wonderful stories. My research career was directed by Drs. McKhann and Price; in fact, Dr. McKhann not only directed my research, he supported it through lean funding times. It was Dr. McKhann who suggested that I should be a pediatric neurologist. During my time at Hopkins, I took a sabbatical in Dan Lane's laboratory, a wonderful experience.

Despite being away for 28 years, I have always felt that Hopkins Neurology was my second home.

Thanks, Dr. McKhann, for all your advice and help, and for forming such a wonderful Department of Neurology full of great people.

1970

Larry E. Davis, M.D.

Distinguished Professor, University of New Mexico and Chief, Neurology Service, Veterans Affairs Health Care System, Albuquerque

My wife and I came to Baltimore following a two-year stint in the U.S. Public Health Service. During that time, I worked for the Centers for Disease Control chasing Midwest outbreaks of "encephalitis," which were mainly foci of viral meningitis. Midway through that stint, I was sent on three-day notice to the jungles of (civil war-torn) Nigeria to work with the International Committee of the Red Cross; famine had developed. That experience was an eye-opener, as I worked in grass clinics with only a stethoscope around my neck, seeing 200 Nigerians per half-day with a limited number of medicines. My only research effort was to develop a rapid method, not requiring clinicians or nurses, to measure children with significant malnutrition; I called it the "Left Arm Circumference Method." To my amazement, 40 years later on a trip to Ethiopia, I discovered the method is still in widespread use throughout Africa.

On arrival to Baltimore in the fall of 1970, my wife and I got Hopkins simple rental housing and I started off to work as a resident. I knew Guy McKhann from my days as a medical student at Stanford, and really liked his approach to teaching about patients. I actually knew Dick Johnson during my internship year at Cleveland Metropolitan Hospital, and was impressed by the quality of his research. We were the first group of residents and discovered that there were no experienced residents above us except for a few young research faculty spending their time in the labs. Mornings were spent on the small neurology inpatient ward, and afternoons were spent seeing neurology consults throughout the Hospital. Our attendings would spend one hour a day, several days a week, seeing our most interesting patients and teaching us the basics of their neurologic illness. This was the era of no internet, and the medical library was in a separate building across the campus, so reading the neurology literature was a challenge. Whenever I goofed up on the inpatient ward, Guy would call me to visit him in his office, and we politely discussed what the problem was. It was a long time before I discovered how Guy rapidly knew about my screw-ups: It turned out that he met every morning with the head nurse, and she told him!

Guy was excellent at examining, especially children, and asking challenging questions during rounds; Dick Johnson and Dan Drachman had an amazing fund of both basic science and practical knowledge on caring for the patient. Those attending rounds sent me to the library: I was not afraid to show my lack of knowledge to the attending, but (felt) discomfort demonstrating it to my very bright fellow residents. I had the privilege of attending Dick Johnson's weekly research meeting; however, Dick made it clear that he did not want me to start any research laboratory adventures until after I had completed my Neurology residency. I did that, and am grateful for his advice to become a strong clinical neurologist before starting a research lab. In Dick's lab, I had the opportunity to work with excellent researchers and learn the basics of cell cultures, doing good animal studies, and writing grant proposals. Dick was wonderful at "reviewing" my manuscripts and always nicely improving them.

One lesson I learned was that major medical schools often had powerful fiefdoms. I had discovered an immunodeficient pediatric patient who had received the oral polio vaccine – but sadly, the vaccine back-mutated to the wild virus and was causing chronic poliomyelitis. When the Pediatric Department discovered what I had found, the chair politely informed me that they did not want my services any further and they would control the patient. When the child died, the on-call pathologist was a friend of mine and quietly let me know that the autopsy would be at 7:30 a.m., and I was welcome to collect any autopsy samples I wanted.

This became the first documentation that the polio vaccine could back-mutate in an immunodeficient individual.

Years later, when the HIV epidemic came, many cases of clinical poliomyelitis started to appear from a back-mutation of the vaccine leading to our now using only the killed polio vaccine. (After my residency), Guy invited me to remain on the junior faculty. He offered me $20K. I told him that I was already making $21K, since I was moonlighting at a local clinic on the weekends. He responded by stating he would match it. Unfortunately, homes in Baltimore were way out of my salary range, I had accumulated no money in a bank account, and now had a wife and two young children to support. Since I was studying how viruses infect the inner ear as well as other illnesses that crossed into medicine, surgery, and pediatrics services, I knew I had to find a medical school that was young and had not developed fiefdoms. This is how I found my home in New Mexico, at their brand-new medical school in Albuquerque.

William J. Logan, M.D.
Professor Emeritus, University of Toronto

During my service time at NIH, I decided to be a Pediatric Neurologist. Guy McKhann was starting a new Pediatric Neurology training program at Stanford with John Freeman that sounded appealing. I was accepted and spent the first two years of Pediatric Neurology training in Palo Alto. I then moved with Guy and John to Johns Hopkins. I finished my clinical training in 1970, and with Guy's help was accepted as a research fellow with Sol Snyder. This was a productive time, and with the excellent clinical training received in Guy's programs, I was well prepared for my academic career. My first faculty position was at The University of Virginia, where I established a Neurochemical laboratory and became Head of the Pediatric Neurology Service and training program. Six years later, I was recruited as Head of Neurology at The Hospital for Sick Children and Professor of Paediatrics and Medicine at the University of Toronto. The final phase of my career arose from my sabbatical year at Massachusetts General Hospital, where I learned fMRI basics and applied these to language localization in children. More recently I developed clinical fMRI techniques for assessment of cerebrovascular reactivity in children with cerebral vascular disease; this work is continuing at The Hospital for Sick Children. I was very fortunate to have been able to train with Guy, and to be at the start of an exciting new development at Hopkins. I have very positive memories of my experiences, of my fellow trainees, of the staff that Guy assembled and of his leadership and mentorship. Guy continued to be very supportive after I graduated, and for this I remain very appreciative and thankful. Congratulations to Guy on his great achievements.

David S. Zee, M.D.
Professor, Department of Neurology, Johns Hopkins Hospital

I was a resident from 1970 to 1973 as a member of the first full complement of trainees in Guy's new Department of Neurology. My training here laid the groundwork for my career as a physician-scientist and ultimately as an educator, largely through my exposure to my clinician mentors (my co-residents in that first class, especially Jack Griffin and Larry Davis), my scientific mentor (David A. Robinson at the Wilmer Eye Institute) and my academic mentors (Guy McKhann and the faculty he brought to Hopkins). Eye movements, vertigo and ataxia have been my clinical and scientific interests ever since.

The guiding principles I learned as a resident included: ameliorating disease of our patients is always the ultimate focus of our research: there is always something one can do to improve a patient's lot; and unselfishly giving a boost to those early in their careers is one of the most rewarding services we can do as mentors.

I will always be indebted to my chief residents, Gihan Tennekoon and Alan Percy, who taught me so much about all aspects of life, personal and professional.

Diane E. Griffin, M.D., Ph.D.
University Distinguished Service Professor, Molecular Microbiology and Immunology, Medicine and Neurology; Johns Hopkins University Schools of Medicine and Public Health. Vice President, National Academy of Sciences

Jack and I were medical students and then internal medicine residents at Stanford. In 1970, Guy McKhann recruited Jack to join the first group of neurology trainees in the new Neurology department at Johns Hopkins. I had completed a Ph.D. in immunology at Stanford and was interested in research on immune responses to virus diseases. Amongst the new JH Neurology faculty was Dick Johnson, who had a research focus on virus infections of the nervous system and was looking for postdocs. Dick's philosophy for pathogenesis research involved assembly of people with multiple types of expertise. I became the immunologist. Others in the initial Traylor Building research group included faculty Les Weiner (neurology, virus-induced demyelination) and Bob Herndon (neuropathologist) and postdocs Henry McFarland (neurology, immunology), Opendra (Bill) Narayan (veterinarian, virology) and Howard Lipton (neurology).

I began working on encephalomyelitis in mice caused by Sindbis virus, a mosquito-borne virus that Dick had studied while he was in Australia.

This has continued to be a fruitful model for dissecting the interactions between virus-infected neurons and the immune response. During a visiting professorship in Lima, Peru, Dick noted many patients who had developed encephalomyelitis as a complication of measles. Thus began our studies on the pathogenesis of measles and its complications, which I have continued in Zambia and in experimentally infected macaques. I joined the faculty in the Infectious Diseases Division with a joint appointment in Neurology in 1973. From 1994 through 2014, I was chair of the Department of Molecular Microbiology and Immunology in the School of Public Health.

Robert Ouvrier, A.C., M.D., FRACP
Emeritus Professor, The Children's Hospital at Westmead, Parramatta, Australia

I was born in Perth, Western Australia, but have lived in Sydney for most of my life. (After medical school at Sydney University), I interned at the Royal Prince Alfred Hospital, which has had a long association with Johns Hopkins Hospital since the Second World War. I spent six months in Papua New Guinea, working as a general pediatrician. My initial training in pediatric neurology commenced in Melbourne, under the tutorship of Ian Hopkins – who, himself, had been trained at Hopkins Hospital. I then trained in pediatric neurology with David Clark in Lexington, Kentucky. After 18 months working with Clark, Michael McQuillen and Doug Jamieson, I was accepted in the new Neurological department at Hopkins in 1970, working with Guy McKhann, John Freeman, Dan Drachman, and a group of very enthusiastic trainees in adult and pediatric neurology. In

both Lexington and Baltimore, my family and I received a warm and generous welcome, excellent support and supervised autonomy in learning the art and science of Neurology with excellent training in the ancillary skills of the specialty, such as neuroradiology: we performed angiography, PEGs, nerve conduction studies and EEG interpretation. In the laboratory of Paul Lietman, I did some early work on assays of serum anticonvulsant levels.

Another major opportunity was Frank Walsh and David Knox's Saturday morning sessions on Neuro-ophthalmology in the Wilmer Institute: these excellent teaching sessions stimulated my interest in the field and led to several papers.

Johns Hopkins also kindled an interest in basic research, which I continued on my return to Sydney: at first in anticonvulsant assays, but later in neuromuscular research, focusing particularly on peripheral neuropathies. I have written a textbook on these conditions in childhood, assisted by Professors James McLeod and John Pollard in Sydney, where I returned in 1972. Due to the confidence that training in medicine at The Johns Hopkins Hospital creates, I was appointed to the first Chair of Pediatric Neurology in Australia. There is no doubt in my mind that Johns Hopkins has played a key part in my personal evolution and development. I will never forget my debt of gratitude!

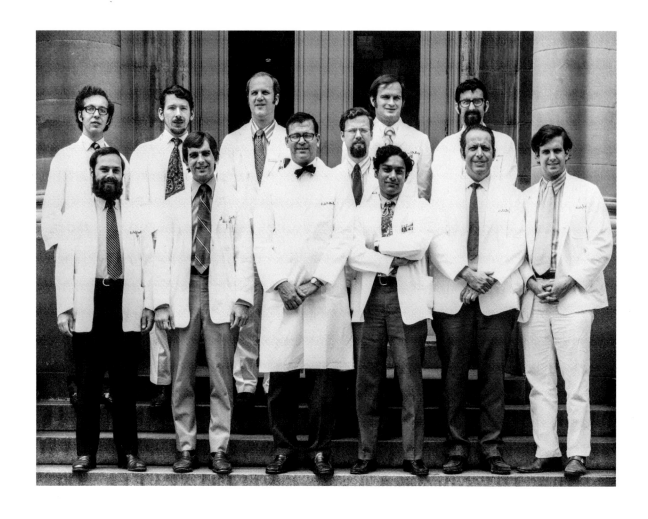

1970-1971

Front Row:
M. Molliver
D. Ginter
G. McKhann
G. Tennekoon
E. Myer
D. Zee

Second Row:
E. Sperber
R. Haller
L. Davis
D. Benjamins
A. Percy
R. Ouvrier

"The research and mentorship experience in pediatric neurology and neuroscience I have received from faculty in Neurology and other departments at Hopkins have had an indelible effect on my career." – Michael V. Johnston, M.D.

1971

Michael V. Johnston, M.D.

Professor, Departments of Neurology, Pediatrics and Physical Medicine and Rehabilitation, Johns Hopkins Medicine; Blum Moser Endowed Chair for Pediatric Neurology; and Director, Neuroscience Laboratory, Hugo Moser Research Institute, Kennedy Krieger Institute

I was a resident in pediatrics at Johns Hopkins from 1971 to 1974 when I met Guy McKhann, during one of his mesmerizing teaching sessions in pediatric neurology. He made a strong impression on me, and influenced me to go into pediatric neurology. After spending two years in research in the U.S. Army in Washington, D.C., I returned to Hopkins to begin my residency in Pediatric Neurology under the direction of John Freeman and Guy. I was impressed by the focus on research in adult neurology at Hopkins, and I decided I wanted to prepare for an academic career combining pediatric neurology with neuroscience research. In addition to Guy and John, I discussed my interests with Hugo Moser at the Kennedy Institute, Paul Lietman in Clinical Pharmacology, and Joe Coyle in Psychiatry and Pharmacology, all at Hopkins. Guy worked out a plan in which I could combine training in adult and pediatric neurology with research in basic and clinical neuropharmacology over four years. This experience was very successful. At the end of my training, Gary Goldstein recruited me to join him in his new pediatric neurology program at the University of Michigan in Ann Arbor and start my own lab. After seven years at Michigan, I was promoted to the rank of Professor, and the following year, Gary was recruited to become the President of the Kennedy Krieger Institute. I joined him in the move to Baltimore as the Chief Medical Officer and Executive Vice President of Kennedy Krieger, a position I held for 30 years. The research and mentorship experience in pediatric neurology and neuroscience I have received from faculty in Neurology and other departments at Hopkins have had an indelible effect on my career.

Vernon D. Rowe, M.D.

President and CEO, Rowe Neurology Institute, Lenexa, Kansas, President and CEO, Neurrow Pharamceuticals, Inc., Adjunct Professor of Neurology, University of Kansas School of Medicine

My time at Duke, Hopkins, and the NIH helped hone a vision for what a physician-scientist can be. After completing my Neurology residency at Hopkins in 1977, I joined the faculty of the University of Kansas School of Medicine, combining clinical practice with a basic research program using primary cultures of pineal cells and sympathetic neurons. After rising through the academic ranks, I founded the independent Rowe Neurology Institute in Lenexa. The Rowe Neurology Institute has three arms: clinical practice, including sleep laboratory and neuroimaging, a nonprofit research foundation which does basic and clinical research, and a drug development incubator. The clinical practice is a tertiary referral center specializing in multiple sclerosis, headache, sleep, and hypermobility syndrome – the latter arising from our observed links among migraine, sleep disorders and joint hypermobility. With my wife, Elizabeth Rowe, Ph.D., M.B.A., I founded Verrow Pharmaceuticals, which recently sold to Ligand Pharmaceuticals, Inc. Its first product, a kidney-safe iodinated contrast agent, is slated to enter the clinic in early 2019. Neurrow Pharmaceuticals is focused on neurodegenerative disease. We have two sons and five grandkids, and our hobbies include flying, sailing, bluegrass music, cowboy mounted shooting, and writing.

Saty Satya-Murti, M.D.

Formerly, Professor of Neurology, Albany Medical College, Albany, New York; Health Policy Consultant, Santa Maria, California; Medicare Medical Director, panelist and Vice-Chair Medcac (Medicare Evidence & Coverage Advisory Committee

My medical school and residency training urged us to follow, not question, and learn from extraordinary and talented preceptors.

Hopkins Neurology Department, barely two years old in 1971, chose its fellows carefully. The emphasis was on independent inquiry and creative autonomy.

This environment, antipodal to my background, raised both hope and anxiety. My mentor, Dan Drachman, advised and encouraged – but left all details to me. This was a new culture, and I struggled. Dan was generous with his praise and mild with criticisms. He discouraged the effortless way out: declining to get me a digital averager, or a technician for processing histochemistry slides. He supervised my motor-point biopsies, key to our myasthenia gravis studies, without micromanagement. He let me develop our "rodent ICU" to keep our cobra-toxin-blockade rats alive for 12 hrs. Little did I realize that he was watching me develop confidence for independent research. This mindful guidance with a light touch was the key to develop and sustain my enthusiasm for the rest of my career to explore, learn, fail, and succeed. It was a giddy time. All this learning to the accompaniment of Mozart's A major clarinet concerto, exposure to colleagues' research projects and Wednesday late neuromuscular rounds!

Marjorie E. Seybold, M.D., MPIA
Retired Adjunct Professor of Neurosciences, University of California, San Diego

I had the pleasure of working at Hopkins from July 1970 to December 1972. The first year, I was a fellow in neuro-ophthalmology at the Wilmer Institute, working under Drs. Frank Walsh and David Knox. Since my fellowship was unfunded, I had several moonlighting jobs, including the reading of EEGs under the supervision of Ernst Niedermeyer, one of the most learned and kindest of mentors. Through this job, I also got to know the neurology resident group, including David Zee, Ed Myer, Larry Davis, Jack Griffin, Gihan Tennekoon and Al Percy, all of whom became lifelong friends. After completing my

fellowship, I joined the faculty of Neurology and Ophthalmology, and had the good fortune to work with Dan Drachman in his neuromuscular clinic. I had a previous interest in myasthenia gravis, and Dan kindly shared his patients and expertise. Guy McKhann and Dick Johnson encouraged my use of EMG, a tactic that wasn't widely used at Hopkins at that time. I carried this acquired experience to my next job at the new University of California-San Diego, Medical School, where I was able develop both neuro-ophthalmology and EMG services.

1972

Alan Pestronk, M.D.
Professor, Departments of Neurology and Pathology & Immunology; Director, Neuromuscular Clinical Laboratory, Washington University School of Medicine, Saint Louis

I was a medical student at Johns Hopkins in 1969 when Guy McKhann arrived. At our teaching conferences that year, Guy reaffirmed to me that Neurology was an interesting and rewarding specialty. He eliminated unnecessary formality by removing our *de rigueur* striped ties to test optokinetic nystagmus in patients. I was a member of the second class of residents in Guy's Neurology Department; I trained with wonderful senior residents Dave Zee, Jack Griffin and Larry Davis, and co-residents Ron Haller, Ray Roos and Allan Krumholz. Guy recruited Dan Drachman, my mentor, to head our neuromuscular group. Over 15 years, Dan taught me the importance of hard work and honesty, and the joy of scientific and clinical neuroscience, neuromuscular pathology, and teaching. Our neuromuscular teaching program at Washington University has trained over 100 fellows since I arrived in 1989. We also developed the Neuromuscular Disease Center website, an online resource that is visited each day by over 1,000 medical professionals from 100 countries.

Ian John Butler, M.B., B.S., FRACP

Professor, Departments of Pediatrics and Neurology, McGovern Medical School at The University of Texas Health Science Center, Houston

My background included training as a pediatrician (Australia) and in both pediatric and adult neurology (Australia, United Kingdom). I was instructed by Queen Square London-trained neurologists and electromyographers and was taught that myasthenia gravis was a "presynaptic disorder" based on electrophysiological parameters. Imagine my surprise after rotating with Dan Drachman and assisting him in performing "motor point biopsies" when I realized that my knowledge base was incomplete! Shortly thereafter as a resident, I had an unique opportunity to collaborate with established investigative biochemists and geneticists while describing a new neurometabolic disorder. With encouragement and advice from faculty (Guy McKhann, John Freeman, Mark Moliver) and a couple of years of concentrated effort, we demonstrated the pivotal role of defective biogenic amine metabolism and designed specific innovative treatment. After several false starts, Dan Drachman encouraged submission of my first basic neuroscience manuscript to one of his favorite journals. I finally could call myself a "triple threat" in academic neurology! In 1976, I transported my wife, Patricia, and three children to Houston to establish the Division of Child Neurology at this new medical school in Houston, Texas. I persuaded Harvey Singer to take over my Tourette Syndrome clinic in Baltimore. We continued to collaborate long-distance; our cerebrospinal fluid studies of biogenic amines were beginning to be fruitful. Initially, I was concerned at moving to an academic position in a new and growing medical school. Fortunately, my extensive training, particularly my formative experiences at Johns Hopkins, enabled me to grow and thrive in this dynamic environment in the largest medical center in the world (Texas hyperbole).

Allan Krumholz, M.D.

Professor Emeritus, Department of Neurology, University of Maryland School of Medicine

In 1970, I came for an internship at the former Baltimore City Hospitals, and one of my rotations was Neurology at Hopkins. This led to my entering the Hopkins Neurology residency. I shared wonderful experiences with co-residents including David Zee, Jack Griffin, and Alan Pestronk. Caring faculty such as John Freeman and Ernst Niedermeyer cultivated my career in epilepsy care and electroencephalographic studies. Later with Guy McKhann's support, we established a Hopkins-affiliated Neurology program and residency at the Sinai Hospital of Baltimore. We were fortunate to recruit two great Neurology faculty just starting their academic careers, Howard Weiss and Barney Stern.

Together, we built a special Hopkins-affiliated community academic neurology program and had great fun.

In 1989, Greg Bergey recruited me to the University of Maryland's Epilepsy Center, and later I became the Director of the Epilepsy Program when Greg returned to Hopkins. I continued to enjoy valuable collaborations with current and former Hopkins colleagues such as Bob Fisher and Greg Krauss. I enjoy fond memories of my productive times at Hopkins and continued positive associations.

Natan Gadoth, M.D.

Chairman of Neurology, Maynei Hayeshua Medical Center, Bnei Barak and Professor (Emeritus) of Neurology, Sackler Faculty of Medicine, Tel-Aviv University, Israel

I had already a keen interest and some clinical experience with rare neurological disorders in specific ethnic groups in Israel when I started my residency in Pediatric Neurology with Dr. J. Freeman. While learning the secrets and perils of clinical neurology, even without the help of CT, MRI, DNA sequencing etc., I obtained the clinical skills to continue my main field of interest: hereditary and genetic disorders. This was a period blessed with the privilege to be guided by "John" (Dr. Freeman) and learn from Dr. G. McKhann, Dr. Ian Butler and my fellow residents, some of whom I am still in touch with. My time with Dr. McKusick at the Moore clinic was indeed the determinant of my career and research after returning to Israel.

In the years to come, I was able to outline a few neuro-hereditary disorders among specific ethnic groups in Israel, and also, together with a few colleagues, to build the first steps toward establishing Pediatric Neurology as an independent specialty in Israel.

Harvey S. Singer, M.D.

Professor, Neurology and Pediatrics, Johns Hopkins University

After completing my military obligation, I came to the Johns Hopkins Hospital in 1972 as a pediatric neurology resident under the mentorship of Dr. John Freeman. Fully recognizing the enormous clinical and research benefits of this Institution, I am pleased to note that I never left. During my tenure, I have had the honor and privilege of advancing the field of child neurology, serving in various roles including Director of Child Neurology at Johns Hopkins for 20 years, President and Secretary–Treasurer of the Professors of Child Neurology, Secretary-Treasurer for the United Council of Neurological Specialties, and within the Child Neurology Society; Chairman of the Resident Match and Training Committees, and Secretary–Treasurer. My clinical research interests have included movement disorders, especially Tourette syndrome and stereotypies, as well as several proposed autoimmune disorders.

Under my leadership, Johns Hopkins Hospital was selected as a Tourette Association of America Center of Excellence.

In the laboratory, translational research-oriented activities have focused on the neurobiology of human movement disorders, the pathophysiology of repetitive movements in animal models, and autoimmune mechanisms in autism and PANDAS. With the support of multiple colleagues, residents, and technicians, NIH funding, and private philanthropy, I have authored numerous articles, chapters, and three books; the latest, a must-read text, entitled *Movement Disorders in Childhood*. Enjoyable activities include biking, travel, visiting my five grandchildren, and work.

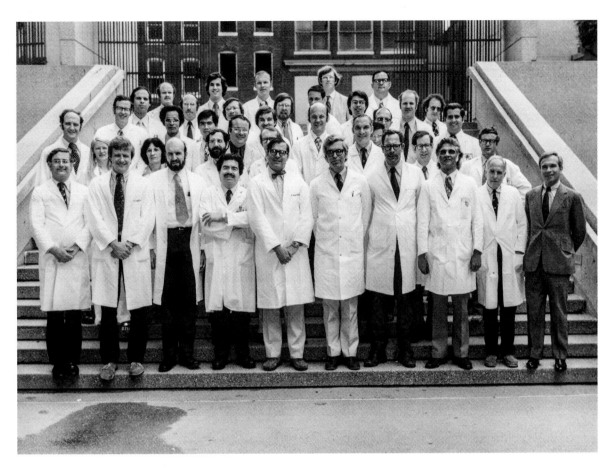

1974-1975

Front Row:
L. Weiner
D. Price
R. Herndon
O. Marin
G. McKhann
R. Johnson
J. Freeman
T. Preziosi
J. Magladery
H. Moses

Second Row:
A. Zimmerman
M. Oster-Granite
M. Mazlo
R. Morrell
R. Haslam
H. McFarland
M. DeLong
D. Drachman
R. Roos
N. Gadoth

Third Row:
S. Goldstein
B. D'Souza
L. Kao
K. Toyka
J. Burks
D. Jackson
C. Lao-Velez
K. Hennessey
E. Niedermeyer
L. Davis
S. Cohen
R. Polinsky

Back Row:
D. Bachman
W. Leahy
H. Singer
B. Gordon
R. Skoff
M. Graves
R. Moxon
T. Sprinkle

1974

Barry Gordon, M.D., Ph.D.

Therapeutic Cognitive Neuroscience Professor; Professor of Neurology with a Joint Appointment in Cognitive Science, Johns Hopkins University and Medical Institutions

My training, experience, and colleagues at Hopkins (1974—present) have been critical in helping me crystalize several goals and make progress in achieving those goals: to understand human cognition at the micro-architectural level, and how operations at this level relate to neural processes; to understand what goes wrong in developmental and acquired disorders from this perspective; and to devise solutions using any methods possible. Originally, my work focused on aphasia and memory disorders, including amnesia and the dementias. For the past 20-plus years, it has also encompassed autism and related developmental disorders. To these ends, I established the subdiscipline of Cognitive Neurology, within Behavioral Neurology, to emphasize the need to take cognitive operations per se into account. I founded the Cognitive Neurology/Neuropsychology Division and Memory Clinic of the Neurology Department at Hopkins (with Ola Selnes, Barbara J. Mroz, Deborah Hasenauer, and John Hart) to foster collaboration between clinical and research efforts. Most recently, I created an educational program for individuals with low-functioning autism with the indispensable assistance of educators such as Jessica O'Grady and Olivia Pullara. Among the many teachers and colleagues I most deeply appreciate for my training and experience at Hopkins are: Oscar Marin and Guy McKhann; Alfonso Caramazza and Rita Berndt; Ronald Lesser; Walter Stewart; and Dana Boatman. My patients and research subjects continue to be inspiring, motivating, and humbling as well.

Ronald J. Polinsky, M.D.

Vice President & Scientific Director, Global Clinical Neuroscience, AstraZeneca Adjunct Professor of Neurology, Ohio State University College of Medicine, Columbus, Ohio; Chief, Clinical Neuropharmacology Section, Clinical Neuroscience Branch, NINDS, Bethesda (retired)

My training in neurology at Johns Hopkins (1973-1977) provided me with a solid foundation for a successful career in clinical research at the NINDS, and later within the pharmaceutical industry research environment. The attending physicians who most influenced my career interests in degenerative neurological disorders were Guy McKhann, Oscar Marin, and Tom Preziosi. While at the NIH, I developed a world-class neuropharmacology research program focused on neurotransmitter and neuropeptide function in autonomic disorders, including multiple system atrophy. Using a variety of neurochemical and pharmacological strategies, I demonstrated that it was possible to distinguish between central and peripheral forms of autonomic failure. My program on autonomic disorders also led to a collaboration with Sir Roger Bannister; together, we published the first large, multinational experience in these relatively rare disorders. In addition, I became interested in the dominantly inherited form of Alzheimer's disease and began a longitudinal study of clinical, biochemical and imaging markers in affected and at-risk members from the large pedigrees under investigation. Most importantly, I organized the first international collaboration that successfully linked a region on chromosome 21 with the disease in four very large pedigrees with the disorder. After assuming a leadership role in pharmaceutical research, I participated in the selection of research targets and guided the clinical development of therapeutic strategies for treating a variety of neurological disorders, including Alzheimer's disease.

Andrew W. Zimmerman, M.D.

Professor, Pediatrics and Neurology, UMass Memorial Medical School, Worcester, Massachusetts

Over the 40 years since neurology training at Johns Hopkins, my appreciation has increased for the faculty and the culture they developed for thoughtful patient care and scholarship.

The spark and drive of our mentors inspired my own commitment to the field. This led me on a circular route to UConn, to practice in Tennessee, back to Kennedy Krieger and Hopkins, then MGH and finally, UMass. Along the way, I have come to appreciate first-hand the value of having pediatric neurology training incorporated within the Department and closely associated with our adult colleagues – as at Hopkins, which emphasizes the fundamentals of neurology and neuroscience throughout the lifespan. In practice, I cared for adults as well as children, and became interested in autism (which was "discovered" at Hopkins by Leo Kanner, literally across the wall in child psychiatry, but I rarely saw it!). With colleagues I have investigated immunological and metabolic features of autism. This led to collaboration with Paul Talalay and colleagues at Hopkins on studies of sulforaphane in the treatment and search for biomarkers in autism. Today, the neuroscience of autism is foremost in this lifelong disorder, which underscores the continuum between pediatric and adult neurology.

1975

Gavril W. Pasternak, M.D., Ph.D.

Anne Burnett Tandy Chair of Neurology, Laboratory Chair, Molecular Pharmacology Program, Memorial Sloan Kettering Cancer Center, New York

Having received my undergraduate, M.D. and Ph.D. degrees from Hopkins, I consider myself fully "Hopkins Trained." The training I took with me is heavily based upon both my scientific and clinical years. My tutelage under Dr. Solomon H. Snyder and the chemists in the Department of Pharmacology gave me the tools to study the chemical biology of opioids and their receptors for more than 40 years. Our work has established the importance in alternative gene splicing in G-protein coupled receptor function and uncovered a new molecular target that is leading to safer, more effective analgesics. What has set my group apart has been our focus on integrating our molecular observations with behavior and physiology. My training in neurology provided me with a general understanding of the nervous system and an appreciation of the complexity and subtlety of sensation. I brought this to Memorial Sloan Kettering Cancer Center, where I integrated my clinical work in neuro-oncology and pain with my laboratory work, providing a unique perspective that proved invaluable in establishing the direction of research.

Life is like a jigsaw puzzle – each piece is needed to form a complete picture. Hopkins has provided many of the pieces of my life that comprise that picture.

1976

Klaus V. Toyka, M.D., FRCP

Emeritus Professor and Chair of Neurology, University of Wurzburg, Germany, Adjunct Professor of Neurology, Johns Hopkins University

My time as a neuromuscular fellow in the lab of Daniel B. Drachman (1974-1976) was instrumental in my career as a clinician-scientist. The experimental work in myasthenia gravis initiated a new translational research strategy, identifying pathogenic autoantibodies in putative human autoimmune disorders. This became the focus of my clinical and experimental work after returning to Germany: in several neurological disorders, autoantibodies could be defined as partly or entirely causative pathogenic agents. We also tested various treatment strategies in rodent models elucidating disease mechanism. This occasionally paved the way toward clinical applications, including new modes of plasma exchange, new drugs, and target-specific antibodies. After (my) mandatory retirement in 2010, John W. (Jack) Griffin and Justin McArthur invited me to return as part-time faculty for collaborative projects. In addition, the e-book on Neurological Examination was inspired by Logan Schneider at Hopkins Neurology and was published online in 2016, becoming a practical source in Europe and beyond. My connection with Hopkins for over four decades was instrumental in my professional life. My separate field of interest was playing and performing chamber music as an amateur violinist, starting in 1974 with Daniel Drachman, an amateur clarinetist. This activity ultimately led to serving the Neurology Department with music performances at various occasions, lately together with Peabody pianist Arno Drucker.

1977

R. John Leigh, M.D.

Blair-Daroff Emeritus Professor of Neurology, Case Western Reserve University, Cleveland, Ohio; Adjunct Professor of Neurology, Johns Hopkins University

My time as a Neurology Fellow/Faculty at Hopkins (1977-1983), under the tutelage of mathematician-biologist David Robinson and clinician scientist David Zee, was the formative period of my scientific career. I established the foundations of my field of research – which overlaps neurology, ophthalmology, and computation neuroscience – and had my first successful research projects, developing models for periodic alternating nystagmus (providing insights for treatment), eye movements in Huntington's disease (with Susan and Marshall Folstein), and eye movements in unconscious patients (with Daniel Hanley). My subsequent career as a clinician scientist at Case Western Reserve University built upon these interests, focusing on how the rotational and translational vestibulo-ocular reflexes serve vision during natural activities, and malfunction in neurological disease; evaluating treatments for pathological forms of nystagmus; and applying the advantages offered by eye movements to better understand diseases ranging from myasthenia gravis to multiple sclerosis to Parkinsonian disorders.

This interest in translational research, shared with my Hopkins mentor, David Zee, led to the publication of five editions of our book, The Neurology of Eye Movements. *Thus, my time at Hopkins not only prepared me for my career but also led to lasting, productive friendships.*

Hamilton Moses III, M.D.

Founder and Chairman, The Alerion Institute, Charlottesville, Virginia; Adjunct Professor of Neurology, Johns Hopkins University School of Medicine

Johns Hopkins, in his 1873 bequest, set clear hopes for the institutions' clinical and academic programs: Because we will always be surrounded by human suffering, they must afford the best care. Because new knowledge will be necessary, they must find it. Those expectations have underpinned neurology for the past half-century. My contribution has been to help sustain and strengthen the ability to do so. By the early 1980s, it had become evident to Guy McKhann, Donlin Long, and Robert Heyssel that the primary challenges for medicine would come from the outside: whims of insurers, growing dependence on the NIH, limitless demand for care, and challenging economics. They reasoned that internal organizational limitations, paradoxically strong at the very best hospitals, would hinder their ability to realize the promise of burgeoning scientific opportunities. My career has been built on those observations, as chief physician of the JHH (1988-1994), as an early architect of the Massachusetts General-Brigham-Partners system in Boston (1995-1998, alongside JH alumni Eugene Braunwald, Samuel Thier, Anne Young), and latterly as head of the science and technology practice of The Boston Consulting Group, a large international strategy firm.

The JH Neurology tradition of, "act first, ask permission later" has served well.

Randall R. Long, M.D., Ph.D.

Dartmouth Hitchcock Neurology, Keene, New Hampshire

My ten years at the Hopkins (1970-1980; M.D., Ph.D., Neurology residency) provided a liberal education in the biomedical sciences and an excellent foundation in clinical Neurology. I have subsequently been at times a teacher, at too many times an administrator, often a clinical neurophysiologist, but always a general neurologist. I enjoyed 28 years on the University of Massachusetts medical faculty, the final six years as interim chair. It was my pleasure to span the David Drachman and Robert Brown eras at that institution. For the past decade, I have been a country neurologist, living and working in the Monadnock region of southwestern New Hampshire. I will retire the end of this calendar year. I have loved every minute of neurology practice.

1978

Orest Hurko, M.D.

Senior Clinical Consultant, Vertex Pharmaceuticals; Associate Professor, Sackler School of Graduate Biomedical Sciences, Tufts University; Professor (Hon.) of Medicine, Nursing and Dentistry, University of Dundee

By the time that I came to Johns Hopkins as resident /faculty (1978 – 1998) I had already realized that success demanded choices. However, I hadn't yet framed them correctly. Dan Drachman, Mahlon Delong, John Leigh, Hugo Moser, Victor McKusick, Harvey Singer, Guy McKhann, David Zee, Neil Miller, Tony Murphy, David Valle, Marshall and Susan Folstein taught me that there needn't be a conflict between clinical and scientific excellence, neuroscience and genetics, self-advancement and compassion. Rather, it was finding that unique niche into which these all fit. With Guy's unflinching support, I devoted my time both to the Neurology and Genetics Clinics, as well as neurogenetics rounds with Richard Kelly and SakkuBai Naidu at the Kennedy-Krieger. My next major revelation occurred two decades after my arrival in Baltimore. Translating understanding of pathophysiology of neurogenetic diseases into effective therapies required greater resources than I was able to marshal as an academic. Following the example of Dennis Choi, I swallowed my pride and joined the satanic mills of industry, where I have contributed to the registration of two novel medicines and am now designing gene therapy trials for neurodegenerative disorders of infants. I no longer have my own patients but do teach.

Raymond S. Kandt, M.D.

Hospital Neurologist, Howard County General Hospital Johns Hopkins Medical Institutions

My neurology residency at Hopkins included an additional three months as chief resident on adult neurology and occurred concurrently with a fellowship in developmental pediatrics at the Kennnedy-Krieger Center (Hugo Moser, director). John Freeman and Hugo Moser helped me craft a program as the first jointly trained neurodevelopmentalist at Hopkins. One of my mentors, Gihan Tennekoon, triggered my interest in neurocutaneous diseases. I then joined Michael Johnston and Gary Goldstein as a child neurologist at the University of Michigan in Ann Arbor. Recruitment to Duke Med Center by Bernie D'Souza, who had been a faculty mentor at Hopkins, allowed me to explore neurogenetics with Allen Roses. This led to genetic discoveries in tuberous sclerosis complex. My next phase was Chief of Child Neurology at Wake Forest Medical Center in Winston-Salem, NC. A 14-year interlude of private-practice adult and child neurology in central North Carolina preceded my return to Wake Forest neurology faculty. Prior to my first grandson, I returned to Baltimore and my position as an adult neurohospitalist at Howard County General Hospital.

The rigorous clinical training, enthusiastic joy of discovery, and flexibility at Hopkins formed the underpinning for my career.

Peter J. Whitehouse, M.A. (bioethics), M.D., Ph.D.

Professor, Neurology, Psychiatry, Neuroscience, Cognitive Science, and Organizational Behavior, Case Western Reserve University, Cleveland, Ohio; Professor of Medicine (Neurology) University of Toronto

After undergraduate work in the now Bloomberg School of Public Health and obtaining my M.D.-Ph.D. at Johns Hopkins with field work at Harvard and Boston University, I was fortunate to complete a Neurology Residency followed by a Fellowship in Neuroscience and Psychiatry and an initial faculty appointment at John Hopkins. My early work at Hopkins with a team led by Don Price and others involved studies of the basal forebrain and other subcortical nuclei in Alzheimer's, Parkinson's and Huntington's followed by discoveries of associated neurotransmitter losses in the same conditions and others. I was then recruited to Case Western Reserve University to start what became the second-best funded Alzheimer's program in the U.S., with both NIMH and NIA Center designations. I directed the center for ten years and worked internationally to develop the first-generation Alzheimer's drugs. After further training in bioethics and organizational development, I became critical of overly reductionist biomedical conceptions of dementia. I assumed leadership positions in geriatrics, ethics, and then public health. In 2000, my wife (also a Hopkins graduate) and others founded the world's first public intergenerational schools serving inner-city Cleveland children and elders, some with cognitive impairment. Currently, I am focusing on prevention and health consequences of environmental deterioration, such as pollution and climate change, using for me a new set of tools from the arts and humanities, including narrative, history, photography, videography, music, dance, and performance art (my character, Sylvanus is a metaphorical transdisciplinary Tree Doctor). I remain a scientist as well, but a skeptic of scientism and a critic of neoliberalism.

1979

Gregory K. Bergey, M.D.

Professor, Department of Neurology, Johns Hopkins School of Medicine; Director, Johns Hopkins Epilepsy Center

I came to Hopkins to do my Neurology residency (1979 to 1983) after a postdoctoral fellowship in neurophysiology with Phil Nelson at the NIH.

Those were the days before a resident match, and Neurology was still a relatively new department at Hopkins.

I was impressed not just with the energy of the faculty, but also with their commitment to academic neurology. Even the best researchers were great clinicians and attendings. Because I was initially a cellular physiologist, after residency I moved across town to the University of Maryland departments of neurology and physiology, where I later helped establish the Maryland Epilepsy Center and worked with Alan Krumholz, among others. I was fortunate to be able to return to Hopkins Neurology in 1999, then chaired by Jack Griffin. By then, my clinical interests had developed and my research had evolved from cellular physiology to studies of human seizure dynamics, something that fit well with my clinical investigations of closed loop neurostimulation. I have been active in the American Epilepsy Society as a Board member and am one of the founding editors of their successful journal, *Epilepsy Currents*. Here at Hopkins, over the past two decades, over 75 percent of our epilepsy fellows have gone on to full-time academic positions, reflecting the continued mission of Hopkins Neurology.

William C. Mobley, M.D., Ph.D.

Florence Riford Chair for Alzheimer's Disease Research, Distinguished Professor of Neurosciences, University of California-San Diego

The Hopkins Neurology residency showed me what an extraordinarily rich environment can accomplish for teaching how to care for neurology patients, and the importance of linking basic and translational research advances to care. Critical to the Hopkins experience were devoted faculty mentors including Guy McKhann, Dick Johnson, Dan Drachman, Jack Griffin, Don Price, Mike Johnston and John Freemen. The lessons taught, and the support provided, continue to guide me. Indeed, the direction for my research was influenced by discoveries made during residency. Two were critical: first, Mike Johnston and Joe Coyle showed that the nucleus basalis neurons were responsible for cholinergic innervation of the cortex; second, Peter Whitehouse and Don Price showed that these neurons degenerated in Alzheimer's disease. Studies suggesting that nerve growth factor NGFa protein, which I studied as an M.D.-Ph.D. student at Stanford under Eric Shooter, could be a trophic factor for these neurons inspired me to explore this topic.

Now, many years later, the answers to the many questions raised at that time have been answered in part, as my lab and many others continue to explore a role for failed neurotrophic factor support in the pathogenesis of Alzheimer's disease, including Alzheimer's in Down syndrome.

Amy (Fremion) Chappell, M.D.

Vice President (Neuroscience), Pharmaceutical Product Development (PPD), Naples, Florida

In 1979, I suddenly found myself with a year between completing years of a pediatrics residency at JHH and beginning a neurology residency at Indiana University Medical Center. John Freeman invited me to be his first-ever pediatric epilepsy fellow. What initially seemed like a setback in my career became one of its best years ever! In addition to teaching me about the care of pediatric seizure patients,

John Freeman encouraged me to be courageous and to challenge the status quo. Patti Vining demonstrated for me humility, empathy and ways to find humor in even the most heart-breaking situations.

Diana Pillas exemplified for me excellence in patient care and advocacy. Ernst Niedermeyer taught me how to read EEGs. I established a network of experts and friends in Neurology that has been invaluable throughout my career. Since leaving Hopkins in 1980, I completed a neurology residency, became an assistant professor in Neurology (Child), and worked for Eli Lilly and Company for 25 years, conducting clinical trials in all phases of drug development across a broad array of neurological indications. I have continued to practice clinical neurology throughout my career and continue to volunteer now at The Neighborhood Health Clinic in Naples, Florida. In 2017, I passed the inaugural Lifestyle Medicine board examination, and facilitate The Complete Health Improvement Program at the Greater Naples YMCA.

1980

Robert S. Fisher, M.D., Ph.D.

Maslah Saul Professor of Neurology, Stanford University Medical Center

When I interviewed for Johns Hopkins Neurology residency, I had already made up my mind to go elsewhere. But a snowstorm prevented my return to California. As I was snowed in, Guy McKhann drove me back to his house and he and his wife gave me a drink in front of his fireplace, fed me dinner, and late that night drove me to the airport. He was chair and I was one of dozens of nameless applicants. So I spent the next 12 years at Hopkins. I opened my first lab at Hopkins studying hippocampal slices and epilepsy in 1983. Hopkins Neuroscience was so dominated by the pioneering extracellular sensory physiology studies of Vernon Mountcastle that my tiny lab was one of the only intracellular labs at the Medical Center. Over time, I moved away from studying epilepsy drugs and towards epilepsy devices. Together with the late surgeon, Sumio Uematsu, we performed the first controlled trial of deep-brain stimulation for epilepsy. Decades later, this has contributed to neurostimulation becoming available as a new therapy (in several flavors) for refractory epilepsy. On the clinical side, I watched my advisor, John Freeman, resurrect both the ketogenic diet and with Ben Carson, Patty Vining and a group of very courageous parents, hemispherectomy. We performed the first receptor PET scans on patients with epilepsy. With Al Krumholz, we set out guidelines for driving and epilepsy. We tied for first report of high-frequency EEG at start of a seizure. I participated with Ron Lesser and Greg Bergey in opening one of the early epilepsy monitoring units in the U.S. Initially, the unit ran continuous paper EEGs, which we clipped each morning to retain the segments with seizures. One day, the custodial staff had me called before the hospital administrator for abuse. Apparently, the trashcan in the epilepsy monitoring unit weighed 70 pounds each morning. We solved that problem, first with multiple trash cans and then with digital EEGs. Watching all those videos of seizures induced an interest in distinguishing epileptic from nonepileptic seizures. That interest later led to a role in defining and classifying epilepsy. Together, we trained fellows who are now epilepsy leaders, including Brian Litt, Greg Krauss, Nathan Crone. The late, great electroencephalographer, Ernst Niedermeyer, trained me, but at the start of my fellowship, Ernst immediately took a 6-month sabbatical to Dusseldorf, leaving me to muddle through the EEGs. I commented that I was not yet trained to read them, and he replied, "It's mostly on-the-job training anyway." Somehow, Patti Vining and I kept the ship afloat until he returned. A few years ago, I returned to Hopkins to give Neurology Grand Rounds. During my talk, I did what I always do – calling on residents in the audience for their opinions. However, the interaction was not working. Only later did I realize that those residents were now all professors and vice-chairs, not used to being called on until at least three other people had opined. Time passes.

David Buchholz, M.D.
Associate Professor of Neurology,
Johns Hopkins University

Post-residency, I joined the faculty of the Department of Neurology at Johns Hopkins as an Assistant Professor, and was later promoted to Associate Professor, a title which I retain. From 1983 to 1997, I served primarily as a dedicated clinician, practicing and teaching general neurology, and secondarily in a number of outpatient and quality assurance administrative roles, with clinical research activity particularly in the field of neurogenic dysphagia and related publications, as well. Over the years, my main interest became migraine; not migraine as I was taught (including in my neurology training at Johns Hopkins) but migraine radically redefined both diagnostically and therapeutically. In

1997, I left my full-time faculty position and set up a solo private practice at Johns Hopkins at Green Spring Station, where I remain today. My proudest accomplishment is the publication of *Heal Your Headache: The 1-2-3 Program for Taking Charge of your Pain* (Workman Publishing, 2002) which, over the past 16 years, has become by far the most widely read book ever written on the subject, now in its 18th printing with over 200,000 copies in print.

Ronald J. Tusa, M.D., Ph.D.
Emeritus Professor of Neurology, Emory
University, Atlanta

In 1959, prize winners David Hubel and Torsten Wiesel physiologically mapped the central portions of the visual field in area 17-19 in cat at Johns Hopkins Hospital. For my doctorate thesis at University of Pennsylvania, I examined the peripheral portions of the visual field in those areas and ultimately found 13 separate representations of the visual field in cat cortex. For my Neurology residency, I wanted to come to Johns Hopkins University to work with David Zee, my mentor, on the cortical control of eye movements. It was one of the best decisions that I made. I stayed on through 1993 and had the opportunity to work with some of the greats in eye movements, vestibular function and control systems, including R. John Leigh and David Robinson. With Dr. Zee's leadership, we started seeing patients with vestibular defects and dizziness. This new focus was the start of a new future for me. With the help of Susan Herdman and Dr. Zee, a new area of vestibular rehabilitation became a fruitful area of research and a very practical form of treatment for the dizzy patient. We ultimately brought this interest with us to the University of Miami and then Emory University, where we established research labs and dizziness programs. I will be forever grateful for the expertise, guidance and collaboration that I received at Johns Hopkins University.

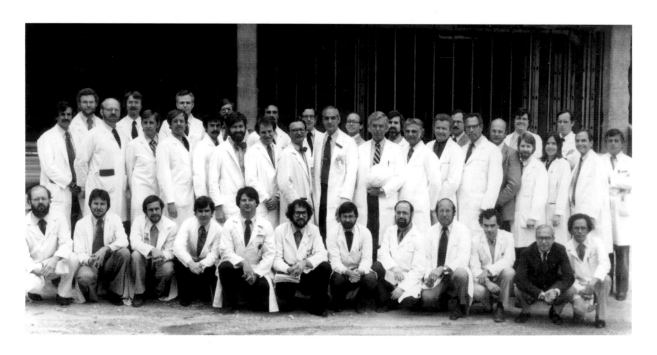

1980-1981

Front Row:
D. Hilt
R. Kuncl
R. Tusa
A. Seay
R. Patchell
R. Fisher
J. Wolinsky
S. Shinner
H. Singer
J. Troncoso
H. Moses
B. D'Souza

Second Row:
D. Zee
B. Brooks
J. Leigh
S. Stein
E. Stanley
C. Andrew
A. Pestronk
O. Hurko
D. Drachman
R. Johnson
T. Preziosi
D. Price
J. Freeman
M. DeLong
R. Kandt
M. Bleecker
H. Moses III
A. Arregui

Third Row:
A. Clark
G. Uhl
W. Mobley
D. Buchholz
R. Bailey
J. Griffin
H. Weiss
B. Gordon
B. Stern
P. Whitehouse
D. Hanley

"Guy McKhann instinctively lit a fire under me as a new instructor, as he probably did for many of us, saying, 'You'll do EMG with Dave Cornblath if you want to put food on the table.'" – Ralph W. Kuncl, Ph.D., M.D.

Stephen J. Peroutka, M.D., Ph.D.

Vice President and Global Therapeutic Head, Neuroscience, PPD, Inc., Carmel, California

My first visit to Hopkins was via the Emergency Room at the age of five days.

I stayed a week, but never really left. In fact, I am still actively working on a new collaboration with Hopkins. In between those two events, I spent eight of nine years at the Johns Hopkins University School of Medicine, first as an M.D.-Ph.D. student in Sol Snyder's lab and then as a Neurology resident. Those years both shaped and guided the rest of my career and life: Assistant Professor of Neurology and Pharmacology at Stanford; Chief, Neurology Service at the Palo Alto VA Hospital; first Director of Genentech's Department of Neuroscience; and Founder of Spectra Biomedical, a company focused on migraine genetics. For the past 20 years, my work has focused on clinical drug development as both CMO of small biotech companies and via clinical research organizations. All of this has resulted in more than 300 publications and 100 guest lectures at universities and institutes, a body of work that is due largely to the outstanding education and training that I was fortunate to receive at Johns Hopkins.

Ralph W. Kuncl, Ph.D., M.D.

President, Professor of Biology, University of Redlands, California

Many of us heard Dan Drachman advise, "You have to have more than one string in your bow," using both an archery and musical metaphor about career breadth. First string: Hopkins Neurology began for me when Dan, Jack Griffin, and Alan Pestronk hired me as neuromuscular clinical and research fellow because of my interest in the pathology of drug-induced myopathy. Second string: Guy McKhann instinctively lit a fire under me as a new instructor, as he probably did for many of us, saying, "You'll do EMG with Dave Cornblath if you want to put food on the table," inspiring a path in clinical-pathological correlation in neuromuscular disorders. Third string: ALS became a passion when it was clear in 1983 that those patients were among the neediest, yet physicians used placebos on them and offered little family support or cogent research – hence the then-new frontier of translational work in motor neuron pathology and mechanisms of degeneration/regeneration. Fourth string: This emerged with Dick Johnson's request that I become Director of the Clinical Neuromuscular Laboratory, as steward of the lab Dan had founded. After some 20 years of research, a philosophical dilemma was set up for me: Drachman ("One should never retire, as the chase of research is too intriguing") vs. Griffin ("The beauty of an M.D. is that you can do almost anything with it.") I chose being Associate Editor of the *Annals of Neurology* with Dick Johnson and Dave Zee, and thus, scholarly editing became a Fifth string. Because research often leads to posing ever more narrowly focused questions, a Sixth string was inevitable: making an impact on an entire institution. So, in 2001, I began as the founding Hopkins Vice Provost for Undergraduate Education. Because of the Hopkins model, I was recruited to the University of Rochester (designed as a mini-version of Johns Hopkins University), and there became Provost, Executive VP, and Chief Research Officer. One accomplishment was as founder of a three-way corporate-university-government alliance with IBM and NY State to create a $100-million, high-performance computer facility, the Health Sciences Center for Computational Innovation. In 2012, I was chosen as the 11th president of the University of Redlands. You couldn't graph my career on a PowerPoint, because as Alan Pestronk taught me, "Any chart with more than three arrows on it is never right." Well, it all makes perfect sense to me, if it's traced back to JHU Neurology.

Michael A. Rogawski, M.D., Ph.D.

Professor of Neurology and Pharmacology,
University of California-Davis, Sacramento

After completing the Neurology residency at
Johns Hopkins in 1985, I moved back to NIH,
where I had been a postdoctoral fellow, to
begin a career as an NINDS intramural scientist.
Beginning as a senior staff fellow (assistant
professor equivalent) in the NINDS Medical
Neurology Branch, I achieved tenure in 1990,
becoming a senior investigator and chief of the
Epilepsy Research Section. I remained at NIH
until 2007, when I left to chair the Department
of Neurology at the University of California-
Davis School of Medicine. My research focuses
on neuropharmacology and the mechanisms
of action of drugs used to treat epilepsy. In
recent years, an increasing amount of my time
has been spent on academic drug discovery
and development. In addition to the usual
responsibilities of an academic neurologist, I
teach courses in drug discovery at UC-Davis
and help companies to develop novel treatments
for epilepsy, several of which are now FDA-
approved. With Barb Slusher, director of Johns
Hopkins Drug Discovery, I teach a short course
on neurotherapeutics discovery that has been
funded by NINDS since 2012. Among those
with a Hopkins Neurology connection whom I
had the honor of hosting in my lab at NIH were
Nick Maragakis, while he was a student at the
University of Utah, and Adam Hartman and
Gholam Motamedi, when they were fellows.
While rotating in child neurology, I naïvely asked
John Freeman how the ketogenic diet works
to treat epilepsy. I got the sense that he didn't
seem to think it made a whole lot of difference,
as it clearly worked. He brushed me off with
the challenge: "Why don't you find out." Years
later, Adam Hartman came to my lab and made
a go of it, but the mechanism of the diet is still

largely a mystery. I lucked into a collaboration
with Sol Snyder when Angel Parent, the wife
of Gopal Thinakaran, joined my lab. Angel and
Jean-Pierre Mothet, a postdoc with Sol, collected
convincing evidence to support Sol's iconoclastic
belief that D-serine (along with glycine) is an
endogenous co-agonist of the NMDA receptor.
The report, published in *PNAS*, is one of my most
highly cited papers. Over the years, I have been
active in the American Epilepsy Society. Greg
Bergey and I were among a group of four who
created, and for 11 years edited, *Epilepsy Currents*,
AES's journal.

Justin C McArthur, M.B.B.S., M.P.H.

John W. Griffin Professor, Director, Department
of Neurology, Johns Hopkins University School
of Medicine

I initially came to Hopkins to do internal
medicine and then cardiology, but fell in love
with Neurology after rotations as a medical intern
with chief residents Dan Hanley and Bob Fisher,
and attendings Dick Johnson and Guy McKhann.
After completing the Neurology residency at
Johns Hopkins in 1985, I had no real idea of what
I wanted to do, but Guy and Dick encouraged me
to dive into NeuroAIDS. Hopkins had just begun
clinical and research programs for this brand-new
disease that was ravaging Baltimore and other
cities. After fumbling unsuccessfully in the lab
for a few months, I enrolled in an M.P.H. and this
gave me the training to submit grants to study the
neurological complications of AIDS: dementia,
neuropathy, and opportunistic infections. The
first decade was an incredible time. We were
seeing the full-on impact of the epidemic without
any treatments until after 1987, but effective
combination therapies were not introduced until
1996. Initially, everyone died, usually within a few
months, and it was an ugly, painful death.

Gradually, the treatments improved to the
point that we were regularly seeing the

'Lazarus' effect, where cachectic people riddled with various infections started antiretrovirals and then regained their health. HIV became a chronic manageable disease, and people with HIV starting living a close-to-normal lifespan.

Dick Johnson had completely shifted the focus of his laboratory from measles to studying HIV, and he helped establish a NeuroAIDS Center and the Center for AIDS Research. He engaged several of us in this effort, and a number of us are still working collaboratively to understand the mechanisms of NeuroAIDS and to develop new therapies. Longtime collaborators in this include Janice Clements, Ned Sacktor, Glenn Treisman, Marty Pomper, Norm Haughey, Amanda Brown, many from Infectious Diseases, and more recently, the JHU Drug Discovery unit, led by Barb Slusher. I have led an NIMH Center for drug discovery since 2006, and we are now engaged in a trial of intranasal insulin for HIV-associated neurocognitive disorder, as well as using an ecoHIV murine model of neuropathogenesis. During this time, I learned the importance of collaboration, both at JHU and outside. HIV is a great example of the necessity of interdisciplinary interactions to achieve results. My greatest contribution has been to define the neurological complications of HIV/AIDS, based on my own clinical observations, and to define the critical role of sustained and damaging inflammation in NeuroAIDS. I believe that I could never have had this opportunity anywhere else. The encouragement that I received from Neurology and ID mentors was enabling and empowering, and the milieu for combining discovery and excellent care was unsurpassed. Another unexpected contribution, stimulated by Jack Griffin, was the development here of the technique of punch skin biopsy as a method to evaluate epidermal innervation in a variety of sensory neuropathies. This technique has now been used in many clinical trials for both HIV-positive and diabetic neuropathies, and has entered clinical practice as a useful tool to assess neuropathies. I was the founding director of the JHU Cutaneous Nerve laboratory, which became the first in the U.S. to obtain CLIA certification for punch skin biopsies.

1983

Bernard L. Maria, M.D., M.B.A.

Division Chief of Child Neurology and Developmental Medicine, Atlantic Health System; Professor of Pediatrics and Neurology, Sidney Kimmel Medical College, Thomas Jefferson University

I joined the Hopkins pediatric neurology residency program in 1983 after completing my pediatrics training at McGill University. I had rotated as a medical student with opportunities to learn from John Freeman, Harvey Singer, Guy McKhann and many others. The best way to describe the impact of my training at Hopkins is to say "it is the only place I never left." I learned to appreciate the art of the exam and to formulate a working clinical hypothesis. I came to appreciate the importance of reaching out to other experts, no matter where they are in the world. I learned to move the field forward. One of the most influential faculty was Bernie DeSouza, who was a gifted teacher and an encyclopedic neurologist. Bernie introduced me to neuro-oncology before leaving for Duke University; that was my foundation of a 30-year career in pediatric neuro-oncology. In 2004, I had the privilege of introducing my primary mentor, John Freeman, for the Hower Award, the Child Neurology Society's highest Honor. I would like to think that I lived up to John's and Hopkins' expectations as the 2018 Hower Awardee. I am deeply grateful to Drs. McKhann and Freeman for taking me on as their first Canadian trainee, and I continue to enjoy the benefit of Oslerian values bestowed by a tradition of Hopkins Neurology excellence.

1984

Eva L. Feldman M.D., Ph.D.
Russell N. DeJong Professor of Neurology; Director, Program for Neurology Research and Discovery; Director, ALS Center of Excellence at Michigan Medicine, University of Michigan, Ann Arbor

My time as a Neurology resident (1984 to 1987) at Hopkins established my scientific and clinical career path, my lifelong mentors and wonderful colleagues. I entered residency with the intent of becoming a stroke neurologist, until I met Jack Griffin. He informed me I was "misdirected" and "I must become a friend of the Schwann cell!" In parallel, Hopkins was a trial site for early plasma exchange in GBS, and as an eager resident, I followed the trial patients. Soon I was working in Jack's lab and the EMG lab. As chief resident, I also spent time with Guy, who taught me the art of the neurological examination with an added twist: how to interest your patients in the tripartite mission of neurology so they will partner with you to fund research and education. As I established my career as a neuromuscular clinician scientist at the University of Michigan, I had a "hotline" to Hopkins, speaking nearly weekly at first with Jack and Guy.

Twenty years later, having spent my career at Michigan, I received a $100 million-dollar donation from a patient to begin a research institute; the first person I called was Guy—who replied "Great work, kid!" I smiled.

Colin R. Kennedy, M.B.B.S., M.D.
Professor in Neurology and Paediatrics, Faculty of Medicine, University of Southampton; Hon. Consultant in Paediatric Neurology, University Hospital Southampton NHS Foundation Trust

My time as a Neurology fellow at Johns Hopkins (1985-1987) provided me with access to the

generous guidance and disciplined examples of John Freeman, Harvey Singer and many senior colleagues across the entire Department of Neurology. I also took on the role of interim joint lead of the Pediatric Neuro-Oncology service. These experiences set the direction for my subsequent research efforts, which followed a path of enquiry through clinical trials and cohort studies.

On my return to the UK, I was appointed to be the founding provider of an NHS paediatric neurology service for the 3.5 million population of central southern England.

Over the subsequent 30 years, a progressively increasing proportion of my working life has been devoted to organization of the specialty at a UK national and European level and research. Over the last ten years, I have also put energy into the reduction of disparities in the standard of care of children with neurological problems between Eastern and Western parts of the WHO European region.

1985

Jerrold L. Vitek, M.D., Ph.D.
McKnight Professor and Chair of Neurology Department, University of Minnesota Medical School, Minneapolis

My research involves close collaboration with other neurologists, neuroscientists, neurosurgeons, neuroimaging and biomedical engineers.

The roots of my collaborative, multidisciplinary approach to research originated at Hopkins, where I trained with Mahlon R. DeLong, doing systems neurophysiology in nonhuman primates.

This work evolved into intraoperative mapping of deep brain structures with both Dr. DeLong and Dr. Fred Lenz in the neurosurgery department at JHH, which I have continued to this day. My work has provided new insight into the pathophysiology of movement disorders, the therapeutic mechanisms of deep brain stimulation (DBS), and has contributed to the application of DBS to other neurological and psychiatric disorders. I am the Chair of the Neurology Department and the Director of the Neuromodulation Research Program at the University of Minnesota. I have held faculty positions at The Johns Hopkins University and Emory University, where I assisted in the development of the functional neurology/neurosurgery programs and conducted research on the pathophysiology of movement disorders and mechanism(s) underlying the beneficial effects of DBS. I also previously served as the Co-Director of the Center for Neurological Restoration and Center Director of the Neuromodulation Research Center Director at the Lerner Research Institute of the Cleveland Clinic Foundation, developing functional surgery and DBS techniques for the treatment of neurological disease.

1986

Allan I. Levey, M.D., Ph.D.

Goizueta Foundation Endowed Chair for Alzheimer's Research; Betty Gage Holland Chair, Department of Neurology, Emory University, Atlanta

My experiences as a resident and junior faculty member at Johns Hopkins launched my career and fueled my passion for academic neurology. I was initially attracted to Hopkins for neurology training by the pioneering work of Don Price, Mahlon DeLong and Joe Coyle, identifying a role for the cholinergic system in Alzheimer's disease, as my own research as an M.D.-Ph.D. student was the mapping of central cholinergic pathways in

brain. As a resident, my passion for cognitive and behavioral neurology evolved as natural link to my research interests, and I was fortunate to have Ola Selnes and Barry Gordon teach me an enormous amount of neuropsychology and cognitive neuroscience. Following residency, I integrated additional clinical training with them as a cognitive neurologist and concurrently retooled as a bench researcher. With the support of a K08 award, I learned molecular biology at the NIH with daily commutes from Baltimore to Bethesda, and then returned full-time to Hopkins Neurology and Neuropathology, becoming part of the Alzheimer's Disease Research Center. In this group led by Don Price, the foundation for my career as an Alzheimer's disease researcher was established, learning deeply about neurodegenerative disease while also forming deep friendships and collaborations with so many great colleagues. I also obtained my first R01 studying Alzheimer's disease. I relocated to Emory in 1991, along with many other Hopkins Neurology colleagues, when Mahlon DeLong assumed the role of Chair at Emory (aka, Hopkins South!).

My activities have continued to span basic to clinical aspects of Alzheimer's disease and related disorders, and I have also attempted to create a Hopkins-like culture as Chair of the Emory Neurology Department.

William R. Tyor, M.D.

Professor, Department of Neurology, Emory University School of Medicine; Neuroscience Academic Coordinator, Atlanta VA Medical Center, Decatur, Georgia

I was a post-doc and faculty member in the Department of Neurology at Hopkins from 1986 through 1992. My mentors were Richard Johnson and Diane Griffin, I had many friends

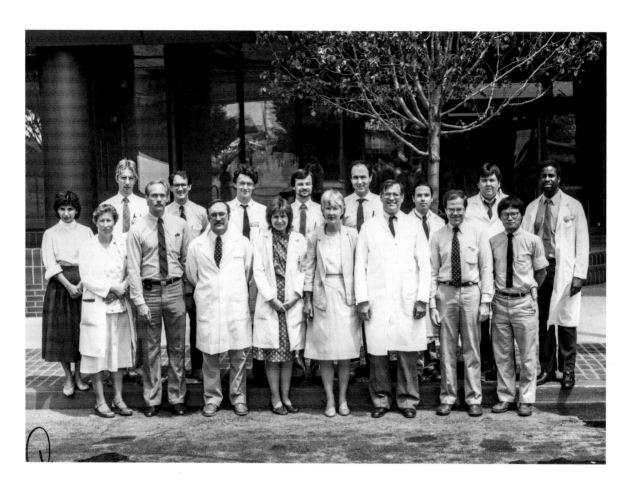

1985-1986

Front Row:
N. Dalos
L. Empting
M. Mabry
E. Feldman
C. Meyd
G. McKhann
K. Marek
C-M Tang

Second Row:
S. Kitttur
C. Kennedy
S. Kinsman
J. Ashe
J. Vitek
D. Galasko
J. Vornov
J. Hart
W. Royal

"I found that the incredible amount of clinical responsibility placed on our shoulders drove me to learn neurology in a hurry and to develop my clinical judgment." – Richard F. Lewis, M.D.

and collaborators, and they contributed to this most exciting and inspiring period of my academic life. I have fond memories of me (singer), Walter Royal (saxophone) and Orest Hurko (piano) entertaining folks at the annual party in Dick Johnson's home. Although my work on mouse Sindbis virus (SV) encephalitis while at Hopkins is less cited than my work on HIV encephalitis, fundamental discoveries made, such as lifelong SV infection of neurons, remain underappreciated, particularly as the concept may relate to multiple sclerosis. Dick and Diane guided the neurovirology group to investigate HIV encephalitis pathogenesis, and I was fortunate enough to be part of a seminal paper describing the brain inflammatory cytokine reaction of HIV encephalitis in humans. The lack of a small animal model for HIV encephalitis prompted me, Chris Power and Dick Markham to invent one. To this day, I still have two active federal grants using an updated version of this model to investigate pathogenesis and novel treatments for HIV-associated neurocognitive disorders (HAND).

1987

Avinoam Shuper, M.D.
Professor Emeritus in Pediatrics, Tel-Aviv University, Israel; Former Director, Pediatric Neurology, Schneider Children's Medical Center of Israel

When I came for training in Hopkins, I was already a senior pediatrician at Beilinson Hospital, a major hospital in Israel. It was after five years of Israeli residency in pediatrics, including frequent night shifts, and seven more years through which night shifts were as well required. Being newcomers to the States, a time period to acclimate was naturally required. A situation of residency at Hopkins with a busy night shift every third day, with full working day afterwards, and in adult wards, was quite hard. And getting used to the English slang and

abbreviations... I must mention with love my very understanding and helpful Seniors: the late John Freeman, Dave Zee, Patty Vining. Later on, it was a great pleasure for me to meet the guys from Hopkins upon their visit to Beilinson: Oh, what a different situation! After my return to Israel, I became the head of Neurology in the Schneider Children's Medical Center of Israel, the major children's hospital in the country. I used a lot all that I learned in Hopkins wards, Epilepsy Monitoring Unit and clinics. I retired upon 2014, that's the law in Israel, and continue now with medical work on a free-lance basis. I am a professor Emeritus of Tel-Aviv University.

Marina AJ (de Koning-) Tijssen, M.D., Ph.D.
Professor and Head of the Movement Disorder section of the Neurology Department, University Medical Center Groningen (UMCG), University of Groningen, the Netherlands

In 1987, I worked as a medical student in David Zee's lab, together with Chiara Straathof. I did a research project, "Optokinetic after-nystagmus in humans: normal values of amplitude, time constant, and asymmetry," that was published as my first paper in 1989. We were named Dutch, and as Europeans we introduced the highly appreciated tea-time in the lab. Following my period at Hopkins, I did my Neurology Residency at the University of Leiden and the Institute of Neurology and Neurosurgery, London, UK, and wrote my thesis on hyperekplexia. Subsequently, I established an internationally renowned movement disorders group in Amsterdam. My research has always been focused on hyperkinetic movement disorders, with a research line covering clinical and translational research in relation to jerky movements and dystonia. To facilitate clinical diagnostics using new genetic possibilities, I published diagnostic algorithms for dystonia and myoclonus. In 2012, I started as professor in Groningen, with dedicated time for movement disorders and the opportunity to build a new research group. As secretary of the EU section of the International Parkinson and Movement Disorder Society, the main society in my field, and chair of the Groningen European Movement Disorders Expertise Centre, I have created a unique platform to train young clinicians and researchers and explore the fascinating field of hyperkinetic movement disorders.

Richard F. Lewis, M.D.

Associate Professor, Otolaryngology and Neurology, Harvard Medical School; Director of the Jenks Vestibular Diagnostic and Vestibular Physiology Laboratories, Massachusetts Eye and Ear, Boston

I spent 12 years in the Neurology Department at Johns Hopkins (resident 1987 to 1990, fellow 1990 to 1994, and faculty 1994 to 1999) before moving to Harvard. I feel strongly that both my clinical and scientific careers were defined by my time at Hopkins. Regarding my residency, I found that the incredible amount of clinical responsibility placed on our shoulders drove me to learn neurology in a hurry and to develop my clinical judgment. I was inspired by my amazing trio of chief residents (Allen Levey, Jon Glass, and Jeff Rothstein) whose knowledge was only surpassed by their enthusiasm. During fellowship with David Zee, I was taken by his ability to make clinical problems so interesting, an attribute that I have tried to emulate in my career with varying success. On the research side, I was given enormous latitude, which led to many short-term failures as I tried to figure things out, but ultimately drove my development as a vestibular clinician-scientist. Again, I was always amazed by David's ability to find scientific meaning in clinical problems, which I have also tried to emulate, as my research focus has gradually shifted from basic science to more translational topics. He was always so generous with his time even though he was incredibly busy, and I appreciate him now more than ever. I was also lucky to find the vestibular field, since my background in physics didn't serve me well in

many medical specialties, but was a perfect fit with this one. I consider my time at Hopkins as the crucible that formed my career, with medical school and college mere distractions. For this, I am very thankful.

1988

Stephen G. Reich, M.D.

Professor of Neurology, The Frederick Henry Prince Distinguished Professor in Neurology, Department of Neurology, University of Maryland School of Medicine

I came to Johns Hopkins as a fellow in 1987 to work with Mahlon DeLong, having discovered in my residency that the basal ganglia were where I wanted to be. I started out in the lab doing single unit recording in MPTP monkeys. I also spent time in the clinic with Mahlon and others in the movement disorders group. It did not take long for me to appreciate that my first love was clinical neurology, especially movement disorders, and not the lab. It was with great trepidation and a sense of disappointment when I went to tell Mahlon that I did not want to continue in the lab. To my surprise and relief, Mahlon was completely understanding and supportive, and for that I remain grateful. I have subsequently had similar experiences with mentees and have used Mahlon's reaction to my change of plans as a guidepost. One of the highlights of my fellowship was initiating use of botulinum toxin for cervical dystonia; it is hard to appreciate now that this really was a miracle for these desperate patients. Toward the end of my fellowship, Hamilton Moses, who headed the Parkinson's Clinic, became VP for Medical Affairs, leading to a great opportunity for me to take over. For the next 14 years, I was very busy clinically, teaching and doing clinical research. In 2002, I was recruited to the University of Maryland by the new chair, William J. Weiner. At Maryland, I have continued to focus on clinical care, clinical research and teaching with a particular interest in parkinsonian syndromes, including PSP. I am very grateful to Johns Hopkins for setting me on what has been, and continues to be, a very rewarding career path, and especially for a long list of valued Hopkins friends and colleagues.

1989

Gerald Dal Pan, M.D., M.H.S.
Director, Office of Surveillance and Epidemiology, United States Food and Drug Administration

My time at Hopkins was exciting and formative from the very first day.

My first rotation was the inpatient pediatric neurology service – a real shock after having just completed a three-year residency in Internal Medicine, especially since most of the patients on the Pediatric Neurology service were under one-year old (or so it seemed).

I was very intimidated by Harvey Singer's encyclopedic knowledge of inborn errors of metabolism and all the eponym-based pediatric neurological diseases. I was intrigued by John Freeman's sit-on-the-floor-and-play-with-the-child method of the neurological exam. Harvey and John were two of my most valued teachers. By far the most important happening during my residency occurred in the Fall of 1989 (just a few months into our first year), when Russ Margolis, then a Hopkins Psychiatry resident and now a Hopkins Professor of Psychiatry, and his wife Leslie (both college classmates of mine) gave me the name of someone they thought I might like meeting. I called Kathi on a Sunday evening while on call at Key (now Bayview). We've been together ever since, and have now been married for 24 years. After residency, I completed a Master of Health Science in Clinical Epidemiology at the Johns

Hopkins School of Hygiene and Public Health and fellowship in Clinical Neurovirology at Hopkins with Justin McArthur. I joined the Neurology faculty at Hopkins, where I remained through late 1995. I then went to a small pharmaceutical company in Baltimore, where I learned an immense amount about drug development. In 2000, I joined the Food and Drug Administration, where I started as a clinical reviewer of centrally acting analgesics. In 2003, I moved to a managerial position in the FDA drug safety office and became the director of that office in 2005, a position I've held since then. Running FDA's post-market drug safety monitoring office, where I am responsible for a staff of over 350 physicians, pharmacists, and scientists who monitor the safety of all marketed human medicines and therapeutic biologics in the United States, has been as challenging as it's been rewarding. Since 2008, I also have served as one of two co-chairs of the World Health Organization's Advisory Committee on the Safety of Medicinal Products. I've been fortunate to maintain academic endeavors through research projects and publications at FDA, including mentoring Masters- and Ph.D.-level dissertations in the area of drug safety. I'm still on the part-time faculty in Neurology at Hopkins, where I teach residents, though not as much as I'd like. I also am involved in the Hopkins Center for Drug Safety and Effectiveness.

1990

David N. Irani, M.D.
Professor of Neurology, University of Michigan Medical School, Ann Arbor

As a research fellow (1988 to 1990), house officer (1990 to 1993), and junior faculty member (1993 to 2007) at Hopkins, I developed a passion to better understand the pathogenesis of inflammatory disorders of the CNS. Research (Diane Griffin, Dick Johnson) and clinical mentors (Jack Griffin, Dick Johnson, Justin McArthur) taught me how to exploit animal models for this purpose, but also never let me forget the importance of learning directly from my patients themselves. Along with fellow junior faculty members Carlos Pardo and Doug Kerr, I helped established the world's first Transverse Myelitis Center at Hopkins in 1997, which still exists today. Our interactions with many patients having a wide range of neuroinflammatory disorders naturally led us to establish a large repository of clinical samples, including a sizable bank of cerebrospinal fluid (CSF) specimens (>600) from people with well-characterized clinical and radiographic disease. This sample repository has yielded numerous studies that have shed light on the pathogenesis of multiple sclerosis, acute transverse myelitis, and HIV dementia. It also stimulated the idea that an updated book on human CSF would be a welcome addition to our field. Although *Cerebrospinal Fluid in Clinical Practice* (2009) was finalized after I moved from Hopkins to the University of Michigan, the ideas and all of the chapter content have deep ties to the Johns Hopkins Neurology Department.

Kyra J. Becker, M.D.

Professor Emeritus, Neurology & Neurological Surgery, University of Washington School of Medicine

I was a Neurology Resident (1990 to 1993) and Neurocritical Care Fellow (1993 to 1995) at Hopkins, during which time my clinical interests were nurtured by Daniel Hanley and my research interests by Richard Traystman and Patricia Hurn. My time at Hopkins shaped my career; in fact, my first significant publication (oral tolerance for the treatment of stroke) was inspired by a journal club presentation by one of my co-residents. This paper was written during my time as a research fellow at NINDS, after which I moved to Seattle and had a career as a vascular neurologist at the University of Washington (UW). While at UW, I started the stroke program and ran a translational research laboratory that focused on the contribution of the post-ischemic immune response to stroke outcome.

In fact, it was the inspiration from that journal club at Hopkins that laid the foundation for my entire line of research – that antigen-specific immune responses occur after stroke, and that these responses can be manipulated to improve outcome.

I will be forever thankful for the friends and colleagues I developed during my six years at JHH, and I value these relationships every day.

1991

Laura J. Balcer, M.D., MSCE

Professor of Neurology, Population Health and Ophthalmology, Vice Chair, Neurology, NYU School of Medicine New York; Adjunct Professor of Neurology and Epidemiology and Biostatistics, University of Pennsylvania

I currently co-lead national collaborative clinical and research efforts in the neuro-ophthalmology of multiple sclerosis (MS) and concussion. My research at Johns Hopkins (M.D.'91) focused on basic science and animal models of myasthenia gravis in the laboratory of Daniel Drachman. During the past 20 years, my research has focused on development of visual function tests for clinical trials in MS. Our team, including Peter Calabresi, received the 2015 Barancik Prize for Innovation in MS Research. More recently, we have investigated new vision-based tests for sideline diagnosis of concussion. I have mentored more than 80 trainees, and lead a PI site for a U01 proposal to investigate biomarkers for chronic traumatic encephalopathy (CTE) among retired football athletes. My time at Johns Hopkins and subsequent training have thus led to an enjoyable and productive career of research and mentoring, lifelong clinical learning and much-treasured collaborations.

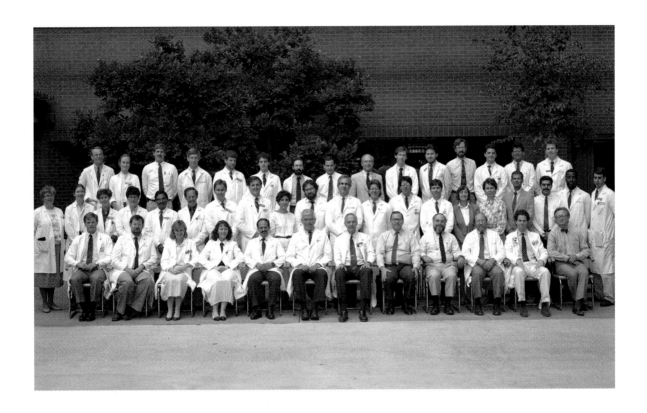

1990-1991

Front Row:
B. Litt
E. George
A. Corse
S. De Rossett
M. Al-Lozi
R. Johnson
D. Drachman
G. McKhann
M. Molliver
H. Singer
R. Shapiro
O. Hurko

Second Row:
E. Vining
E. O'Hearn
C. Hart
K. Becker
V. Chaudhry
R. Tusa
J. McArthur
G. Dal Pam
C. Kawas
R. Fisher
B. Gordon
A. Levey
J. Rothstein
J. Glass
P. Talalay
M. Hardwick
B. Mondell
W. Royal
R. Elfont

Third Row:
O. Selnes
K. Andreasson
D. Johns
D. Cornblath
B Rabin
A. Blum
J. Vornov
A. Cole
J. Moses
W. Tyor
R. Kuncl
G. Krauss
S. Attoyo
R. Ratan
R. O'Brien

"My current efforts in AAV-based gene therapies for neuromuscular and neuro-degenerative disorders are feasible because of curiosity, skills, and enthusiasms developed as a trainee at Hopkins." – Kevin M. Flanigan, M.D.

Kevin M. Flanigan, M.D.

Director, Center for Gene Therapy, and Robert F. & Edgar T. Wolfe Foundation Endowed Chair in Neuromuscular Research, Nationwide Children's Hospital; Professor of Pediatrics and Neurology, Ohio State University, Columbus

My years as a neurology resident and neuromuscular fellow at Hopkins profoundly influenced my entire career. It was at Hopkins that I was exposed to role models who were both excellent clinicians and profoundly productive researchers, who have had lasting impacts on their fields. Although an adult neurology resident, I spent significant time with Harvey Singer and Tom Crawford – quite fortunately, as my primary appointment now is at a pediatric hospital. While a resident, I gravitated to the dynamic personalities of the neuromuscular division, and as a fellow benefited from the great teaching of Dan Drachman, Jack Griffin, Ralph Kuncl, David Cornblath, and Vinay Chaudhry. Having learned to extract DNA and pipette during a couple of elective months, I went on to a fellowship in Human Molecular Biology and Disease at the University of Utah, pursuing mapping of genetic diseases. There we developed a method for the rapid sequence analysis of the DMD gene that led to a large collaborative project addressing genotype/phenotype correlations and identifying other genes that modify the Duchenne phenotype. My current efforts in AAV-based gene therapies for neuromuscular and neurodegenerative disorders are feasible because of curiosity, skills, and enthusiasms developed as a trainee at Hopkins.

Elliot M Frohman, M.D., Ph.D., FAAN, FANA

Professor of Neurology and Ophthalmology; Director, Multiple Sclerosis and Neuroimmunology Center, The Dell Medical School at The University of Texas at Austin

Residency, Chief Residency, and Fellowship at Johns Hopkins uniquely prepared me for fulfilling my goals of becoming a master clinician for patients with MS and complex neuroimmunological disorders, developing my skill sets as an educator, and as a scientist focused upon discovery by using the eye as a 'Window' into the brain for purposes of dissecting the pathobiological underpinnings of MS, and translating these into innovative neurotherapeutic interventions. Mentoring by David Zee, David Cornblath, Jack Griffin, and Dick Johnson convinced me that high-precision characterization of eloquent tract systems (e.g. the MLF in INO and the optic nerve in optic neuritis) into their structural and functional pathophysiologic signatures would potentially provide innovative methods for translational discovery initiatives focused upon neuroprotection, myelin repair, and performance enhancement.

1992

Neil R. Holland, B.Sc., M.B.B.S., M.B.A.

Neurology Chair, Neuroscience Institute, Geisinger, Danville, Pennsylvania; Professor of Clinical Medicine, Geisinger Commonwealth School of Medicine, Scranton, Pennsylvania

My first experience of Hopkins was in 1991 as a student, when I was lucky enough to meet Justin McArthur. We wrote a paper together on CMV encephalitis. Justin encouraged me to come back to Hopkins as a Neurology resident in 1993. I stayed on as an EMG fellow, working with Vinay Chaudhry and David Cornblath. We wrote two papers on small fiber neuropathy. I became involved in intraoperative neuromonitoring and we wrote some papers. I left Hopkins in 1998 for an internship at York Hospital, followed by a faculty appointment in Neurology at Oklahoma University and the Oklahoma City VA Medical Center.

We reported some patients with heretofore unknown neurologic complications caused by copper deficiency.

From 2001 to 2014, I was in private practice in Monmouth County New Jersey, where I started the Neuroscience Institute at Monmouth Medical Center, developed an outpatient TIA clinic, and worked on my MBA from UMass. While at Monmouth, I held an academic appointment and did some educational research at Drexel. I moved to Geisinger in 2014, where I have been responsible for growing the department, increasing access to neurology care for members of the Healthplan, and educating students and residents.

1994

Valina L. Dawson, Ph.D.

Director, Neuroregeneration and Stem Cell Programs, Institute for Cell Engineering; Professor of Neurology, Neuroscience and Physiology, Johns Hopkins University School of Medicine

I was recruited into the department of Neurology by Richard Johnson in 1994 and was given additional appointments in the departments of Neuroscience and Physiology. In this rich academic environment, I have focused on understanding the cellular signaling events that underlie neuronal injury in stroke, Parkinson's disease and other neurodegenerative diseases, with the goal of finding new clinical therapies.

In collaboration with Ted Dawson, we discovered neurotoxic signaling pathways in familial and sporadic Parkinson's disease that are leading to drugs to halt the disease.

We found the receptor responsible for the cell-to-cell transmission of pathologic alpha synuclein, and that blocking this receptor is neuroprotective. We defined poly (ADP-ribose) signaling and Parthanatos as key mediators of neuronal cell death. We discovered that genomic DNA cleavage in Parthanatos is mediated by macrophage migration inhibitory factor (MIF) nuclease, and discovered MIF nuclease inhibitors that are neuroprotective. Recently, we discovered how healthy A2 astrocytes are converted to reactive toxic A1 astrocytes, and identified a drug that blocks this conversion. I became Professor in 2001; in 2002, I was asked to co-direct the Neuroregeneration and Repair Program, and in 2009 the Stem Cell Program in the Institute for Cell Engineering.

Ahmet Höke M.D., Ph.D.

Professor of Neurology and Neuroscience, Johns Hopkins School of Medicine; Director of Daniel B. Drachman Neuromuscular Division, Department of Neurology, Johns Hopkins School of Medicine

Apart from two years away as a neuromuscular fellow, I've been at Johns Hopkins since 1994, when I came as a junior resident of neurology. I can't think of a better place to train and grow as a clinician-scientist neurologist. Dick Johnson was my attending on my first month and inoculated me with his infectious curiosity in tackling challenging cases, but my true mentor has been Jack Griffin.

Although I was trained as a scientist ready to tackle CNS regeneration, Jack persuaded me to see peripheral nerve diseases and regeneration as a more fun way to spend a career.

After I completed my fellowship in Canada, he recruited me back to Hopkins and gave me opportunities to grow as a scientist and neurologist. Quickly, I was able to establish a program on mechanistic studies using models of peripheral neuropathies, initially focusing on HIV-associated sensory neuropathy and later on diabetic and chemotherapy-induced neuropathies. I've also been working on peripheral nerve regeneration with special emphasis on chronic denervation changes in Schwann cells and role of Schwann cell heterogeneity in dictating specificity of nerve regeneration.

Dominik Straumann, M.D.

Associate Professor, Department of Neurology, University Hospital Zurich, University of Zurich, Switzerland

My time as a postdoctoral research fellow (one year in 1994/95) and later as a visiting scientist (two to three months each in 1998, 1999, 2001, 2003) at David Zee's laboratory decisively influenced my further work in clinic and research. Since this fruitful time at Hopkins, David Zee has always been a role model to me in how one can combine dedicated clinical neurology with excellent research that is inspired by observations at the bedside. So far, there are 27 publications (papers, chapters, proceedings) that have both David Zee's and my name on the authors' list. In all these contributions, normal or abnormal eye movements in humans are in the center of the research. Besides the intellectual aspects, one important reason to join David Zee's lab was the presence of an exceptional instrument for recording eye rotations in three dimensions (horizontal, vertical, and torsional). The three-dimensional search coil system – invented by David Robinson, constructed by Adrian Lasker and programmed by Dale Roberts – was an indispensable tool to study 3-D ocular kinematics in healthy human subjects and in patients with eye movement disorders. David Robinson, the pioneer in applying control theory to better understand the neural control of eye movements, although already retired, gave an unforgettable private multi-session seminar on the mathematics of ocular motor physiology and pathophysiology in the fellows' room. The lab's two outstanding engineers, Adrian Lasker and Dale Roberts, were later immensely helpful in expanding my own lab back in Zurich. Graciously, they made us a copy of the three-dimensional search coil system, which we were using for many studies in the years to come. In 2009/10 Alexander Tarnutzer, a first-class neurologist and researcher in my lab, also spent a postdoc year at David Zee's lab and excelled thanks to the Hopkins collaborations. In conclusion, I cannot think of my further clinical and scientific career without the wonderful time at Hopkins and the continuous collaboration, support, and friendship with David Zee and many of his co-workers, whom I could not all list in this short abstract.

Jeremy N. Rich, M.D., M.H.S., M.B.A.

Professor, Department of Medicine, Division of Regenerative Medicine, University of California, San Diego; Director, Neuro-oncology, Director, Brain Tumor Institute

During my Hopkins Neurology residency (1994 to 1997), I had the honor of learning to serve patients with the highest ethical standards and greatest intellectual depth. Not only was I exposed to world leaders in Neurology every day through interactions with the faculty, but my fellow residents set daunting standards that drove me to learn and implement the best approaches for my patients. From Dick Johnson, I learned the power of stories and personal connections. He recognized something in me that I did not when he suggested that I consider basic science training after residency. I demurred that I would never be a "gene jockey," but 11 years later, I became a Chairman of a basic science department. Jack Griffin would gently ask questions naïvely, only to show in the most humble way that he knew everything. John Freeman would throw money on the floor then diagnose children with amazing accuracy.

While the world has lost these giants, they live on in my love for caring for patients, not diseases. Two decades later, few days pass without recalling my Hopkins experiences as influences on my life.

Donald L. Gilbert, M.D., M.S., F.A.A.P., F.A.A.N.
Professor of Pediatrics and Neurology, Cincinnati Children's Hospital Medical Center, University of Cincinnati College of Medicine

My time as a Child Neurology resident at Johns Hopkins (1993 to 1998) provided a clinical foundation for my subsequent work in pediatric movement disorders, motor physiology in pediatric neurobehavioral disorders, and graduate medical education. My clinical and academic mentors, Harvey Singer, John Freeman, Paul Fisher, and Justin McArthur, impressed upon me the importance of establishing a clinical niche as well as obtaining formal training in research methodology, which I ultimately obtained as part of my K23 award. My relationship with Harvey Singer resulted in opportunities for multi-center studies in genetics, epidemiology, clinical trials, and physiology in Tourette Syndrome as well as two editions of our book, *Movement Disorders in Childhood*. After developing expertise in transcranial magnetic stimulation, my complementary interests with Martha Denckla and Stewart Mostofsky at the Kennedy Krieger have led to several highly productive NIH grants. Finally, as I enter my 10th year as child neurology residency program director at Cincinnati Children's, I appreciate the extent that child neurology has evolved clinically and scientifically since my residency. In the mold of my Johns Hopkins mentors who worked for change, I play an important role in advancing innovation in child neurology training to better prepare us to improve the health of children with neurological problems.

1995

Nicholas J. Maragakis, M.D.
Professor, Department of Neurology, Johns Hopkins University

My decision to come to Johns Hopkins for my neurology training was greatly influenced by my impressions of the senior neurology residents and the camaraderie they shared with one another. During my neurology residency training (1995 to 1998), I had the privilege of training with outstanding residents, with whom I continue to share friendships, scientific interests, and clinical interests. At the suggestion of Dr. John Griffin, I spent my post-residency scientific training with Jeff Rothstein, a mentor and collaborator to this day.

I was fortunate to begin my research career at the time human stem cells were just being discovered.

I had the opportunity to investigate the potential for using glial progenitor cell transplantation into models of Amyotrophic Lateral Sclerosis as a potential strategy for modulating motor neuron cell death. This work has continued to evolve to include the derivation of induced pluripotent stem cells (iPSC) from the ALS patients in our clinic. Our hope is to use these iPSC to understand cell-specific contributions to ALS and to identify potential therapeutic targets. I am, perhaps, most proud of being part of a larger Hopkins vision to try to translate discoveries in our laboratories to meaningful therapies for the ALS patients seen in our clinic.

Gretchen L. (Dike) Birbeck, M.D., M.P.H., D.T.M.H.
Epilepsy Research Director and the Edward A. & Alma Rykenboer Professor of Neurology, University of Rochester, Rochester, New York

I arrived in Baltimore (1994 to 1998) fresh from several months working in a rural Zambian hospital. Having decided that my life's work was meant to be in Africa, I initially struggled to conceive of how I could possibly carve out an academic neurology career based there. "RTJ" helped me see the way. With his support and the kind flexibility of my fellow residents, I was able to spend several months of my chief year in Zambia. I never looked back. My overarching professional goal is to elucidate the mechanisms of common neurology disorders in sub-Saharan Africa, and identify risk factors for the secondary medical and social morbidities resulting from these conditions – so that feasible, affordable, evidence-based interventions aimed at preventing or ameliorating neurologic illness/injury can be evaluated and, if warranted, broadly implemented. With so few neurologists in the region, there is a lot to do. My research program encompasses observational epidemiologic studies of new-onset seizure in people with HIV and clinical trials of neuroprotective interventions for pediatric cerebral malaria. My mentees study TB meningitis, coma, nutritional neuropathies, health-related stigma, and mHealth apps to track Ebola outbreaks. A bit chaotic but never boring!

1996

Isaac E. Silverman, M.D.

Vascular Neurologist; Associate Clinical Professor of Neurology, University of Connecticut School of Medicine; Chief, Neurohospitalist Division, The Ayer Neuroscience Institute, Hartford HealthCare Partner, Hartford Neurology

I feel fortunate to have worked at Johns Hopkins as both an Osler Medical Service Intern at Hopkins Hospital (1995 to 1996) and then a Neurology Resident (1996 to 1999). It was a time of great enthusiasm for emergent treatment of acute ischemic stroke, with IV tPA NINDS publication and an array of neuroprotective trials ongoing. My primary mentors at Hopkins were stroke clinicians, Bob Wityk (JHH) and Chris Earley (Hopkins Bayview). The greatest teachers, I felt, were my fellow residents, who had strong clinical and basic science backgrounds and tremendous academic aspirations. I also am indebted to the chairmen during my time at Hopkins, Richard Johnson and Jack Griffin, who were outstanding role models. In fellowship years at Yale-New Haven Hospital (1999 to 2001), I spent a year in Clinical Epidemiology in the Robert Wood Johnson Clinical Scholars program, and then a second year there as a Vascular Neurology fellow with Pierre Fayad and Larry Brass as mentors. When I moved from the New Haven area north to Hartford, in central Connecticut, I began my early attending career as a clinician educator and stroke clinical trialist. In 2001, I was the founding co-Medical Director and lead vascular neurologist of the first Primary Stroke Center in New England, recognized in 2004 by the Joint Commission (JC), situated at Hartford Hospital (HH), the primary teaching institution for the University of Connecticut (U-Conn) School of Medicine's neurology residency. I took the first version of the ACGME vascular neurology boards in 2005 and have been recertified. We pioneered – by working closely with Interventional Neuroradiology – some of the early aspiration and mechanical thrombectomy devices for endovascular therapies for large-vessel acute ischemic stroke.

I currently enjoy a hybrid existence: most of my clinical time (about 60 percent) is as a hospital-based vascular neurologist here at HH. I stepped down as Medical Director of the Stroke Center in 2015. In the hospital, I regularly teach our U-Conn Neurology Residents and other visiting neurology residents and medical students on both the Inpatient Neurology/ Stroke Service and the Consult Services. Every year, I sponsor neurology residents who choose fellowships in vascular neurology and related fields, in particular neurocritical care and interventional neuroradiology. As chief of a new Neurohospitalist Division since mid-2017, I direct two teaching conferences: a didactic Academic series on topics that combine hospital neurology with other medical fields (e.g. psychiatry, cardiology, rheumatology, geriatrics) and a second NH Case Conference CPC at our Neurology Department's Grand Rounds, presented with Audience Participation Software. The other parts of my practice include a busy outpatient private practice clinic, where

I follow-up recently hospitalized stroke patients as well as see general neurology patients. Finally, I do clinical trials adjudication work for stroke and large cardiovascular clinical trials, and also participate in medicolegal case reviews on topics in stroke medicine and hospital neurology.

Nathaniel Carter, M.D.

President/CEO Maryland Center for Neuro-Ophthalmology & Neuro-Otology, PC, Columbia, Maryland

Two of my first three years as postdoctoral fellow (1994-1997) were spent studying axonal transport with a truly brilliant and scholarly scientist, Paul Hoffman. This exposure gave me an appreciation for bench research and an understanding of the various challenges facing the faculty, and basic science and clinical post-docs.

As an active member and later as the first physician President of the Johns Hopkins Postdoctoral Association, I had first-hand knowledge of post-doc fellow concerns while having the unique honor of working directly with a legendary civil rights activist, pioneer in cardiothoracic surgery, and Dean of Postdoctoral Fellows, Levi Watkins, Jr.

My clinical training as a subspecialty neurologist was enhanced under the tutelages of Neil Miller (neuro-ophthalmology) and David Zee (neuro-otology). Working with these two iconic clinicians/scientists has resulted in numerous enduring personal and professional friendships. The intellectually stimulating years at Hopkins provided me with tools to have a fulfilling and unique career as a multi-subspecialty neurologist in private practice.

Argye E. Hillis, M.D., M.A.

Professor and Deputy Director, Department of Neurology, Johns Hopkins University School of Medicine

I decided to become a neurologist while collaborating with Guy McKhann, Ron Lesser, Barry Gordon, and others in the Mind-Brain Institute when I was an Associate Research Scientist in Cognitive Science at JHU and a speech-language pathologist. Guy continued to mentor me throughout medical school and residency in neurology at Hopkins (1995 to 1999), and as a faculty member (1999-present). As I completed residency, with wonderful colleagues who have remained lifelong friends, including Lauren Moo (now at Harvard), Louise McCullough (now Chair at University of Texas), and Carlos Pardo (Hopkins), the field of stroke changed dramatically.

New imaging in stroke, including diffusion and perfusion MRI, demonstrated that there was an opportunity to intervene to reduce the damage and improve function in acute stroke, and trials showed the efficacy of IV tPA as one mechanism to restore blood flow.

Robert Wityk was recruited to start a cerebrovascular division at Hopkins to treat acute stroke. Bob mentored me in clinical stroke treatment and my early research, using diffusion and perfusion MRI in acute stroke to reveal regions of the brain critical for important cognitive functions, before reorganization or recovery. Together we built the stroke program, and I now direct the division of 14 faculty members, two clinical fellows, and numerous research post-docs. I am also excited to have the opportunity to develop innovative methods to improve stroke recovery, as the Director of the Center for Excellence in Stroke Detection and Treatment, with an endowment from the

Sheikh Khalifa foundation. Throughout my career at Hopkins, I have had rewarding clinical work, exceptional trainees to help educate, and outstanding collaborators in research. My greatest joy has been in mentoring students, residents (including as residency program director for nearly a decade), postdoctoral fellows, and junior faculty.

1997

Lauren R. Moo, M.D.

Site Director, VA New England Geriatric Research Education and Clinical Center (NE GRECC), Bedford, Massachusetts; Staff Neurologist, Cognitive Behavioral Neurology division Massachusetts General Hospital; Assistant Professor of Neurology, Harvard Medical School, Boston

My years as a resident, fellow, and junior faculty member at Johns Hopkins were formative for me in terms of both my formal training in neurology and my interests in cognition and behavior.

I entered residency without a clear focus within the field, and I can point to an experience watching John Hart examine a teenage patient with an unusual aphasia due to a left hemisphere abscess as a turning point for me.

My fellowship in Cognitive Neurology and Neuropsychology allowed me to work not only with John Hart but also Ola Selnes, and cemented my interest in studying brain-behavior relationships. Upon moving to Massachusetts General Hospital and Harvard Medical School, and more recently joining the Bedford division of the NE GRECC, I came to appreciate the close-knit nature of the JHH residency program. My current research and clinical innovation projects center primarily around dementia, and I still look back on my time at Johns Hopkins as important in laying the foundation for my neurology career and as the source of many of the friendships I still cherish.

1998

Gene Sung, M.D., M.P.H.

Director, Division of Neurocritical Care and Stroke, University of Southern California

I was a fellow and then faculty member in the Neurosciences Critical Care Division (1994 to 1998). This was truly an inspirational time for me, as I learned, and then taught, the basics and intricacies of caring for critically ill patients with the severe neurological and neurosurgical diseases. This field was new and unique and multi-disciplinary, with neurologists, neurosurgeons, anesthesiologists working closely together with nurses, respiratory therapists, dieticians, and rehabilitation specialists on a daily basis. As a clinical researcher, I also benefited from the ability to learn skills at the School of Public Health, just across the street from my office. My research was varied, but primarily dealt with cerebral reperfusion (I helped study and gain FDA approval for the first mechanical embolectomy device for acute ischemic stroke) and neuroprotection (particularly hypothermia). Dan Hanley, as a mentor, always showed me the way in advancing both the science and the profession. Developing and organizing acute neurological care became a passion for me as I helped start and run three different professional societies: the Western States Stroke Consortium, the Los Angeles Stroke Society and perhaps most importantly, the Neurocritical Care Society. The new field of Neurocritical Care needed a voice and 'home,' which is what the Neurocritical Care Society has become. With its own journal, guidelines, educational programs and research, it is the only society solely for the field and now has members from over 40 different countries. My experience at Johns Hopkins set the spark and motivation for helping me to be a leader in my field.

Mark Walker, M.D.

Associate Professor of Neurology, Case Western Reserve University, Cleveland, Ohio

I was introduced to the Department of Neurology at Johns Hopkins as a third-year medical student almost 30 years ago. An elective rotation with Justin McArthur confirmed my intent to pursue neurology as a career. After residency, I returned to JHU as a postdoctoral fellow and then junior faculty member in the laboratory of my clinical and scientific mentor, David Zee. I found the Department of Neurology to be an ideal place to begin an academic career. Its strengths were mirrored in Dr. Zee's own laboratory – a place where intense scientific curiosity could be paired with compassionate care of patients with neurological disease; where both professionalism and excellence were highly valued; and where mentorship meant collaboration, advocacy, and real support of career development. David Zee taught me how to take interesting clinical observations into the laboratory and to apply rigorous experimental and modeling tools to elucidate underlying mechanisms and to improve diagnosis and treatment. At Hopkins, my research focused on the effects of cerebellar disease on eye movements and vestibular reflexes. This work laid the foundation for ongoing study of vestibular physiology and rehabilitation.

Jose I Suarez, M.D., F.N.C.S., F.A.N.A.

Professor and Director, Division of Neurosciences Critical Care, Departments of Anesthesiology and Critical Care Medicine, Neurology, and Neurosurgery, The Johns Hopkins University School of Medicine

I was a fellow in the Neurosciences Critical Care Division (1996 to 1998). Prior to joining the fellowship, I spent a month as a rotating resident and quickly learned that coming to Johns Hopkins would be a great opportunity for me. I thoroughly enjoyed the clinical and scientific training I was exposed to.

I can say without a doubt that my fellowship training was the key to my future career in academic neurocritical care and laid the foundations for what I was to accomplish in the future.

I worked under the tutelage of Daniel Hanley and John Ulatowski. My main areas of research interest were subarachnoid hemorrhage, cerebral edema, and neurocritical care outcomes. My subsequent career as a clinician-scientist at Case Western Reserve University and the Baylor College of Medicine built upon the solid foundations established during my time at Hopkins. I have participated in several NINDS-funded clinical trials and research initiatives: PI for the ALISAH Multicenter Pilot Study and the ALISAH II International Multicenter Phase II clinical trial; co-PI for the IMPACT and SPLASH clinical trials; member of the Executive Committee for ATACH and ATACH 2 clinical trials (PI is Adnan Qureshi, who was my co-fellow); PI for the Neurocritical Care Research Conferences (five total); co-Chair for the NINDS CDE project for Unruptured Cerebral Aneurysms and SAH and a member of the Stroke CDE Project. I am also the President of the Neurocritical Care Society and the Founding and Past Chair of the Neurocritical Care Research Network (NCRN), which encompasses 230 sites from 47 countries. I have been so grateful for what I learned at Hopkins that I returned in 2017 to become the Director of the Neurosciences Critical Division and continue with my research endeavors.

1999

Grace C.Y. Peng, Ph.D.

Director for Mathematical Modeling, Simulation and Analysis Programs at the National Institute of Biomedical Imaging and Bioengineering at the National Institutes of Health

I was a postdoctoral fellow in Hopkins Neurology from 1996 to1999, and then part-time faculty until 2007. I came to work with David Zee to apply biomedical engineering to clinical applications in the vestibular system. David provided encouragement to me during my Ph.D. on cross-axis adaptation of the vertical vestibular ocular reflex and modeling the vestibular colic reflex for head and neck control; and he became a wonderful mentor to me at Hopkins. My fellowship experience exceeded all expectations. I was deeply engaged in clinical research through rich collaborations with stellar researchers from all over the world. I learned to conduct and communicate science with rigor, and gained extraordinary appreciation for the patients who allowed me to measure and study their eye movements. The environment truly reflected the positive spirit of the people around me. I had the honor of working with clinicians who embraced quantitative approaches in research and medicine – decades ahead of their time! My Hopkins experience inspired me to promote modeling as a culture change to the broader research community, once I became a program director at NIH in 2002. As a steward of the government (e.g. funding grants, coordinating working groups within and outside the government), I strive to promote rigorous discourse with diverse disciplines to adopt model-driven science. Slowly but surely, the "Hopkins mentality" is taking hold in the multiple communities I serve.

Adam S. Fleisher, M.D., M.A.S.

Chief Medical Officer, Avid Radiopharmaceuticals

The years I spent training at Hopkins during my Internship and adult Neurology residency (1998-2002) were unquestionably the foundation for my clinical and research career. Aside from the amazing clinical experience including Chairman Rounds with Jack Griffin, it is where I first learned to use Powerpoint to present at grand rounds and the newest medical tools, like the PalmPilot (AKA Personal Digital Assistant). I recall diagnosing an ALS patient who presented with frontal temporal dementia to Dr. Griffin, which solidified by path towards becoming a cognitive neurology researcher. I spend many hours at Kennedy Krieger Institute, learning about volumetric imaging as a tool to understand brain neuromorphometry. Subsequently, I spend the next several years at the University of California-San Diego, laying the groundwork for a career in clinical trials and biomarker development for Alzheimer's disease and other cognitive disorders. I completed a dementia research and clinical fellowship in 2002, and a Master's degree in clinical trial research in 2007, publishing my first paper in functional MRI of AD risk in 2005. My subsequent career as a clinician scientist focused on working with cognitive neurodegenerative disease patients in the memory clinic at the Banner Alzheimer's Institute in Arizona. There I continued to work on clinical therapy trials for Alzheimer's disease, while leading research programs to further develop diagnostic tools such as amyloid and tau PET imaging.

We were proud to publish some of the first works on amyloid PET in pre-symptomatic autosomal dominant Alzheimer's disease patients, and to do foundational work in both amyloid and tau PET imaging.

With a passion for clinical research and a quest toward finding a cure for Alzheimer's disease, I eventually took on a role at Eli Lilly to develop and lead international treatment trials in Alzheimer's disease, and now continue to work on treatment trials and diagnostic imaging development, staying close to my original passions that were rooted at John Hopkins.

2000

Stefano Ramat, Ph.D.

Associate Professor of Bioengineering, University of Pavia, Pavia, Italy

I arrived in Baltimore in June 2000 to start as post-doc fellow in neurology with David Zee, whom I had met in my hometown in 1997. I had a background in biomedical engineering and was fascinated by the modeling of eye movements, which I had dealt with during my Master thesis on vestibular nystagmus. The starting idea for my postdoc was that of attempting to develop a test of the otoliths, the utricle in particular, that would parallel the head thrust test for the semicircular canals. Together with Adrian Lasker, we devised a "head sled" for delivering small, abrupt interaural head translations to our subjects while preventing the head from rotating on the neck. The translational VOR became an important topic for my scientific career, and at Hopkins we investigated both interaural and fore-aft responses, understanding how they were tightly coupled with saccades and could be regulated both by context and expectation. A patient of John Leigh's, presenting with saccadic oscillations in spite of a lesion involving the fastigial nuclei, was the occasion to start collaborating with Lance Optican (NIH) on the modeling of the saccadic system, while I had become a Research Associate with the Neurology Department after two years as a fellow. Overall, the three years spent at The Johns Hopkins University were undoubtedly the most formative

in my career. Thanks to my mentor, David Zee, I learned how to do research, its ethics and the value of collaboration, while making friendships that have accompanied me ever since.

David E. Newman-Toker, M.D., Ph.D.

Professor, Department of Neurology, Johns Hopkins Hospital

After having completed my neurology residency and first fellowship in neuro-ophthalmology in Boston, I came to Johns Hopkins in 2000, as a fellow in vestibular neurology under David Zee's mentorship. During my two-year clinical vestibular fellowship, I also began my graduate work in clinical research methods at the Johns Hopkins Bloomberg School of Public Health. I received my K23 grant award and joined the Neurology department faculty in 2002. After this, I completed my doctoral dissertation on new approaches to diagnosing acute dizziness and vertigo in the ED, receiving my Ph.D. from the Graduate Training Program in Clinical Investigation in 2007.

Preventing diagnostic errors, particularly related to acute neurological illnesses, has been my ultimate career goal.

I have had the great good fortune of having mentors and advocates willing to indulge my unique career path linked to improving clinical diagnosis in frontline care settings. In my role as Director of the Armstrong Institute Center for Diagnostic Excellence, and as President of the Society to Improve Diagnosis in Medicine, I am privileged to work with countless junior trainees who have expressed a long-term career interest in better diagnosis.

2001

James B. Brewer, M.D., Ph.D.

Professor and Chair, Department of Neurosciences; Director, Shiley-Marcos Alzheimer's Disease Research Center, University of California-San Diego

My time at Johns Hopkins from 2001 to 2004, with my co-residents, Rebecca Gottesman, Sarah Berman, Jeff Rumbaugh, and Andy Mammen as well as the Child Neurology co-residents, David Leiberman and Lori Jordan, was formative and a time of tremendous growth for me. I remember the nights and days before the new work hour rules were instituted in our final year. They were tough times, but filled with remarkable neurology cases, and our faculty heroes were always engaged and supportive.

I see it as a huge honor to have trained under these giants of neurology, and will long value the education that they and my co-residents provided.

I applied for a K award in my final year of residency, and moved it to UC-San Diego upon completing my training. At UC-San Diego, I started a lab, where my outstanding Neurosciences graduate students pushed me toward productivity. The lab started as a cognitive neurosciences lab and morphed to an Alzheimer's neuroimaging biomarkers laboratory, where I continue my work in directing the Alzheimer's Disease Research Center P30 grant, which was just renewed for its 35th-40th years. I recently also began the role of Department chair here, which reminds me of the times before work hour rules were instituted. I will never forget the times I had and the colleagues I met at Hopkins.

Rebecca F. Gottesman, M.D., Ph.D.

Professor of Neurology and Epidemiology, Johns Hopkins University

As a medical student at Columbia University in New York, I was initially discouraged from spending a month on a visiting rotation at Hopkins, being told that most visiting subinterns usually "end up offending someone." Undeterred by this advice, I spent a month during my last year of medical school as a visiting medical student sub-I in late 1999, and worked with Louise McCullough (as my chief resident), Bob Wityk (as my attending) and Vinay Chaudhry (as my attending, who I managed to impress with my memorization of the brachial plexus anatomy). Needless to say, this team, and the other residents and faculty I met during my visiting rotation, convinced me that Hopkins was where I wanted to be, and fortunately I convinced the group that I would be a valuable member of a residency class. During residency, I received extraordinary mentorship from Argye Hillis, who in many ways is the reason I chose a career in stroke, and from Guy McKhann. We were extremely supported during residency by Justin McArthur, as my then-residency director (and Rafael Llinas as associate program director), and by Jack Griffin as our chair. After residency, I completed a stroke fellowship while pursuing a Ph.D. in the Graduate Training Program in Clinical Investigation, and branched out to study not only cognition after stroke, stroke and cognition after cardiac surgery, but the epidemiology of stroke and vascular cognitive impairment.

My initial exposures to a true "research team" studying neurologic complications of cardiac surgery, with Guy and Ola Selnes, Maura Grega, Bill Baumgartner, and Scott Zeger, among others, solidified my understanding of what science should look like, how it should be conducted, and how the sum (several investigators working together) was better than the parts.

My work remains extraordinarily collaborative: now I work primarily with colleagues at the Bloomberg School of Public Health in Epidemiology, to conduct research on the vascular contribution to cognitive impairment and dementia, mostly as part of the Atherosclerosis Risk in Communities (ARIC) cohort study. My favorite part of my job is mentorship: I mentor a number of trainees, ranging from undergraduates to medical students, residents, fellows, and junior faculty, and my NIH K24 award supports this time as a mentor. I was asked recently if I entered residency expecting to play a major role in mentorship as a faculty member. I answered no, and cannot identify any one point when I decided that I wanted to take on a more major role as a mentor: rather, I blame this evolution of my career entirely on the mentorship I received at Hopkins. My experience at Hopkins has been, without question, career-defining, and I hope to assist future trainees and residents in having the same career progression and positive opinion of their time in training and on faculty.

2002

Benjamin M. Greenberg, M.D., M.H.S.

Cain Denius Scholar, Distinguished Teaching Professor, Department of Neurology, University of Texas Southwestern, Dallas

I began my Neurology residency at Hopkins in 2002 when Justin McArthur was Program Director and Jack Griffin was Chairman. The environment was exceptional, blending teaching, mentorship and camaraderie. The culture blended a commitment to clinical excellence and academic curiosity that integrated our tripartite mission: clinical care, research and education.

We were surrounded by incredible examples of "triple threats" and challenged to contribute.

It's hard to imagine a more comprehensive training program or better faculty. I transitioned onto the faculty and into a research fellowship with Diane Griffin in 2005. With Dick Johnson, Doug Kerr and Peter Calabresi as mentors I began to forge a career in neuroimmunology translational research. With a focus of transverse myelitis and neuromyelitis, I began work in biomarkers research and clinical trials. I was recruited to the University of Texas-Southwestern in 2009 to lead programs in Transverse Myelitis, Neuromyelitis Optica and Pediatric Demyelinating Diseases. My work in these conditions has led to identification of various biomarkers of demyelinating disease, and has led to the first FDA IND for a stem cell trial in transverse myelitis. The trial is slated to begin by 2019, and will bring together many of the lessons learned from my time at Hopkins. We are all familiar with the outstanding, historic, international reputation of Johns Hopkins Medicine, but my time there and my time away made me understand why it deserved such a reputation: the people.

Adam L. Hartman, M.D.

Program Director, Division of Clinical Research, National Institute of Neurological Disorders and Stroke, NIH, Adjunct Associate Professor of Neurology & Pediatrics, Johns Hopkins School of Medicine

I had the privilege of training in Child Neurology (2002 to 2005), Clinical Neurophysiology/ Pediatric Epilepsy (2005 to 2007), and serving as faculty (2007 to 2016). My mentor, Eileen P.G. Vining, was critical in facilitating my career. Patti introduced me to JH Neurology Residency alumnus, Michael Rogawski at NIH, who helped me identify a new animal model to study mechanisms of the ketogenic diet. When I joined the faculty, I was mentored by JHBSPH Bodian Professor J. Marie Hardwick. Data from our lab (generated with Child Neurology trainees and Neurology Diversity program students) showed that the acute antiseizure effects of the ketogenic diet are distinct from intermittent fasting; the ketogenic diet was initially designed to mimic the effects of fasting, so this was a surprising result. Intermittent fasting is now being studied in a variety of neurological disorders. In related work, we identified the atypical amino acid D-leucine as a potential antiseizure agent. In clinical research, ketogenic diet observations led to studies published with Eric Kossoff and Mackenzie Cervenka. Dr. Vining also introduced me to hemispherectomy outcomes research. Results of a multicenter collaboration showed that hydrocephalus can occur years after hemispherectomy, which has changed the long-term management of these children. Our Center for Pediatric Rasmussen Syndrome was established in collaboration with Carlos Pardo and Neuroradiology. I also was a founding co-director of the Neurosciences Intensive Care Nursery, a collaborative effort with Neonatology and the Kennedy Krieger Institute. Johns Hopkins provided a wealth of opportunities and brilliant colleagues.

Daniel S. Reich, M.D., Ph.D.

Senior Investigator and Chief, Translational Neuroradiology Section, National Institute of Neurological Disorders and Stroke, National Institutes of Health, Bethesda; Adjunct Professor of Radiology, Neurology, and Biostatistics, Johns Hopkins University

I was the second of two trainees in the short lifespan of the combined neurology, radiology, and neuroradiology ("2-2-2") residency program (2002 to 2009). This training was ideal preparation for a career as a clinician-scientist focused on neuroimaging. I met Peter Calabresi as a junior resident, and together we built a natural history cohort to study the relationship between functional system MRI findings and clinical outcomes in multiple sclerosis. That project, still ongoing 15 years later, spurred several dozen papers, and the cohort has been invaluable in the training of many clinical and research fellows (in neurology, radiology, biostatistics, etc.) who followed me. Peter's mentorship and trust lured me into his field, and in 2009, I was fortunate to be hired into a tenure-track investigator position in the Neuroimmunology Branch at NINDS, where I built my lab and passed on (I hope) many of the precepts of good medicine and science that I learned at Hopkins. I continue to maintain an adjunct appointment at Hopkins, facilitating collaborations and keeping me close to my intellectual roots. Although these days my clinical practice is in neuroradiology, the approach to patients and to the integration of science and medicine that I learned while a resident in Neurology continue to guide me.

Watching the ever-increasing success of my co-residents and professors — many now close friends — is deeply inspiring.

Jaishri Blakeley, M.D.

The Marjorie Bloomberg Tiven Professor of Neurofibromatosis; Professor of Neurology, Neurosurgery and Oncology, Johns Hopkins University School of Medicine

I was attracted to Johns Hopkins University Neurology residency (2002 to 2005) by a sense of both community and inventiveness that I thought would be perfect for molding me into a neuro-critical care specialist. During residency, my plans shifted after I cared for a patient with glioblastoma, and I was drawn to Neuro-Oncology. I established relationships with John Laterra, Skip Grossman, and Henry Brem and committed to being the first neurologist on the NCI T32 Neuro-Oncology training fellowship (2005 to 2007). During this time, I worked in the Hunterian Laboratory, where I learned invaluable skills for assessing intratumoral pharmacokinetics (PK) but also learned that my talents are not in bench science. I did, however, find my passion for writing and conducting early-phase therapeutic trials using both biologic and functional endpoints.

In 2007, I joined the faculty and launched the Johns Hopkins Comprehensive Neurofibromatosis Center (JHCNC).

JHCNC is now one of the pre-eminent clinical and research centers for neurofibromatosis (NF) in the world and a major contributor to national and international discovery initiatives. In 2012, the Neurofibromatosis Therapeutic Acceleration Program (NTAP) was founded to harness intellectual power, essential resources and strategic collaborations to develop therapies for the peripheral nerve sheath tumors afflicting patients with NF1. Through NTAP, I oversee research projects ranging from basic discovery to clinical trials. My greatest academic impact has been in advancing therapeutics for rare oncologic diseases affecting the nervous system through clinical-translational research. However, my greatest contribution overall has been pulling together both learners and experts from many areas to address the most urgent health needs of people with NF and neuro-oncologic disease, both in the clinic and in the lab, through innovative, collaborative programs like NTAP. There is no question that this intense focus on collaboration and patient-centered research is a direct result of being "raised" as a clincian scientist in the Hopkins Department of Neurology. My original novice impression that Hopkins neurology places emphasis on patients and community 17 years ago has been proven true time after time. That environment has led to extraordinary discovery benefiting people with neurologicdisease in real time.

2003

Scott D. Eggers, M.D.

Consultant, Department of Neurology, Associate Professor, College of Medicine & Science, Mayo Clinic, Rochester, Minnesota

My clinical and research fellowship at Johns Hopkins (2001 to 2003), under the mentorship of David Zee, laid the groundwork for my career as an academic clinician in the field of ocular motor and vestibular disorders. Dr. Zee's infectious joy of learning, dedication to continuously advancing the field, and generosity with his time and knowledge provided an aspirational career model. At Mayo Clinic, I work within our Division of Education, spending considerable time teaching neurology residents in clinic as well as spending years chairing the neuroanatomy course and clinical competency committee. My clinical work focuses on patients with vestibular disorders, nystagmus, diplopia, and other ocular motor disorders as part of our multi-disciplinary integrated neurotology team. My research interests have included the diagnostic boundaries and management of vestibular migraine, ocular motor manifestations in degenerative and autoimmune conditions, and the pathophysiology of saccadic palsies. I am medical editor for AskMayoExpert, an internal online tool that supports practice standardization by providing concise, reliable, actionable answers to clinical questions at the point of care using Mayo-vetted, consensus-driven, evidence-based best practices. In everything I do, my time at Hopkins, and the great people I had the privilege of working with there, continue to influence me.

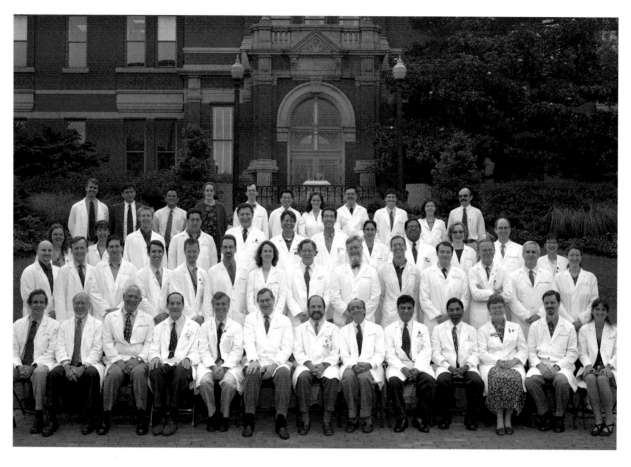

2003

Front Row:
D. Zee
H. Singer
J. Freeman
D. Drachman
R. Llinas
J. Griffin
P. Kaplan
J. Laterra
A. Bhardwaj
V. Chaudhry
E. Vining
N. Crone
A. Hillis

Second Row:
D. Newman-Toker
M. Walker
A. Mandir
E. Kossoff
C. Gibbons
J. Rosenberg
K. Wagner
G. Bergey
C. Andrews
J. De Groot
Unidentified
O. Selnes
B. Gordon
B. Murinson

Third Row:
U. Wesselman
D. Chung
S. Eggers
D. Irani
J. Sepkuty
J. Rothstein
N. Maragakis
L. Moo
S. Sinha
A. Ardelt
A. Mammen

Back Row:
R. Minahan
G. Ricaurte
R. Geocadin
E. Ritzl
T. Reimschisel
T. Nguyen
R. Gottesman
R. Wityk
D. Lieberman
A. Comi
P. Franazczuk

Arun Venkatesan, M.D., Ph.D.

Associate Professor, Neurology; Associate Program Director, Neurology Residency, Johns Hopkins University School of Medicine

The entirety of my training in neurology and subsequent career have taken place at Johns Hopkins (2003 to present). I came to Hopkins for residency, attracted by strengths in neuroinfectious diseases and by the promise of academic career development. With the support and mentorship of many in the Richard T. Johnson Division of Neuroimmunology and Neurologic Infections, and in particular Avindra Nath, I have been able to develop and sustain a research program centered on neurologic injury and protection in the setting of infection and neuroinflammation.

The collaborative nature of our department led to the founding of the Johns Hopkins Encephalitis Center, which represents multiple disciplines including neuroimmunology, epilepsy, and neurocritical care devoted to patient care and research, and which I have the pleasure of heading.

I have also been afforded ample opportunities to engage my deep interests in education – an example is my involvement in the residency program – and have truly enjoyed working closely with and learning from the residents as well as master clinician-educators such as Rafael Llinas.

Michael S. Rafii, M.D., Ph.D.

Professor of Clinical Neurology; Medical Director, Alzheimer's Therapeutic Research Institute, Keck School of Medicine, University of Southern California

The experiences from my residency training (2003 to 2006) provided me with first-hand exposure to the remarkable acumen of world-class clinicians, who are likewise top-notch researchers and embody the academic excellence for which Hopkins is known. Rotations in neuro-ICU, stroke, and neuromuscular showed me the rich, bi-directional connection that can exist between clinical care and translational research.

My own research focuses on the design and conduct of multi-center clinical trials for Alzheimer's disease, including a genetic form which occurs in Down syndrome.

I am Medical Director of the Alzheimer's Therapeutic Research Institute and the NIH-funded Alzheimer's Clinical Trials Consortium, and have been involved in the coordination of AD clinical trials, spanning phase I-III, for over 10 years. Previously, I served as Medical Director of the Alzheimer's Disease Cooperative Study, Director of the Memory Disorders Clinic, Founding Director of the Adult Down Syndrome Clinic and Director of the Neurology Residency Training program at UC-San Diego. Through all of this, the Hopkins model for a clinician-scientist has served as an inspiration to me.

2004

Katherine B. Peters, M.D., Ph.D., F.A.A.N.

Associate Professor of Neurology, Duke University School of Medicine

I am honored to be trained at Johns Hopkins Hospital for my residency in Neurology and fellowship from 2004 to 2008. During that time, I worked closely with many astute, amazing clinicians who were not only experts in their respective fields but also compassionate, caring providers. My research fellowship with Ned Sacktor in HIV/AIDS-related neurological disorders provided me with the tools to develop meaningful clinical research projects. By Dr. Sacktor's example, I learned the importance of the mentor/mentee relationship and how to be a mentor in academic neurology. I am an associate professor of neurology at the Preston Robert Tisch Brain Tumor Center at Duke. My primary areas of research are quality of life in patients with central nervous system tumors and cognitive dysfunction in cancer patients. I honed these interests in my fellowship at Johns Hopkins and my subsequent fellowship at Duke in neuro-oncology. Educating medical students, residents, fellows, and other medical providers was always paramount at Hopkins and I have continued to hold this mission in high regard. One of my cherished accomplishments during my time at Johns Hopkins was being awarded the Guy McKhann Resident Teaching Award in 2007.

Sindhu Ramchandren, M.D., M.S.
Medical Director-Neurology, Medical Affairs, PRA Health Sciences, Raleigh, North Carolina

I look back fondly at my time as a Clinical Neurophysiology-EMG Fellow at Hopkins (2004 to 2005).

I recall feeling as if I had entered the educational equivalent of Hogwarts when I started at Hopkins: it was a magical place of learning and discovery.

My amazing program director was Vinay Chaudhry, and he and my wonderful clinical preceptors – David Cornblath, Andrea Corse, Tom Crawford, John Griffin, Dan Drachman, Nick Maragakis, amongst others – were instrumental in developing my skills in rare neuromuscular disease. After my fellowship, I completed a Master of Science in Clinical Research Design and Biostatistics at the University of Michigan in Ann Arbor, and then joined the faculty at Wayne State University in 2008. There, I pursued my research interests in developing patient-reported outcome measures for clinical trials with an NIH K23 grant and was the Associate Program Director of their Clinical Neurophysiology Fellowship, as well

as Co-Director of the Neuromuscular Program and Muscular Dystrophy Clinic. I then joined the faculty at the University of Michigan in 2013, where I developed and became director of an externally funded Muscular Dystrophy Care Center Program and the Charcot-Marie Tooth Disease (CMT) Center of Excellence clinic. Our research portfolio was funded by grants from NIH, foundation and industry. In 2018, I joined PRA Health Sciences, with the goal of providing innovative solutions to move drug discovery forward and bring more therapies to the market for patients with rare neuromuscular disorders. I strongly believe every step of my career has been informed and enhanced by the professional and personal growth I experienced at Hopkins and will always be grateful for that.

2005

Aasef G. Shaikh, M.D., Ph.D.
Assistant Professor, Department of Neurology, Daroff-Dell'Osso Ocular Motility Laboratory, Cleveland VA Medical center, Functional Electrical Stimulation Center and Advanced Platform Technology Center, Case Western Reserve University, Cleveland, Ohio

Spending time as a research fellow in neurotology with David Zee (2005 to 2009) was critical for shaping my career as a physician-scientist. In these four years, I accomplished many things. I cannot imagine what I would have been if I were elsewhere during this time. In these four years, I learnt the "art" of science; such training, I believe is hard to find at most places. I came to Hopkins with an open mind; the options were becoming a clinician-scientist in otolaryngology, neurology, or to pursue a career in science without clinical practice. I was quite influenced by my mentor, David Zee, and I ended up choosing a career in academic neurology. During my stay at Hopkins, I also met Hyder (Buz) Jinnah, who influenced my thinking and encouraged me to apply the ideas of neurotology and eye movements to study movement disorders.

This approach to movement disorders was a "game changer" in my academic career.

I started applying old concepts in eye movements and achieved very novel results (and publications) in movement disorders. Very importantly, while at Hopkins, I got to collaborate with my mentor's colleagues, Lance Optican and John Leigh. Spending time with Dr. Optican allowed me to learn the math of science, the computational approach to study human disease. Finally, I chose to move to Cleveland for my residency and working with our collaborator and Hopkins connection, Dr. Leigh. After completing my residency, I again trained with another Hopkins connection, Mahlon DeLong, who heavily influenced my clinical and practical approach to movement disorders. In summary, my training as a physician and scientist was quite influenced by Hopkins – either in Baltimore, or elsewhere working with someone who was at Hopkins.

2007

Rahila Ansari, M.D., M.S.
Assistant Professor of Neurology, Case Western Reserve University School of Medicine; Neurologist, Cleveland VA Medical Center

My research is in device development to restore function to patients with amputations, or with weakness due to pathologies such as myopathies and spinal cord injuries.

My approach to helping these patients utilizes my background in biomedical and polymer engineering, in addition to my clinical training in neurology and neuromuscular diseases. My Neurology residency at Johns Hopkins Hospital laid the groundwork for my clinical understanding of neurological pathophysiology and patient needs. The inspiration for my research came from working with Kathryn Wagner in the Johns Hopkins Muscular Dystrophy Clinic. By using "smart" materials and devices, my goal has been to augment strength and enhance function, while decreasing muscle strain. One of my projects is to restore a safer gait pattern and reduce the risk of falls in patients with inclusion body myositis, by providing mechanical assistance to the quadriceps using microprocessor-based, stance-controlled orthotics. Some of my other projects involve using "smart" materials, where their stiffness or shape adjusts in response to measured pressure and shear forces. I am developing these technologies to construct prosthetic liners that adjust in real time to improve fit, while decreasing the risk of skin breakdown. My other principal research area is Functional Electrical Stimulation (FES). In paraplegic patients with cervical spinal cord injuries, walking can be restored by implanting nerve cuff electrodes. These electrodes have multiple contacts, and depending on which contact is used, specific nerve fascicles can be selectively stimulated, which improves fine motor control. My work within the larger FES Center at Case and the VA focuses on chronic neurophysiologic changes within the nerve and its innervated muscles as a function of stimulation. Additionally, I study the fascicular selectivity and stability of these multi-contact nerve cuff electrodes. Due to the interdisciplinary nature of my work, I have forged multiple interdepartmental and cross-institutional collaborations with basic scientists and engineers, with a common goal of more rapidly translating technology into clinical application. This would not have been possible without the clinical training I received at Hopkins, or without the guidance from my mentors.

Amos A. Fatokun, Ph.D.

Senior Lecturer in Pharmacology, School of Pharmacy and Biomolecular Sciences, Liverpool John Moores University, Liverpool, United Kingdom

I was a postdoctoral fellow in the laboratory of Ted Dawson and Valina Dawson at the Department of Neurology and the Institute for Cell Engineering (ICE) between October 2007 and August 2010. During that time, I obtained an American Heart Association Postdoctoral Fellowship (overall best application within the Mid-Atlantic Affiliate region, which was recognised with a special plaque at an award ceremony) to investigate small-molecule compounds that could elicit neuroprotection by inhibiting the translocation of apoptosis-inducing factor, which is one of the key molecular events that culminate in PARP-mediated cell/neuronal death (parthanatos). Two methoxyflavones, 4'-methoxyflavone and 3',4'-dimethoxyflavone were found to inhibit the parthanatos cascade through their direct inhibition of the PARP-1 enzyme. This and further findings garnered through the detailed characterization of these compounds provoked my interest in investigating the potential of such natural compounds or their derivatives to target specific signaling mechanisms – rather than, or in addition to, merely acting as antioxidants (flavonoids are known to elicit anti-oxidant effects). This focus continues to represent a significant part of my research endeavour.

My training at Hopkins gave me the opportunity to expand my research skills, including in academic drug discovery and molecular and cell biology.

Elisabeth Breese Marsh, M.D.

Associate Professor of Neurology, Johns Hopkins School of Medicine; Director, Johns Hopkins Bayview Comprehensive Stroke Program; Associate Program Director, Neurology Residency; Vice Chair of Clinical Operations, Johns Hopkins Bayview Neurology

My training as a resident/fellow, and faculty member at Johns Hopkins has resulted in a passion for the use of evidence-based medicine to better the quality of care for patients and improve both short- and long-term outcomes. Under the mentorship of Argye Hillis and Rebecca Gottesman, I was awarded an R25 Research Training Award through the NIH to investigate factors associated with increased risk of hemorrhagic transformation of acute stroke. This resulted in creation of the Hemorrhage Risk Stratification (HeRS) score, which quantifies risk of hemorrhagic transformation for hospitalized patients needing anticoagulation. My current role as the director of the Comprehensive Stroke Program has allowed me to design and implement studies that have significantly changed our evaluation and management of stroke in both the inpatient and outpatient setting. Through our multidisciplinary stroke follow-up clinic, we follow stroke survivors over the first year of recovery.

I have focused on the population with small strokes and "good outcomes," who continue to have high rates of depression, fatigue, and cognitive dysfunction.

With Rafael Llinas, my lab uses magnetoencephalography (MEG) to explore the underlying pathophysiology of their symptoms, and runs clinical treatment trials to hasten recovery and improve post-stroke morbidity and quality of life.

Helmar C. Lehmann, M.D.

Professor of Neurology, Department of Neurology, University Hospital of Cologne, Germany

I spent two periods at Johns Hopkins to complete a Research Fellowship in Neurology in 2004, and 2008 to 2009. During my fellowship I had the privilege to work in the Peripheral Nerve Group led by Jack Griffin under the tutelage of Kazim Sheikh and Ahmet Höke. This period was fundamental for my later career in academic Neurology. The research area I was interested in was the Guillain-Barré Syndrome, and during my stay at Johns Hopkins I was trained in various preclinical models, aiming to elucidate pathomechanisms of immune-mediated injury to peripheral nerve fibers. Research projects in which I had the opportunity to participate focused on regeneration after axonal injury that eventually led to several publications. During my stays, I was always deeply fascinated by the clinical and scientific diversity of the staff and the approach of the entire department to combine highest level research with best clinical care for neurological patients. I still remember very well Grand Rounds (with a piano in the lecture hall!) with utmost instructive case presentations as well as scientific lectures, in which basic and clinical research was presented and discussed by highly influential neurologists from Johns Hopkins and from all over the world.

This atmosphere was unique and taught me the true meaning of the term, "clinician-scientist."

After my return to Germany, I finished my clinical education and established my own laboratory, in which I try to pass over some of this inspiring spirit of academic Neurology to my residents and medical students. My clinical and my research interests are still in the field of neuromuscular disorders and neuroimmunology. As such, my time at Johns Hopkins was very formative for my career.

Mackenzie C. Cervenka, M.D.

Associate Professor of Neurology, Johns Hopkins School of Medicine; Medical Director, Johns Hopkins Adult Epilepsy Diet Center; Medical Director, Johns Hopkins Epilepsy Monitoring Unit

My fellowship training in epilepsy and clinical neurophysiology in the Department of Neurology at Johns Hopkins (2008 to 2010) and experience as a faculty member in the epilepsy division after completing fellowship have provided me with a unique foundation, which I have built on to pursue a career as a clinician-scientist investigating the use of ketogenic diet therapies for adult epilepsy.

I have been fortunate to work with inspirational mentors and colleagues, and through their support and encouragement, I began the first Adult Epilepsy Diet Center, a multidisciplinary center to provide ketogenic diet therapies to adults with intractable epilepsy.

Our mission is also to train clinicians and dietitians on management of adults with ketogenic diet therapies to broaden the availability of these effective treatments worldwide. To achieve this goal, our team offers a ketogenic diet training program, and I have become a member of the International League Against Epilepsy Dietary Treatments Task Force. Most recently, I also began conducting clinical trials examining the treatment of refractory status epilepticus with the ketogenic diet. My training and mentorship at Johns Hopkins have provided me with the essential tools to become a leader in the study of ketogenic diet therapies for epilepsy.

2009

Richard Leigh, M.D.

Assistant Clinical Investigator, Stroke Branch, Intramural Research Program, National Institute of Neurological Disorders and Stroke, NIH, Bethesda

My foundations in science began when I was an undergraduate at Johns Hopkins University studying biomedical engineering. I later returned to Hopkins for a postdoctoral fellowship mentored by Peter Barker, during which time I developed a method for imaging the blood-brain barrier (BBB). I subsequently joined the Hopkins cerebrovascular division, working as a stroke-service attending for four years. My early work used MRI to measure changes in BBB integrity during acute ischemia, leading to improved understanding of the role of BBB derangements in hemorrhagic complications of acute stroke treatments. I also worked with Peter van Zijl on developing an MRI method for measuring pH in the brain. When I transitioned to the NIH intramural program, I applied my techniques to a large imaging database collected by the Stroke Branch. We identified fluctuations in BBB permeability early after stroke in humans, and distinguished BBB dysfunction from BBB rupture. Our work identified remote effects of cerebral ischemia on the eye, supporting the notion that there is a systemic response to focal cerebral ischemia.

We also discovered BBB alterations associated with subacute and chronic cerebrovascular disease, leading to new hypotheses for the pathogenesis of vascular dementia.

Thus, throughout my career, I have benefitted greatly from Johns Hopkins and its outstanding mentors.

Angela Wabulya M.B., Ch.B.

Assistant Professor of Neurology, University of North Carolina, Chapel Hill

During residency training (2009 to 2012), and clinical neurophysiology/epilepsy fellowship (2012 to 2014) at Johns Hopkins, I had the pleasure of learning from/with and working amidst inspirational colleagues and faculty.

Having had my initial medical degree in Africa, I dreamt of what medicine in the "first world" would be like. Johns Hopkins not only enabled me to realize this dream but inspired me to strive for excellent patient care, a key principle as a clinician.

The standard that was set at Hopkins is a constant reminder to provide the very best patient care, embrace and implement medical changes, as well as set a cornerstone for my career growth. The Clinical Investigation training at Hopkins (2011 to 2012) provided me the needed skill set and confidence to work with clinical researchers committed to the advancement of epilepsy management; and while modest at this time, I anticipate that my clinical and research career will continue to grow, and hopefully truly reflect, the excellence Hopkins represents. Finally, the time at Hopkins facilitated continued collaborations with far- reaching effects here in the U.S. and across the Atlantic: Johns Hopkins Neurology family- Thank you!

2010

Bridgette "Jeanne" Billioux, M.D.

Staff Clinician, International Neuroinfectious Diseases Unit, Division of Neuroimmunology and Neurovirology, Division of Intramural Research, National Institute of Neurological Disorders and Stroke, National Institutes of Health

My Hopkins training (2010 to 2013) was an incomparable experience that largely shaped the neurologist I am now, and helped lead me down my somewhat unconventional career path. Influenced by many incredible neurologists as well as fascinating and complex patients seen while at Hopkins, I eventually decided upon Neuroimmunology/Neurovirology as my field of choice. In particular, I remember the riveting lectures Dick Johnson gave us, detailing his adventures around the world, piecing together the mysteries of various infectious agents and their effects on the nervous system. At the time, I was frankly awed by his remarkable undertakings and couldn't imagine I'd ever be so fortunate to have such a colorful career, or much less be able to accomplish even a modicum of what he had. Nevertheless, I pursued my Neuroimmunology/ Neurovirology fellowship at the NIH, where I have since studied various viruses and their effects on the nervous system.

Mid-fellowship, I was given the opportunity to study the neurological manifestations of Ebola in Liberia.

This project has expanded, leading to various collaborations and publications, and has cemented my interest in international clinical research. Undoubtedly, I have Dr. Johnson as well as many others at Hopkins to thank for the inspiration and training.

Dan Gold, D.O.

Assistant Professor, Departments of Neurology, Ophthalmology, Otolaryngology-Head & Neck Surgery, Neurosurgery, Emergency Medicine, Johns Hopkins Hospital

If it were not for me being introduced to David Zee as a PGY-2 neurology resident at the University of Maryland, I would not be where I am today. After my first shadowing experience with Dr. Zee, I was completely hooked, and spent every available Friday that I could with him throughout the remainder of my residency. As a PGY-2, I was also introduced to David Newman-Toker's first paper describing the 'HINTS' exam to differentiate benign (peripheral) from dangerous (central) causes of the acute vestibular syndrome. By that point, I knew that I would focus my career on ocular motor and vestibular disorders. I came to Johns Hopkins in 2013 following a neuro-ophthalmology fellowship, and I have had the privilege to work with and be mentored by Drs. Zee and Newman-Toker ever since. I am passionate about clinical care and neurologic education, and have been particularly interested in the rapid diagnosis and treatment of acute neuro-ophthalmologic and vestibular disorders, and in minimizing diagnostic errors by educating frontline providers. In fact, Dr. Newman-Toker and I have created and implemented a 'Tele-Dizzy' consultation service in the Emergency Department using portable video-oculography technology to improve peripheral vestibular and stroke diagnosis. I am constantly stimulated by my excellent colleagues and trainees, and am grateful for the superb mentorship I have received at Johns Hopkins. I look forward to the future and feel honored to be a part of the Department of Neurology.

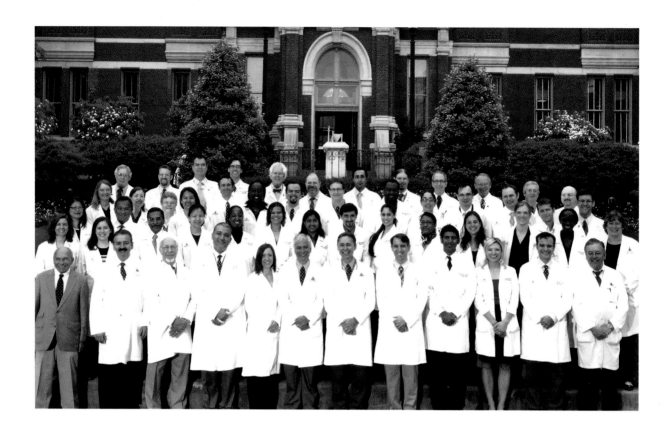

2011

Front Row:
H. Moses
A. Hoke
H. Singer
B. Sahin
L. Jordan
R. Llinas
J. McArthur
E. Kossoff
A. Qureshi
A. Dolce
J. Probasco

Second Row:
J. Blakeley
L. Rosenthal
V. Chaudhry
J. Bang
A. Sharrief
E. Felton
M. Jinka

P. Mohassel
J. Billioux
A. Rao
S. Kelley
E. Marsh
A. Wabulya
L. Clawson

Third Row:
S. Ying
R. Geocadin
S. Jen
A. Owegi
J. Lopez
R. Faigle
M. Arnan
M. Motta
P. Lee Jr.
R. Felling
V. Parfenov
A. Hartman

Back Row:
M. Shins
G. Bergey
M. Cervenka
L. Ostrow
E. Vining
Z. Mari
B. Masselink
A. Puttgen
R. Lesser
T. Crawford
S. Nijjar
R. Leigh
J. Rosenberg
O. Selnes
N. Sacktor
D. Newman-Toker

2011

Carolyn Fredericks, M.D.

Clinical Assistant Professor of Neurology, Stanford University

My time at JHH as a Neurology resident formed the foundation for my still-nascent career as a clinician-scientist in behavioral neurology. I often draw on the experiences I had as a resident on the wards, and many of the connections I made at Hopkins have become lifelong friendships. After my time at Hopkins, I went to the University of California-San Francisco, where I served as Chief Resident, and then completed my fellowship in Behavioral Neurology at UCSF's Memory and Aging Center. In 2016, I accepted a position on the faculty at Stanford University, where I am currently preparing to submit a career award proposal. My research focuses on understanding the neural networks disrupted in preclinical and clinical Alzheimer's disease, including less common Alzheimer's variants.

I also have a strong clinical interest in rapidly progressive dementia and autoimmune encephalitis, inspired by a patient I saw at JHH in 2011 with NMDAR encephalitis.

I'm so grateful to remain in contact with many of my co-residents and colleagues from my Hopkins years: this community is a continual source of mentorship and inspiration.

Jing Xu, Ph.D.

Assistant Research Scientist, The Malone Center for Engineering in Healthcare, Whiting School of Engineering, Johns Hopkins University

My work at the Johns Hopkins Neurology Department as a post-doc fellow has laid the foundation for my career in neurorehabilitation. I became the lead research fellow in 2011 for the Study of Motor Learning and Acute Recovery Time Course in Stroke (SMARTS), under the guidance of John W. Krakauer. We tracked over 50 patients at three centers (Johns Hopkins Hospital, Columbia University, and University Hospital of Zurich) for a one-year period from acute to chronic stages, using motor kinnect/kinematics behavioral and neurological assessments, brain stimulation (TMS), and imaging techniques (fMRI, DTI, and ASL). The study was fruitful, with multiple research articles coming out. Our TMS results challenge the currently dominant theory of inter-hemispheric competition model for motor recovery. For the first time in humans, our kinematic and imaging results show two critical components of the hand function, strength and dexterous finger control, recover separately, and that dexterity is the most difficult to regain. Based on these findings, my colleague, Kevin Olds, and I have developed a new device, using highly sensitive force sensors to detect finger forces in 3-D, in order to deliver portable efficient assessment and therapy for dexterity recovery to the most impaired patients at their bedside.

Peter B. Marschik, Mphil., Dphil., DMsc., Ph.D.

Associate Professor, Medical University of Graz, Austria and University Medical Center Goettingen, Germany; adjunct to the Karolinska Institutet, Stockholm, Sweden

My time as a postdoc fellow at Hopkins (2011 to 2012) was a formative period of my scientific career. Based at JHU and the Kennedy Krieger Institute, I established the foundations of my field of research: interdisciplinary Developmental Neuroscience. Our interdisciplinary research focuses on neurodevelopmental disorders, rare genetic disorders, neurophysiology, development of neural functions, neuroethology, neurocognitive research/cognitive brain research, neurolinguistics/psycholinguistics, development of laterality, general movement assessment, genetic disorders, communication disorders, speech and language development. During my time in Baltimore I had my first successful research projects, developed models and achieved new insights for the study of rare genetic disorders, specifically Rett syndrome and fragile X syndrome. I am very grateful for the fruitful cooperation and guidance of Michael V. Johnston, Walter E. Kaufmann, and Rebecca Landa during my stay. My stay at Hopkins boosted my subsequent career as researcher and translational scientist. My time at this special place not only prepared me for my scientific endeavors, but also led to lasting, productive friendships, in the U.S. but also worldwide.

Overall a brain-gain-brain-drain experience, extremely valuable and eye-opening.

Atul Kalanuria, M.D., F.A.C.P.

Assistant Professor of Neurology, Neurosurgery, Anesthesia and Critical Care Director, Penn Neurocritical Care Fellowship Program; Director, Penn Neurocritical Care Clerkship; The Hospital of The University of Pennsylvania, Perelman School of Medicine

I spent two years (2011 to 2013) as a fellow in neurocritical care at The Johns Hopkins Hospital, and those years were the turning point of my career. I was part of the opening of the new hospital building, and remember being in the old unit one day and new one the next. I worked alongside some amazing colleagues and forged valuable friendships. One of the best things that I learnt during my time at Hopkins was the teamwork among all the care providers. My training at Hopkins prepared me extremely well for the real-world setting, both clinically and from a research standpoint. Some of my best work so far was published during my days at Hopkins. I can also never forget the immense help and advice I received from the faculty, especially Justin McArthur. It's an honor to have

graduated from a program that has produced some of the best neurointensivists there are. I will always be proud that I am part of the Hopkins legacy.

Logan D. Schneider, M.D.

Staff Neurologist, Stanford/VA Alzheimer's Center, Palo Alto; Sierra Pacific VA MIRECC Research Fellow in Sleep and Neurocognition, Palo Alto, Clinical Instructor, Stanford Center for Sleep Science and Medicine, Redwood City, California

During residency training at Hopkins (2011 to 2014), I had the pleasure of working amidst a cohort of inspirational colleagues and teachers, which laid the groundwork for my current career as an academic clinician-scientist in the field of sleep neurology. My current projects uniting sleep and neurocognitive function would not have been possible without the foundations and mentorship provided throughout my neurology training. In building relationships with, and being supported by, such exemplary clinician-educators, I sought to contribute back to the community through sharing with others the world-class training offered in Hopkins' hallowed halls. This endeavor began on two fronts during my residency training. The first was through an international collaboration on a neurology physical exam syllabus with Pf. Dr. Klaus Toyka. This project burgeoned into a free eBook (*Manual of the Neurological Examination for Neurologists in Training*) that is being translated into multiple languages for training neurologists on three different continents. The second began with my election as the AAN's Consortium of Neurology Residents and Fellows Chair. This endeavor to improve the standards of residency training across the country has grown into a leadership role within the AAN's Graduate Education Subcommittee and collaborative projects to uniformly integrate Sleep training into neurology residency training.

2012

Amir Kheradmand, M.D.

Assistant Professor, Departments of Neurology and Otolaryngology-Head & Neck Surgery, Johns Hopkins University

I started at Hopkins as a joint research and clinical fellow under mentorship of David Zee. During this time, my work focused on understanding the neural mechanisms of spatial orientation, with an emphasis on the role of cerebral cortex in processing vestibular inputs. I subsequently joined the Neurology faculty at Hopkins in 2014 as a clinician/educator/researcher. In my lab, we have developed psychophysical paradigms to study neural mechanisms of sensory integration for spatial orientation, and how their dysfunctions can lead to vexing symptoms such as those in patients with vestibular migraine. We have pioneered the use of transcranial magnetic stimulation (TMS) in probing cerebral cortical networks involved in spatial orientation. Our work has shown a functional role of the temporoparietal cortex in sensory processing for perception of spatial orientation. We have also developed a new clinical test of vestibular function based on a novel video-oculography method that can accurately measure torsional eye position. Overall, my academic goals are aimed at translational integration of our research findings into new diagnostic techniques and treatment strategies for the incapacitating symptoms of patients with dizziness and spatial disorientation. Through this path, I have benefited from the outstanding collegial environment at Hopkins, which has nurtured my growth as a clinician-scientist.

Anthony O. Asemota, M.D., M.P.H.

Department of Neurosurgery, Johns Hopkins Hospital

During my time as a senior research coordinator, and subsequently as a postdoctoral research fellow (2012 to 2014) in the Neurology department at Johns Hopkins, I had the exciting opportunity of managing the accelerated cure project (principal investigator, Arun Venkatesan), a multicenter study investigating potential factors associated with development of multiple sclerosis and other demyelinating diseases. I maintained a repository of blood/serum samples for the Johns Hopkins arm of the study, and was also charged with collating and organizing relevant patient data following closure of the study. In addition, I participated in various projects where I applied my knowledge of statistics and honed my expertise in studying various neuro-inflammatory and neuro-infectious diseases, which led to publications in high-ranking journals and presentations at national meetings.

I completed a general surgery/oncology research fellowship, and I am presently undertaking a research fellowship in pituitary/skull base neurosurgery at the Johns Hopkins Department of Neurosurgery, and aspiring to complete residency training in neurosurgery.

In the current era of big data, my exposure and time in neurology department certainly helped advance my skills and awareness in conducting data-driven research for understanding some of the very challenging and complex epidemiological associations pertinent to neurological diseases.

Michelle C. Potter, Ph.D.
Associate Director, Translational In Vivo *Models, Sanofi, Framingham, Massachusetts*

My two-year postdoctoral fellowship (2012 to 2014) in Barb Slusher's drug discovery lab at the Brain Science Institute (BSI, now Johns Hopkins Drug Discovery), as research manager at the Hopkins behavioral core with Mikhail Pletnikov and as a member of the Neurology Department was an invaluable stepping stone in my career, as I transitioned from academia to the pharmaceutical/biotech industry.

Working alongside industry veterans on Barb's team gave me incredible insights into the world of drug discovery, and I quickly realized that was the career path I wanted to follow.

At Hopkins, I learned the value of cultivating a collaborative environment, and have carried this mindset throughout my career path. After two years in Barb's lab, and thanks in large part to the experience I gained at Hopkins, I secured a position as Senior Scientist in Merck Research Labs Neuroscience Department in Boston, working on Neurodegeneration and Neuroimmunology programs for Alzheimer's disease. I recently joined Sanofi as Associate Director in the Translational *In Vivo* Models platform, supporting programs in Neuroscience, Rare Disease and Hematology. I truly appreciate the training and development opportunities I received at Hopkins, as well as the great colleagues, mentors and friends I was lucky enough to work alongside.

Sonja W. Scholz, M.D., Ph.D.
Tenure Track Investigator, National Institutes of Health, Bethesda, Maryland; Adjunct Postdoctoral Research Fellow, Johns Hopkins University

When facing difficult medical questions, an outstanding neurologist relies on five core principles: professionalism, empathy, humility, inquisitiveness, and, above all, persistence. During my Neurology residency from 2012 to 2015, I found that each of these humanistic principles was alive and well.

Indeed, my current research is built on the foundation that I saw practiced daily by my colleagues during my time at Johns Hopkins. Under the mentorship by Dr. Rothstein and Dr. Sumner, I demonstrated that there is a substantial genetic predisposition to Lewy body dementia. This work has given rise to a large-scale, international project to extend gene discovery efforts to this underserved disease. I was fortunate to maintain close ties with the Neurology department following my residency. Attending movement disorders and cognitive neurology clinics has armed me with a comprehensive skill set to tackle these complex syndromes. I am grateful for the inspiring example that my colleagues have provided me with, and believe that they have made me a better physician and a more determined scientist to help those suffering from neurodegenerative conditions. It may take decades to find a cure for these disabling diseases... until then, like Dan Drachman and Guy McKhann, I'll just keep turning up for work.

2013

Jutta Peterburs, Ph.D.
Research Scholar, Heinrich-Heine-University, Dusseldorf, Germany

During my research fellowship (2013 to 2014) in the Department of Neurology, Division of Cognitive Neuroscience, at Johns Hopkins, I had the pleasure of working with an amazing and inspiring group of neuroscientists interested in non-motor functions of the cerebellum (John Desmond, Cherie Marvel, Dominic Cheng). This topic has been one of my core research interests ever since my time as a Ph.D. student at Ruhr-University Bochum in Germany, and my time at Hopkins has allowed me to substantially expand my methodological repertoire and my scientific horizons. My current research is focused on understanding how performance monitoring processes, e.g., error and feedback processing, are impacted by contextual and inter-individual factors, and how especially the cerebellum might contribute by carrying out overarching monitoring and predictive functions. I very much enjoyed the extremely productive, creative, and supportive atmosphere in John Desmond's Neuroimaging and Modulation Lab. While my career path led me back to Germany after completion of my fellowship, I have been maintaining and fostering my ties to Hopkins in my role as a Research Associate.

My time at Hopkins not only shaped and substantially advances my career but it also led to lasting, productive friend-ships and a deep love for Baltimore.

Jorge Otero-Millan, Ph.D.
Postdoctoral fellow, Johns Hopkins University

My time as postdoctoral fellow in the Department of Neurology at Hopkins (2013 to present) has been a period of tremendous growth. Within our group at the Neuro-Vestibular and Visual Disorders divisions, I have been fortunate to work under the mentorship of a diverse group of faculty members such as David Zee, Amir Kheradmand and David Newman-Toker. I arrived at Hopkins after a Ph.D. working at the Barrow Neurological Institute with Dr. Susana Martinez-Conde. My work focused on the small eye movements, called fixational eye movements, that we make when we try to keep our gaze still looking at a small target. During this period, I had the opportunity to collaborate with John Leigh, who was in Cleveland at the time, comparing the characteristics of those eye movements in healthy subjects and neurological patients. This collaboration was my first chance to experience clinical neurology and how eye movements can be useful to study and diagnose diseases. Later, when looking for a postdoctoral fellowship, I decided to follow on this path and joined David Zee, longtime collaborator of John Leigh at Johns Hopkins. At Hopkins, I got to work on studying how our brain maintains an accurate perception of upright despite the continuing motion of our body and eyes. Collaborating with Amir Kheradmand, I developed a method to measure torsional eye movements (rotations of the eye around the line of sight). Lack of a method to measure torsion up to that point had been a roadblock on this line of research. We put this method to good use in multiple studies, ranging from brain stimulation and perception of upright, patients with vestibular loss, and eye movements induced by magnetic fields. Working in this group has also allowed me to collaborate with David Newman-Toker, applying new technologies and data analysis techniques to enable eye movement-based diagnosis of patients with dizziness. In the future, my experience at Hopkins will be key to succeeding as an independent investigator.

2016

Marianna Riello, Ph.D.
Postdoctoral research fellow, Action-Perception Laboratory at the Department of Neuroscience, Biomedicine and Movement Sciences, University of Verona, Italy; Clinical Neuropsychologist in Alzheimer's Disease Centers for Health Care Residences (S.P.E.S) Trento, Italy

During my postdoctoral fellowship at Hopkins (2016 to 2017), I had the pleasure of working amidst a cohort of inspirational colleagues. This laid the groundwork for my current career as an academic clinician-scientist in the field of dementia. I have always sought to combine clinical and imaging data from patients, and I had the chance to do so during my work experience at the Department of Neurology, Neurosurgery and Neurosciences, of Johns Hopkins Medicine under the supervision of Dr. Tsapkini. There, I had the possibility to gain insight on primary progressive aphasia (PPA), by observing patients coming from all over the United States to undergo advanced tools for the improvement of language functions within the National Institute of Health (NIH) research project. Particularly, I had the chance to increase my awareness and expertise about volumetric brain analyses as predictors of worse cognitive outcomes in PPA. In doing this, I have been supported by exemplary clinicians-researcher-educators who wisely supervised my work and shared with me their specialized knowledge. The opportunity to actively contribute to their own research programs, while receiving advanced research training, was invaluable to me. This period was the most formative training of my scientific career. Our productive collaboration has led to a successful publication on predictive model using behavioral and cerebral volumetric data of PPA patients. This postdoctoral experience abroad was highly valued, and I am happy I have been part of such a brilliant environment, one that I tried to share with my country as soon as I came back.

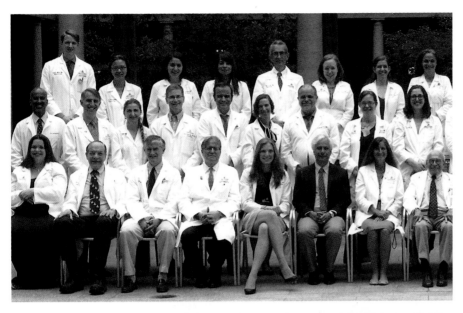

2017

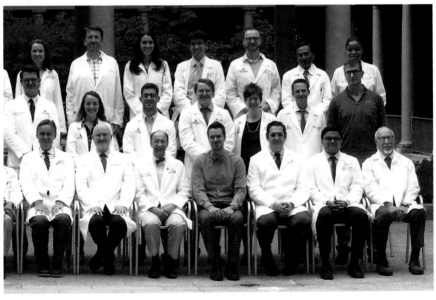

Front Row:
S. Dean
D. Drachman
P. Calabresi
J. Rothstein
E. Marsh
R. Llinas
A. Hillis
H. Moses
J. McArthur
D. Newman-Toker
C. Stafstrom
D. Gold, R. Ricardo
P. Bhargava
H. Singer

Second Row:
A. Venkatesan
E. Kossoff
V. Machairaki
B. Morrison
J. Probasco
T. Johnson
T. Crawford
D. Saylor
J. Orthmann-Murphy
T. Shoemaker
L. Doherty
B. Freund
A. Billnitzer
J. Nance
M. Kornberg
M. Kronenbuerger

Back Row:
K. Mills
J. Bang
L. Gershen
S. Siddiqi
C. Pardo
L. Sun
J. Blakeley
R. Gottesman
P. Dziedzic
B. Kass
W. Tsao
M. Elrick
V. Chaudhry
K-A. Patrice

Images reproduced courtesy of the Alan Mason Chesney Medical Archives of the Johns Hopkins Medical Institutions are shown on the following pages: Facing the Foreword (images of Bodian, Ford, and Mountcastle); pages 3,4, 6, 8,1 1, 12, 14, 17, 21, 25, 28, 31, 32, 34, 37, 44, 50, 52, 53, 59, 62, 98, 123, 125, 134, 138, 142, 144, 147, 156, 161, 164, 190, 196, 201, 210, 216, 221, 236, 244, 251. Images on page 120 are reproduced from Blitz AM et al., Neuroimaging Clinics of North America, 24:1-15, 2014, with permission from Elsevier.

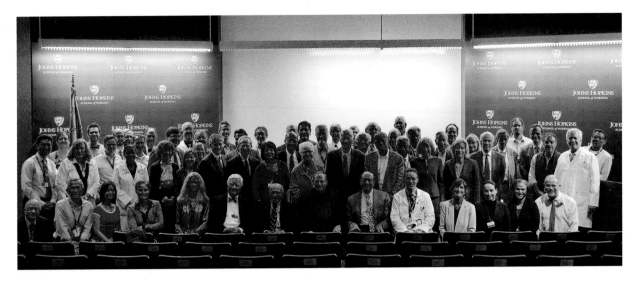

50 Years and Counting: Celebrating the Department of Neurology at Hopkins, May 2019.

AFTERWORD

The idea for this book came from two of the original founders in 1969 of the Department of Neurology, Guy McKhann and Dan Drachman, as we were making plans for a celebration of our Department's 50th anniversary. Rather than make this a comprehensive "history" of Neurology at Johns Hopkins, we wanted to focus on the milieu that has allowed for the evolution, over 50 years, of one of the leading departments in the U.S. – from a nascent unit of fewer than seven faculty members.

Key to this environment has been a culture of scientific discovery that is almost always linked to, and driven by, questions that stem from the clinical arena. The development of an exceptionally strong pipeline of physician-scientists, and of nonclinical Ph.D. scientists, has been critical for us. Our residency program and various career development platforms have ensured the success of this steady flow of disease-oriented scientists. Another vital ingredient has been the robust spirit of collegiality and collaboration that is a hallmark of the Hopkins environment. Always, neurologists at all levels of training and career development have been encouraged to branch out beyond the department for advice, for collaborative scientific projects, and sharing of resources.

Finally, the clinical culture of the Department has always stressed the primacy of clinical care – not only providing it in a compassionate and comprehensive manner, but asking ourselves and each other how we could care for our patients with greater efficacy and efficiency. In telling this story, we hope that this book gives you a glimpse at how the Department of Neurology has developed over the past 50 years, and a sense of our optimism and excitement as we look to the future. In the words of Sir William Osler, "The best preparation for tomorrow is to do today's work superbly well."

JUSTIN C. MCARTHUR, M.B., B.S., M.P.H
John W. Griffin Professor; Professor of Neurology, Pathology, Medicine, and Epidemiology
Director, Sheikh Khalifa Stroke Institute; Director, Department of Neurology, Johns Hopkins
University School of Medicine; Neurologist-in-chief, The Johns Hopkins Hospital;
President-elect, American Neurological Association

INDEX

*Page numbers in **bold** font indicate photographs and portraits.*